Managing Hospital-Based Patient Education

Edited by Barbara E. Giloth, M.P.H., C.H.E.S.

AHA books are published by American Hospital Publishing, Inc.,
an American Hospital Association company

The views expressed in this publication are strictly those of the authors and do not necessarily represent official positions of the American Hospital Association.

Library of Congress Cataloging-in-Publication Data

Managing hospital-based patient education / edited by Barbara E.
  Giloth.
      p.   cm.
    Includes bibliographical references.
    ISBN 1-55648-097-0 (pbk.)
    1. Patient education. 2. Hospital care. I. Giloth, Barbara E.
    [DNLM: 1. Hospital Administration.   2. Patient Care Planning.
    3. Patient Education.   WX 158.5 M266 1993]
    RA975.5.P38M36   1993
    632.1′1′068 — dc20
    DNLM/DLC
    for Library of Congress   92-48394
                                                                                CIP

Catalog no. 070194

©1993 by American Hospital Publishing, Inc.,
an American Hospital Association company

Printed in the USA

Text set in Palatino
2.5 — 03/93 — 0340

Linda Conheady, Acquisitions/Development Editor
Nancy Charpentier and Teresa Cappetta-Kroger, Production Editors
Marcia Bottoms, Assistant Director
Peggy DuMais, Production Coordinator
Luke Smith, Cover Designer
Brian Schenk, Books Division Director

Contents

About the Editor

Barbara E. Giloth, M.P.H., C.H.E.S., was director of health services research for the Hospital Research and Educational Trust of the American Hospital Association in Chicago through 1992. She formerly was program manager, Division of Ambulatory Care and Health Promotion, at the AHA, where she was responsible for managing the association's national policy and program activities in patient education and disease prevention. In addition, she managed a cooperative agreement awarded by the Office of Disease Prevention and Health Promotion to catalyze hospitals' participation in the Healthy People 2000 program, a national initiative to set health promotion and disease prevention objectives for the year 2000. She also was codirector of a national project at the American Hospital Association funded by the Centers for Disease Control to study and improve health education in ambulatory health care settings.

Early in her career at AHA, she was one of three coauthors of a widely used manual entitled *Implementing Patient Education in the Hospital* (1979; now out of print). She coauthored several books for American Hospital Publishing, including *Working with Physicians in Health Promotion: A Key to Successful Programs* (1984) and *Tracking the Impact of Health Promotion on Organizations: A Key to Program Survival* (1988; now out of print), as well as *Consumer Health Information: Managing Hospital-Based Centers* (1991), published by the American Hospital Association, and numerous articles and monographs. She has served on a wide variety of national committees, including the National High Blood Pressure Coordinating Committee, the National Council on Self-Help and Public Health, and the Division Board for Professional Development of the National Commission on Health Education Credentialing.

Prior to coming to AHA, Ms. Giloth served as patient education coordinator at the University of Chicago Hospitals and Clinics. She also worked for three years in community health education as a Peace Corps volunteer in Togo, West Africa.

She holds a bachelor's degree in sociology from the University of Wisconsin, Madison, and a master's degree in public health from the University of Michigan, Ann Arbor.

Contributors

Patricia Agre, M.S., Ed.D., R.N., is the coordinator of patient and family education at Memorial Sloan–Kettering Cancer Center in New York City. In her current position, she planned and implemented a closed-circuit television system for the cancer center. In 1992, she also served as a consultant to Beth Israel Medical Center in New York City to assist the medical center in setting up a hospitalwide patient education program.

Sandra J. Cornett, Ph.D., R.N., has been the patient education coordinator at The Ohio State University Hospitals since 1979 and a clinical assistant professor at The Ohio State University College of Nursing since 1984. As part of her responsibilities, she works with the hospitalwide Health Education Advisory Committee and department-level patient education committees to set and implement strategic initiatives. She has been instrumental in supporting interdisciplinary teams to develop and implement specific patient population education programs. She was a founding member of the AHA/ASHET Patient Education Advisory Committee and has been chairperson of this group for the past two years.

Laura Gilpin, M.F.A., R.N., is national director of educational services for Planetree, a nonprofit organization working to humanize health care. She works as a consultant to many hospitals, conducts nurses' training seminars throughout the country, and lectures widely to both consumer and professional audiences on a variety of topics, including consumer health and patient-centered care.

Virginia M. González, M.P.H., is a health educator and research assistant at the Stanford University School of Medicine, Stanford, California, in the Patient Education Research Center, the Arthritis Center, and the Department of Medicine, Division of Immunology. Ms. González has also worked as a health promotion consultant with college students and with diverse cultural communities.

Bobby Heagerty, M.A., is director of community programs at Legacy Health System's Good Samaritan Hospital and Medical Center in Portland, Oregon. She has spoken and written extensively on family support services, chronic disease management, and care giver research and support. Ms. Heagerty was responsible for developing the Family

Support Center, which provides information, education, respite, and support to families coping with chronic illness. She also manages hospital in-service volunteers as well as several community service volunteer programs.

Salvinija G. Kernaghan is president of Inprint, a Chicago-based firm that provides editorial and communication consulting services and specializes in the health care field. Ms. Kernaghan is the author and editor of numerous books and articles on patient education and health promotion, as well as other issues related to health care policy and management. She is a former editor of *Hospitals*, senior associate editor of *Respiratory Care*, and staff specialist in the American Hospital Association's Center for Health Promotion. Ms. Kernaghan is a member of the American Medical Writers Association.

Leah S. Kinnaird, Ed.D., R.N., is director of oncology nursing and health education at Baptist Hospital of Miami, Florida. She was a member of the first AHA/ASHET Patient Education Advisory Committee and received the Distinguished Achievement Award from the American Society for Healthcare Education and Training for her efforts in patient education. Dr. Kinnaird's research analyzes nurse participation in patient education and sets forth a conceptual framework for promoting patient learning.

Kate Lorig, Dr.P.H., R.N., is a senior research scientist at the Stanford School of Medicine in the Stanford Patient Education Research Center (Stanford University, Stanford, California). Dr. Lorig has developed and evaluated courses on arthritis self-management and chronic disease self-management.

Carolyn E. Maller, M.S., C.H.E.S., R.N., is the patient health education coordinator for the Department of Veterans Affairs Medical Center, Albuquerque, New Mexico. She is a member of the International Patient Education Council, the Sigma Theta Tau Honor Society, the American Public Health Association, the Society for Public Health Education, and the Region 8 Nominating Committee for the American Society for Healthcare Education and Training (ASHET). She is also president of the New Mexico chapter of ASHET. She served on the AHA/ASHET Patient Education Advisory Committee as Region 8 patient education liaison. Ms. Maller has made numerous faculty presentations on patient education topics at the regional and national levels. She also served on national task forces for patient education program planning and development.

Patricia A. Mathews, M.A., F.H.C.E, R.N., is a senior consultant with The Einstein Consulting Group in Philadelphia. She was previously director of health education at Warren Hospital in Phillipsburg, New Jersey, where she developed and managed a comprehensive patient and community health education program. She is former president of the American Society for Healthcare Education of the American Hospital Association, and she is a frequent speaker and consultant on health care subjects. She served as the first chair on the AHA/ASHET Patient Education Advisory Committee.

Kathy L. Menke, M.A., B.S.N., manages staff resource services at the University of Nebraska Medical Center (UNMC), in Omaha. Her past experience includes serving as coordinator of continuity of care and as patient education specialist at UNMC. She was a past chair of the AHA/ASHET Patient Education Advisory Committee.

Annette Rykwalder Mercurio, M.P.H., C.H.E.S., is a health education manager who resides in Simi Valley, California, and currently serves as treasurer of the International Patient Education Council. Her previous experience includes 10 years of experience as director of patient and community health education for the University of Virginia Health Sciences Center. Her projects there included management of a grant designed to train health professionals in development of materials for patients with low literacy skills.

Patricia Dolan Mullen, Dr.P.H., is a professor and associate director for the Center for Health Promotion Research and Development, School of Public Health, University of Texas Health Science Center in Houston. Dr. Mullen has written numerous articles on patient education subjects from both patient and provider perspectives. Her research has focused on the development and evaluation of patient education programs for managing chronic illnesses and reducing risk factors among individuals free of illness. Currently, she is a leading researcher on smoking cessation and postpartum maintenance programs for pregnant women.

Rose Mary Monaco Pries, M.S.P.H., C.H.E.S., is the national coordinator of patient education for the Department of Veterans Affairs, and she works from the Department of Veterans Affairs Continuing Education Center in St. Louis. Her past experience includes serving as patient education coordinator at St. Louis County Hospital and Health Department in St. Louis and at Ellis Fischel State Cancer Hospital in Columbia, Missouri.

Dorothy A. Ruzicki, Ph.D., R.N., is the director of the Department of Educational Services at Sacred Heart Medical Center in Spokane, Washington. She helped establish and develop the framework for patient education at Sacred Heart Medical Center, serving as patient education coordinator from 1982 to 1989. She has published articles and spoken widely in the United States and Canada on the topic of patient education. She also served on the first AHA/ASHET Patient Education Advisory Committee.

Louise A. Villejo, M.P.H., C.H.E.S., is the director of the Patient Education Office at the University of Texas M. D. Anderson Cancer Center in Houston. She is responsible for the strategic planning of hospital- and clinic-based patient education services and the implementation, evaluation, and management of these services. Ms. Villejo is also the president of the Board of the International Patient Education Council. She is a frequent consultant to national health care organizations, hospitals, and private industry and has spoken and published extensively in the area of patient education and the cultural aspects of health care.

List of Figures and Tables

Figures

Tables

Acknowledgments

This book represents a decade of experience in the management of hospital-based patient education. The contributors have not only produced individual chapters for this book, but they have also contributed hundreds of hours to national educational programs, mentoring efforts, professional association committees, policy development meetings, and other activities to move the patient education field forward. They each deserve a personal and heartfelt thank-you. Hundreds of other patient education managers who have attended the AHA national patient education programs since 1983, participated as patient education liaisons in the AHA/ASHET patient education liaison program, or provided examples to one or more of AHA's patient education publications have contributed to the experience of this book even though they are not acknowledged by name.

It is not possible to thank everyone individually for their contributions; however, I would like to mention a variety of key people without whom this wealth of experience could never have been accumulated. First and foremost, I would like to thank Elizabeth Lee, the first patient education manager at AHA and later the director of the AHA's Center for Health Promotion. She set the stage nationally and in the association for the focus on patient education management that began in the 1970s. She served not only as my primary mentor but also as a resource and source of creative ideas for others in the field. Other staff from the center provided invaluable support and advice—Ruth Behrens, the first director of the Center for Health Promotion; Mary Longe, the manager of community health; Lynn Jones, the manager of worksite health promotion (and now manager, preventive services, AHA Division of Ambulatory Care), and Monica Riley, who directed the employee health program. Sharyn Bills, editor of *Promoting Health*, sharpened my writing skills through patient and substantial editing of my articles.

Special thanks go to the four women who chaired the AHA/ASHET Patient Education Advisory Committee since its beginning in 1983—Patricia Mathews, now a senior consultant with The Einstein Consulting Group in Philadelphia; Kathy Menke, now manager of staff resource services at the University of Nebraska Medical Center; Barbara Schroeder, oncology clinical specialist, Rochester Methodist Hospital; and Sandra Cornett, patient education coordinator at Ohio State University Hospitals. Without their enthusiasm, creativity, and endurance, many of the national patient education activities would never have happened. Thanks also go to Dorothy Ruzicki, a member of the first

Patient Education Advisory Committee, who has provided me with an ongoing creative dialogue about the evolving nature of patient education within hospitals. Thanks are also in order for the ASHET presidents, board members, and staff who supported the collaborative Patient Education Liaison Program.

I would also like recognize a few of the many others who have contributed to the success of national patient education activities and provided invaluable contributions to my own understanding of the patient education field. These people include Scott Simonds, professor, School of Public Health, University of Michigan; Nan Stout, formerly national coordinator for patient education in the Veterans Administration, and now chief of the State Home per Diem Program; Barbara Hebert Snyder, patient health education coordinator, Cleveland REMEC, and chair of the Department of Veterans Affairs National Patient Education Evaluation Committee; Nancy Goldstein, patient education coordinator, University of Minnesota Hospitals and Clinics; Sue Pritchett, president of Pritchett and Hull Associates, Atlanta; Katherine Crosson, director of the Patient Education Program, National Cancer Institute, and a Peace Corps colleague; Jane Zapka, associate professor of health policy and management, University of Massachusetts School of Public Health; Carolyn Speros, director of nursing educational services, Methodist Hospitals of Memphis; and Susan Edgman-Levitan, program director, Picker/Commonwealth Patient-Centered Care Program, Boston. A special note of thanks goes to Joy Lomax Martin, formerly patient education coordinator at Baptist Hospitals of Memphis, whose sense of humor, connection with patients, and storytelling ability continue to remind me of the human reasons to advocate for increased emphasis on patient education services.

And finally a special thanks goes to my family—Fred, Christopher, and Elizabeth—as well as to the families of other contributors who have patiently accepted evening, weekend, and vacation hours devoted to patient education.

Introduction

In a 1990 management advisory, the American Hospital Association reaffirmed its position on the responsibility of hospitals to provide patient education services.[1] In this document patient education services are described as those that "should enable patients, and their families and friends, when appropriate, to make informed decisions about their health; to manage their illnesses; and to implement follow-up care at home." Although it is not a traditional definition of patient education in the sense that the result of patient education rather than the process of patient education is specified, this key statement and the six assumptions that follow provide the underlying conceptual framework for this book:

1. Patients do not exist in a vacuum; they have families, friends, and a cultural context that must be addressed by patient education services.
2. Patient involvement is more important than patient compliance. Even though health care professionals often think they know what patients should do in particular situations, it is important that the patients themselves be provided with information, support, and skills they can use to make decisions about their own health.
3. Although patient education has been shown to have an impact on anxiety, complication rate, recovery time, service utilization, and other health status measures, from an ethical perspective its primary goal should be to enhance patient self-determination. Thus, health care professionals need to accept the fact that some patients are going to make health-related choices that professionals would not recommend and that will not necessarily result in the "best" health outcomes.
4. One important criterion for the success of a health encounter, on either an in-patient or outpatient basis, is whether the patient emerges with a strengthened ability to manage his or her health condition. A recent survey of 6,455 newly discharged patients showed that 20 to 30 percent reported problems with discharge preparation. For example, 30.2 percent were not told about the side effects of their medications, and 26.5 percent were not told about danger signals.[2]
5. Patient education is a multidimensional service that involves a number of strategies and disciplines. Everyone having contact with patients contributes to it. In

addition, patient education occurs in a number of different settings—preadmission, inpatient, outpatient, and home—and comprises cognitive, psychomotor, and psychosocial elements. Isolated, unreinforced patient education activities are rarely effective; instead, their success depends in large part on a combination of reinforcing educational strategies.

6. Patient education is a service that must be managed if it is to be successful. Its pervasiveness and complexity require management at the institutional level, the target population level, and the individual patient level.

The purpose of *Managing Hospital-Based Patient Education* is to capture the management and program development experience of those patient education managers, coordinators, and researchers who have successfully designed and implemented hospitalwide patient education programs during the past decade. (The term *patient education manager* will be used throughout this book to refer to positions whose responsibility it is to manage the patient education function. The actual position title may be coordinator, director, manager, or some other. Although the term *coordinator* is very commonly used, it does not connote the role as well as *manager* does.) From the inception of the American Hospital Association's Center for Health Promotion in 1978 until the present, AHA staff have persuaded dozens of dedicated hospital professionals and patient education researchers to share their growing expertise in patient education management through conferences, teleconferences, monographs, and journal articles. Whereas the AHA's 1979 publication *Implementing Patient Education in the Hospital* set the stage for the development of the patient education manager's role, *Managing Hospital-Based Patient Education* brings together management experiences gained during the 1980s and early 1990s to provide a jumping-off point for patient education during the next century.

Part one of this book addresses the various dimensions of hospitalwide management, including program structure, strategic planning, environmental support, decision-maker support, internal collaboration, risk management, financing, discharge planning, documentation, quality improvement, and staff development. Part two focuses principally on program development, including target population design, the research base, use of technology and print materials, family involvement, and the role of consumer health information resource centers.

Each chapter begins with a list of objectives that it will address, and many chapters provide sample forms and examples of approaches used by patient education managers in hospital settings. In addition, some chapters conclude with specialized bibliographies or lists of resources. A list of national patient education and health promotion organizations and a general bibliography of patient education references are included at the end of the book. The comprehensive approach taken in this book will help everyone involved in patient education to meet current and future challenges.

Health care is in the midst of rapid and inconsistent change, which will have a significant impact on the ways in which patient education is provided. Technology, management incentives, and care delivery options that were unheard of 10 years ago are commonplace today. Although it is not known how patient education will look and feel by the year 2000, it is clear that patient education services can only become more important. As technology pushes clinical care into the outpatient and home settings, patients and their families must take on additional responsibilities. Ethical issues, advance directives, the pervasiveness of chronic disease, and cost containment all force the patient and family to become more involved in health care decision making. It is becoming increasingly obvious that with health care reform must come a restructuring of the health care delivery system, which will move many decisions about how resources are to be used to the community level, thus engaging community members in health care decision making beyond the traditional patient role.

All of these changes require that patients, families, and the public have increased access to educational services and support so that they can take on these new roles. The challenge for hospitals will be to determine how to provide more education and support as they themselves undergo major structure- and service-related changes and as resource constraints intensify.

References

1. American Hospital Association. *Management Advisory, Patient Education Services.* Chicago: AHA, 1990.

2. Cleary, P. D., Edgman-Levitan, S., Roberts, M., Moloney, T. M., McMullen, W., Walker, J. D., and Delbanco, T. L. Patients evaluate their hospital care: a national survey. *Health Affairs* 10(4):254–67, Winter 1991.

Part One

Hospitalwide Management

Chapter 1

Developing Effective Patient Education Management Structures

Barbara E. Giloth, M.P.H., C.H.E.S.

☐ Objectives

The reader will be able to:

- Examine the historical development of patient education management structures
- Identify the range of hospitalwide management structures for patient education
- Suggest a framework for developing appropriate hospitalwide patient education management structures

☐ The Growth of Patient Education Management Structures

Although patient education has been an integral part of health care delivery for centuries, the management of this process is a relatively new concept. Beginning in the late 1960s, documentation of patient education coordinator positions (as they were then known), policies, committee mandates, and other management structures began to appear. National surveys and projects documented the growth of these structures and provided some evidence that their existence had a positive impact on the number of programs and their effectiveness.

The 1980s brought the prospective pricing system, other financial pressures on hospitals to control health care costs, downsizings, reorganizations, and dramatic increases in outpatient services—all of which posed additional challenges to the fledgling patient education management structures that had begun to develop. With the focus on quality, outcomes research, and health care reform, the 1990s further challenge patient education coordinators or managers to develop cost-effective programs that help patients and families to make critical behavior changes and cope with injuries or chronic diseases.

In addressing these concerns, it is helpful for patient education managers (PEMs, the term used throughout this book) to be aware of the evidence suggesting a link between hospitalwide management of patient education and effective program delivery. After

This chapter is adapted from the following article with permission from the publisher: B. E. Giloth. Management of patient education in U.S. hospitals: evolution of a concept. *Patient Education and Counseling* 15(2):101–11, Apr. 1990. Copyright ©1990 by Elsevier Scientific Publishers Ireland Limited.

summarizing some of these results, this chapter provides an overview of various ways that hospitalwide patient education programs can be structured to meet the challenges of the 1990s and the next century.

☐ Historical Perspective

A strong historical thread defines patient education as integral to effective health care delivery and a part of every health care provider's responsibility.[1] Most of the early writings on patient education and the majority of current research have focused on the case level of this process—patient–provider communication and interaction. More recently, this focus has expanded to the target population level—the development of education activities and programs for an identified group such as persons with diabetes or pregnant women. The development of broad patient education programs in hospitals, for example, often grew out of diabetes education programs that expanded rapidly in the late 1960s and early 1970s.

However, it was not until the late 1970s that the institutional management of patient education formally emerged in American Hospital Association[2] (AHA) and American Public Health Association[3] (APHA) publications. The APHA's Model for Patient Education Programming (see table 1-1) is relevant today as a framework for analyzing the three levels of patient education programming.

Recently, because of the growing complexity of the hospital itself, the numbers of health care providers who saw patient education as part of their role, and the increasing number of sites for patient care delivery, it became clear to some managers that if the case-level goals of patient education were to be met, hospitalwide processes to support these activities had to be developed. Thus there was a greater need for policies, committees, monitoring systems, and so forth specifically for patient education programs.

☐ What Hospitalwide Management Looks Like

Two national surveys of hospital inpatient education in 1975 and 1978 conducted by the AHA provide the broadest overview of patient education management structures in hospitals. Both surveys defined *inpatient education programs* as "educational activities with written goals and objectives for the patient and/or family during inpatient hospitalization."[4,5] Review of data from both years shows that the percentage of respondents reporting at least one program rose from 57.4 percent, or 2,680 respondents, in 1975 to 62.4 percent, or 2,921, in 1978 (see table 1-2, p. 8).

Reporting an operational patient education program is directly related to bed size. For example, in 1978, only 19.9 percent of respondents from under-25-bed hospitals reported programs as compared to 95.0 percent of those with 400 to 499 beds and 93.9 percent of those with 500+ beds.

Table 1-3 (p. 8) documents a more important change from the management perspective; the three years from 1975 to 1978 had seen an increase from 45.4 to 68.8 percent of hospitals with operational programs that had designated a coordinating department for patient education. Correspondingly, there was an increase from 38.4 to 56.6 percent of hospitals with operational programs that also had designated a person responsible for patient education (see table 1-4, p. 9).

Data from a 1981 survey that went to all registered hospitals showed a similar percentage—69.4 percent with a coordinating department; however, 60.5 percent of reporting hospitals had a person responsible for coordinating inpatient education. The pattern of designating a coordinating department in 1981 continued to show a substantial bias toward nursing, with 39 percent of respondents designating nursing in-service education, 21 percent nursing administration, 19.6 percent education, and 7.1 percent administration.[6]

It is noteworthy that with regard to both designation of coordinating department and person responsible for patient education, the direct relationship with bed size disappears. In 1978, for example, designation of a coordinating department was most likely

Table 1-1. Schema for Patient Education Program Development at Three Levels of Organization

Program Development Stage	Level of Organization		
	Institutional (Institutionwide System)	Programmatic (Selected Target Groups)	Patient (Individual Patient or Patient Group)
I. Assessment			
1. Objectives	Determine need for policy	Generate specific patient group and disease profiles	Determine knowledge, attitudes, and skill of patients and family
2. Outcome	Facility profile (educational needs and programs)	Priority needs for program development	Learning needs
3. Baseline questions	Policy statement for patient education in the facility?	What are disease characteristics? Prevalence, incidence, clusters	Course of disease, stage, and impact on individual patients?
	Support for patient education?	Who are the patients? Demographic, Psycho/social, Physical levels, Family configurations	Individual patient and family psycho/social and cultural background?
	Perceptions of utility and effectiveness of patient education	Climate for change? Staff readiness and capability	Readiness of patient for learning?
	What organizational units are involved in patient education? Coordination mechanism? Administrative focus for education? Support for creating one?	Are staff knowledge, attitudes, skills sufficient?	Patient's level of functioning—physical, mental, etc.?
	Existing expenditures, resources administrative capacity, staff, funds, etc. Management of resources? Potential for coordinating consolidation?	What are the organization's characteristics? Number of patients, average length of stay, total hours, number of contacts, space, records system	Level of patient–provider interaction?
	Present status of quality of care: morbidity, mortality, disability, etc.?	Resources available Manpower, space, equipment dollars	Are resource and educational materials available, adequate, used?

(Continued on next page)

Table 1-1. (Continued)

Program Development Stage	Level of Organization		
	Institutional (Institutionwide System)	Programmatic (Selected Target Groups)	Patient (Individual Patient or Patient Group)
II. Planning			
1. Objectives	Develop facilitywide plan patient education	Develop program plans for priority needs	Identify individual patient learning objectives or contract
2. Outcomes	Formulation of policy statement Development of goals and strategies Development of organizational structure Identification and establishment of internal and external linkage systems Establishment of data and communication systems	Standard protocols Staff training Educational methods and materials Records and evaluation systems Communication channels	Individual teaching plan for patients and family Plan for follow-up and referral Documentation method
3. Participants	Multidisciplinary task force	Health team members Representatives of community agencies Representatives of patients and family members	Patient Family Provider or team
4. Decisionmakers	Administration Board of Trustees Chief of Services	Chief of Services or Section Chiefs Medical Advisory Committee or equivalent	(Same)
III. Implementation			
1. Organization	Carry out plan Test, revise Use information gained through implementation to refine and improve program	(Same)	(Same)
2. Processes	Testing goals and strategies and adapting as necessary Monitoring: data and communications systems, policies, and procedures	Monitoring program delivery in terms of utility and acceptance of procedures, training, materials, methods, communication patterns, records systems	Monitoring patient learning in terms of utility; acceptance of methods and materials; patient–provider interaction; referral mechanisms; documentation systems; staff communications
3. Communication Mechanisms	Progress reports, staff meetings, and so on	Documentation in medical records, team conferences, etc.	Medical record notes, team conferences, etc.
4. Time frame	Annual	Monthly	Daily or weekly

5. Participants	Multidisciplinary task force	Health team members; Representatives of community agencies; Representatives of patients and family members	Patient; Family; Provider or team
6. Decision-makers	Administration; Board of Trustees; Chief of Services	Chief of Services or Section Chiefs; Medical Advisory Committee or equivalent	(Same)
IV. Evaluation			
1. Focus	Guide policy formulation and administrative management and resource allocation decisions	Guide changes in program design and implementation	Identify alternative approach and methods for communication patient education
2. Outcomes			
a. Effectiveness	Reductions in morbidity, mortality, disability	Improved health status related to patient behaviors, especially utilization (composite indicators/aggregate data) of health sources, acceptance of best medical alternatives, life style changes	Patient demonstration of: self-management; monitoring; reporting side effects and symptoms; problem-solving ability; appointment keeping
	Patient, staff, and community satisfaction	Patient, staff, and community satisfaction	Patient, staff, and community satisfaction
			Staff demonstrated competency in interpersonal skills, teaching, problem solving
b. Efficiency	Appropriate allocation resources to site/population/community	Appropriate utilization of resources—money, manpower, materials, etc.	
		Accomplishment of staff training goals	
3. Time frame	3–5 years (with interim progress reporting and decision making)	Yearly or at completion of specific programs	At time of discharge and/or subsequent follow-up visit
4. Participants	Multidisciplinary task force	Health team members; Representatives of community agencies; Representatives of patient and family members	Patient; Family; Provider or team
5. Decisionmakers	Administration; Board of Trustees; Chief of Services	Chief of Services or Section Chiefs; Medical Advisory Committee or equivalent	(Same)

Source: Reprinted, with permission, from S. G. Deeds, B. J. Hebert, and J. M. Wolle, editors. A model for patient education programming. Special project report, Public Health Education Section, American Public Health Association, 1979.

Table 1-2. Hospitals Reporting Inpatient Education Programs, by Bed Size, 1975 and 1978

	1975 Survey			1978 Survey		
	Total Hospitals Reporting	Hospitals Reporting Operational Programs		Total Hospitals Reporting	Hospitals Reporting Operational Programs	
Bed Size	Number	Number	%	Number	Number	%
U.S. total	4,669	2,680	57.4	4,678	2,921	62.4
Under 25	194	37	19.1	176	35	19.9
25–49	822	236	28.7	795	261	32.8
50–99	1,166	519	44.5	1,125	535	47.6
100–199	1,106	724	65.5	1,111	775	69.8
200–299	593	477	80.4	625	534	85.4
300–399	338	286	84.6	357	321	89.9
400–499	200	178	89.0	222	211	95.0
500+	250	223	89.2	267	249	93.9

Source: American Hospital Association. *Hospital Inpatient Education: Survey Findings and Analyses.* Atlanta: Centers for Disease Control, 1980.

Table 1-3. Hospitals with Operational Programs and a Department Designated to Coordinate Inpatient Education, by Bed Size, 1975 and 1978

	1975 Survey			1978 Survey		
	Number of Operational Programs	With Coordinating Department		Number of Operational Departments	With Coordinating Department	
Bed Size		Number	%		Number	%
U.S. total	2,680	1,218	45.4	2,921	2,009	68.8
Under 25	37	11	29.7	35	22	62.9
25–49	236	107	45.3	261	179	68.6
50–99	519	229	44.1	535	366	68.4
100–199	724	349	48.2	775	566	73.0
200–299	477	244	51.1	534	379	71.0
300–399	286	122	42.7	321	214	66.7
400–499	178	76	42.7	211	138	65.4
500+	223	80	35.9	249	145	58.2

Source: American Hospital Association. *Hospital Inpatient Education: Survey Findings and Analyses.* Atlanta: Centers for Disease Control, 1980.

in hospitals with 100 to 199 beds and 200 to 299 beds, in 1981 the 200–299-bed and 300–399-bed categories topped the list.

More recent AHA health promotion surveys provide less information about management structures and, because of lower response rates (suggesting that the more interested hospitals were likely to respond), may have overstated the extent of hospitals' commitment to the management of patient education. The 1984 survey of Hospital-Based Health Promotion Programs documented that 84 percent of responding hospitals offered at least one inpatient education program with written objectives.[7] A briefer 1987 survey reported that 87.1 percent of responding hospitals reported offering inpatient education services.[8] Both these surveys had substantially lower response rates than earlier patient education surveys. The AHA's annual survey of all registered hospitals, with a response rate of over 90 percent, added patient education to its list of monitored services in 1986. While 64.8 percent of community hospitals said they offered patient education in 1986, by 1990 this percentage had grown to 86.4 percent.[9] (See table 1-5.)

In the spring of 1990, a Patient Education Management Models questionnaire was sent out to all chapter and regional liaisons in the American Society for Healthcare Education and Training (ASHET), as well as to registrants at AHA's 1989 national patient education conference. The purpose of this project was twofold: (1) to collect information on the reporting structures of patient education managers (PEMs); and (2) to collect examples of job descriptions that could be shared with others in the field. Approximately 50 percent, or 116 of those mailed the questionnaire, returned a completed questionnaire. In terms of reporting structure, respondents fell into four major subgroups: hospitalwide education/human resources (37 percent); nursing administration (32 percent); nursing education (20 percent); and hospital administration (11 percent).[10]

Does the existence of these hospitalwide management structures, such as the presence of a PEM, make a difference in terms of the patient education provided? Limited data suggest that they do. The 1975 survey looked at the impact of six management structures (presence of a policy, a committee, a person to coordinate, a budget, an audit mechanism, and an evaluation) on the number of organized patient education programs. Table 1-6 documents the tendency for hospitals with four to six of these variables to offer more programs than hospitals with only one or two. A 1981 study of 200 hospitals documented the positive impact of similar management variables (policy, committee, coordinator, audit, and budget) on the presence of a variety of instructional design components of patient education programs.[11]

Results of the Patient Health Education Profile in Veterans Administration (VA) medical centers, a universe survey of 166 VA medical centers completed in 1985, suggests a

Table 1-4. Hospitals with Operational Programs Reporting a Person Responsible, by Bed Size, 1975 and 1978

Bed Size	1975 Survey: Total Hospitals Reporting			1978 Survey: Total Hospitals Reporting		
	Operational Programs (Number)	Operational Programs with Person Responsible (Number)	Percent of Hospitals with Operational Programs (%)	Operational Programs (Number)	Operational Programs with Person Responsible (Number)	Percent of Hospitals with Operational Programs (%)
U.S. total	2,680	1,030	38.4	2,921	1,625	56.6
Under 25	37	11	29.7	35	21	60.0
25–49	236	91	38.6	261	146	55.9
50–99	519	200	38.5	535	315	58.9
100–199	724	308	42.5	775	483	62.3
200–299	477	202	42.3	534	291	54.5
300–399	286	97	33.9	321	171	53.3
400–499	178	60	33.7	211	114	54.0
500+	223	61	27.4	249	111	14.6

Source: American Hospital Association. *Hospital Inpatient Education: Survey Findings and Analyses.* Atlanta: Centers for Disease Control, 1980.

Table 1-5. U.S. Community Hospitals Providing Health Promotion Services, 1986–1990

	1986	1987	1988	1989	1990
Patient education	64.8%	68.1%	76.3%	78.4%	86.4%
Community health promotion	55.3%	60.3%	67.7%	70.2%	77.2%
Worksite health promotion	34.3%	38.5%	43.9%	47.1%	53.9%
Total Number	5,678	5,671	5,533	5,455	5,056

Source: American Hospital Association. *Annual Survey of Hospitals, 1986–90.* Chicago: AHA, 1990.

Table 1-6. Hospitals with Specified Administrative Variables of Patient Education and Operational Programs, 1975

Variable(s)	Total Response Number	Responses with Fewer Than 7 Programs		Responses with More Than 10 Programs	
		Number	%	Number	%
One or two variables					
Pr	85	53	62.4	15	18.6
C, Pr	12	7	58.3	0	0
A	593	327	55.1	135	22.8
Pr, A	184	93	50.5	47	25.5
Four to six variables					
Pl, C, Pr, B, A	31	1	3.2	24	77.4
Pl, C, Pr, B, A, E	47	6	13.0	32	68.0
C, Pr, B, A, E	22	4	18.1	14	63.6
Pl, C, Pr, A, E	27	4	3.2	17	62.9
Pr, B, A, E	92	20	21.7	44	47.8

Source: American Hospital Association. *Hospital Inpatient Education: Survey Findings and Analyses, 1975.* Atlanta: Centers for Disease Control, 1977.

Note: Variables are abbreviated as: Pl, policy; C, committee; Pr, person responsible; B, budget; A, audit; E, evaluation.

strong link between hospitalwide coordination or management of patient education and effective program delivery.[12]

- The likelihood that a hospital would have a written hospitalwide plan for patient education in VA medical centers was nearly six times greater where a patient education committee was present.
- Only 29 percent of the sites that did not have a PEM had written plans, compared with 42 percent among the sites where coordination functions had been assigned part-time and 68 percent of the sites with full-time managers.
- Sites that had written plans reported 1.9 times as many staff development programs as sites that did not, and sites with committees had 1.8 times as many programs as those without committees.
- Sites with full-time PEMs had 1.6 times as many programs as sites where coordination functions had been assigned part-time and 1.5 times as many as sites with no manager.

One other major national activity adds qualitative evidence to this description of the impact of hospitalwide management structures. In 1982 and 1984, the AHA sponsored a National Patient Education Leaders Award program to recognize hospitals for their achievement in the hospitalwide and target population management of patient education programs.

Analysis of the 18 hospitals winning awards for hospitalwide management showed considerable variation in the way patient education was managed; however, some patterns emerged. For example, although national data consistently showed that nursing departments were overwhelmingly the coordinating department, the coordinating department in the winning hospitals was most likely to be either a separate department or a department of education. This is consistent with later data from the AHA/ASHET Patient Education Liaison Program and suggests that the neutrality of these latter options facilitates coordination among clinical departments, provides easier access to hospitalwide management systems, and increases the visibility of the function. Additionally, 16 out of 18 winners had at least one full-time staff member to coordinate patient education, although all supported the decentralization of the delivery of service. All but one developed and used a variety of committees to achieve broad-based involvement in planning and program development.

Finally, all the award winners had established a process to guide the development of target population programs, and most had achieved at least some success in coordinating print and audiovisual teaching resources for the entire hospital.[13] As might be expected, the hospitalwide goal-setting process was in general weak and the evaluation process usually lacking. The 1984 winners were more likely to show evidence of strategic planning, linking their hospitalwide objectives to hospital goals, perhaps reflective of the pressures of prospective pricing and other environmental changes.[14]

Although the 1990 AHA/ASHET Patient Education Liaison Program data did not collect information on program impact, the survey did ask respondents if they wanted to change their organizational structure. Overall, 61 percent of respondents wanted a change. When comparing four subgroups, the lowest percentage that desired change (53 percent) was for those reporting to hospital administration and the highest percentage (72 percent) was for those reporting to nursing education. The majority of changes that respondents requested fell into the following four categories: (1) establish a PEM position; (2) increase staff allocated to patient education; (3) change reporting structure; and (4) establish a hospitalwide department.[15]

☐ Target Population Programs

The existence of target population programs has been relatively easy to validate, although their effectiveness has been much more difficult to document. In 1984, the most commonly offered inpatient education programs were diabetes, preoperative education, heart attack, cardiac rehabilitation, and nutrition; for outpatients, the top five included diabetes, nutrition, prenatal education, cardiac rehab, and heart attack.[16] Within the VA system, diabetes programs also topped the outpatient list followed by alcoholism, hypertension, special diet instructions, and dental health, suggesting the somewhat different needs of veteran populations.[17]

Respondents to the 1984 AHA survey were also asked to provide more in-depth information about their diabetes programs, including an identification of the populations served by their programs when first initiated and currently. Results document a major shift to provision of services to outpatient and community members, as well as a small percentage of hospitals that provide diabetes education to corporations and businesses in addition to other more traditional target populations. A critical question from the perspective of impact is to what extent the target population has been reached by the program. Often, elaborate systems have to be developed to track patients through various phases of the program.[18] The VA found in its in-depth review of stroke programs that data on the number of stroke inpatients and outpatients were not available.[19]

Concerns continue to be raised about the quality of the patient education programs delivered to target populations. In 1982, the Michigan Department of Public Health and the Michigan Hospital Association launched a project to assess the quality of patient education activities in Michigan hospitals. A list of criteria was developed by an ad hoc committee and used as the basis for a survey instrument that collected information about 280 target population programs (up to three per hospital). Only one of the programs met all the criteria. When project staff selected five basic criteria that were considered minimum (planning/advisory group, written program goals, written content outline of program, written learning objectives, and evaluation of patient progress), only 31 of the programs met these criteria.[20]

The most ambitious attempt to define and ensure the quality of a target population program was organized by the diabetes community under the auspices of the National Diabetes Advisory Board. A multiyear consensus process resulted in the adoption of National Standards for Diabetes Patient Education Programs that incorporate, in addition to clinical content and instructional design elements, most of the critical program management elements identified by the AHA and APHA planning models cited earlier.[21] A pilot study of the proposed recognition process tested the 70 review criteria that had

Barbara E. Giloth, M.P.H., C.H.E.S.

been identified. The average program met two-thirds of the criteria, and there did not appear to be any predictable association between bed size and ability to meet the criteria. Adequate staff time strongly influenced the ability of the 203 sites to meet the criteria; programs having less than one full-time equivalent scored 40 percent of the criteria as unmet.[22]

There has been a relatively large outpouring of research documenting the impact of patient education interventions on knowledge, behavior change, recovery, complications, pain, anxiety, and morbidity, including the increasing use of the meta-analysis strategy to consolidate research findings. (See chapter 14 in this book for the range of specific references.) However, very little attention has been paid to management variables that would help ensure that patient education programs would actually run in a nonresearch setting.

In 1987, Redman and others studied the relationship between organizational variables at the target population level and the completeness of instruction. Hypothesis testing identified three predictor variables as significantly related to patient or provider report of instruction: degree of structure for implementation (for example, teaching guides, sample teaching plans); provider perception of reinforcement for doing patient education; and perceived payoffs from the program.[23] In 1986, Lorenz and others examined the impact of organizational interventions on the delivery of patient education in a diabetes clinic. Having found in earlier research that only a very small amount of time was devoted to patient education, nursing responsibility for managing patient flow was reduced, and an education checklist was included in the medical record. As a result of these interventions, time spent in needs assessment increased by one-half and instruction by nearly two-thirds.[24]

☐ Ways to Develop Effective Patient Education Management Structures

With a research base that points to the need for patient education management but is very unclear about the effectiveness of any particular management structure, the question becomes what type of hospitalwide program to develop. The purpose of this section is to examine the major patient education functions that should be delivered, and to identify the options for hospitalwide management as well as the range of management structures that should be developed. A process for shaping hospital-specific management structures is also suggested.

Patient Education Functions

No matter what the structure of the hospitalwide program, the following functions appear basic to the effective implementation of a hospitalwide patient education program.[25]

1. Coordination of a hospitalwide patient education program through development of management structures (for example, policies, procedures, patient education committees, and so forth) that will enable development of a variety of patient education activities
2. Development of hospitalwide cooperation and support for patient education activities
3. Design and evaluation of patient education programs to meet the educational needs of specific patient populations
4. Acquisition, development, and distribution of patient education materials and media
5. Development of hospital staff's patient education skills through in-service education programs
6. Direct delivery of patient education services as part of ongoing patient care (for example, as part of routine nursing and medical care)
7. Direct delivery of patient education services through group classes or some other means separated from the patient's hospital unit (for example, providing patient education classes in the hospital's ambulatory care center)

8. Development of processes to ensure continuity of patient education service for specific patients or groups as they move through inpatient, outpatient, and home care delivery sites

In general, two major types of roles emerge from analysis of the functions: (1) the PEM's role and (2) a variety of patient educator roles. (Patient educators are those who actually teach the patients and may be nurses, discharge coordinators, or other staff.) Functions 1 through 3 are the core of the PEM's role; functions 6 through 8 are provided by staff in patient educator roles. Functions 4 and 5 are often shared, with the PEM focusing on the management aspects and the patient educators focusing on the clinical, content aspects. What is important to remember is that this is a discussion of roles, not necessarily positions. For example, although the term *patient education manager* is used as a common reference point throughout this book, in different hospitals the person performing this role might have a title such as patient education coordinator, director of education, director of in-service education, director of discharge planning, or health education specialist.

Critical Patient Education Management Processes

Given the above-mentioned patient education functions, there are several major management processes that an organization needs to develop as an infrastructure to support the effective implementation of a hospitalwide patient education program. These include broad-based institutional support; a coordinating mechanism; a committee structure; policy and procedure support; a system to support the acquisition, development, and distribution of patient education materials; and opportunities to develop the staff's patient education skills.

Broad-Based Institutional Support
A broad base of support for patient education is critical if the other management structures and processes are to be effective. Appropriate levels of support, however, are not frequently apparent at the start-up of a patient education program and must be nurtured as the program develops. A little bit of the chicken–egg controversy makes this process somewhat ambiguous. Does strong hospital support produce an effective patient education program, or does an effective patient education program produce strong hospital support? The answer to both sides of this question is yes, suggesting that program development and gaining support are intertwined. Figure 1-1 suggests activities for key target populations that can contribute to the effective implementation of patient education. Although developed specifically for VA facilities, this outline offers a vision of the breadth of institutional support necessary for a patient education program in any type of medical center.[26] (For further information about gaining support from administration, medical staff, and other staff, see chapter 5.)

Coordinating Mechanism
The implementation of patient education across multiple departments, disciplines, and settings requires some type of coordinating mechanism—most likely a person, department, or committee to ensure a reasonable level of consistency, communication, and efficient use of resources. There is some indication, and common sense would support, that the coordinating function is enhanced by having a specific person designated as responsible. The management glue that can keep an active patient education program together means having a person to run meetings, prepare minutes, collect resources, and provide educational consultation. These tasks are often very difficult to accomplish by people who have other full-time responsibilities. However, having a designated PEM may not work if the position is isolated, without a rich array of networks through which to encourage interdisciplinary involvement, program development, and administrative support. (See figures 1-2 through 1-10, pp. 15–27, for organizational charts and samples of PEM job descriptions within different management structures.)

Figure 1-1. Activities of Key Target Populations That Contribute to Effective Implementation of Patient Health Education Services

Top Decision Makers
(Medical Center Director, Assistant or Associate Director, Chief of Staff, Associate Chief of Staff for Research, Education, and Ambulatory Care, and bed section chiefs)

1. Includes patient health education goals and objectives in medical center mission statement and facility planning documents.
2. Promotes concept that patient health education (PHE) is a critical component of quality health care.
3. Supports multidisciplinary approach to planned, coordinated PHE.
4. Supports the establishment and continued operation of a facility multidisciplinary PHE committee.
5. Supports the allocation of resources to PHE.
6. Approves medical center PHE policies.
7. Recognizes/commends service or staff achievement of PHE.

Middle Managers
(Service chiefs and supervisors)

1. Supports concept that PHE is a critical component of quality health care.
2. Supports use of staff time to plan and implement PHE services.
3. Facilitates professional development in patient health education through problem solving, mentoring, continuing education and consultation.
4. Monitors quality of patient education activities performed by their staff.
5. Serves or nominates staff to represent service on facility PHE committees.
6. Supports multidisciplinary planning and implementation of PHE.
7. Recognizes/rewards staff achievement in patient health education.

Physicians

1. Accepts concept that PHE is an integral part of the treatment plan.
2. Refers and encourages appropriate use of patient health education services by patients.
3. Supports multidisciplinary planning and implementation of PHE.
4. Serves on committees to plan target population specific programs.
5. Reviews patient health education materials for content accuracy.

Clinical Staff

1. Supports PHE as a component of quality health care.
2. Uses approved program guides and materials to implement PHE.
3. Selects appropriate teaching methodologies to meet assessed learning needs.
4. Documents PHE and patient response in medical record using accepted format.
5. Serves on program task forces/committees as assigned.
6. Contributes to effective implementation of PHE by supporting active roles of co-workers in PHE.

Veterans Organizations

1. Supports and promotes PHE as part of quality health care.
2. Accepts assignment on appropriate PHE committees and task forces.
3. Contributes volunteer hours and resources to implement PHE programs of interest.

Patient Health Education Committee

1. Defines PHE program priorities for institutionwide programs.
2. Develops PHE plan annually and evaluates progress.
3. Develops approval mechanism to review submitted target population PHE programs.
4. Presents important PHE issues to top decision makers and medical center committees.
5. Provides a forum for discussion and resolution of multidisciplinary issues in PHE.
6. Identifies common staff development needs in PHE.
7. Provides an opportunity to use communication lines between committee members and their respective services.
8. Identifies resources needed to provide PHE at institution, target population and case levels.

Reprinted from VA Patient Health Education Program, Office of Academic Affairs. Facilitator's guide. In: *Patient Health Education: Building Medical Center Commitment.* Washington, D.C.: Department of Veterans Affairs, 1988.

Figure 1-2. Organizational Chart for the Education Office, VA Medical Center, Albuquerque

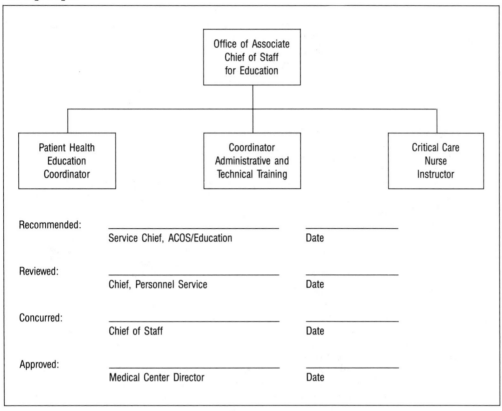

Reprinted from the Department of Veterans Affairs, Albuquerque, New Mexico, 1989.

Committee Structure

Because of the number of people required to implement a patient education program successfully, there should be a series of mechanisms to involve a wide variety of departments and staff from all levels of the organization in planning and monitoring patient education activities. A hospitalwide patient education committee chaired by a powerful person within the organization and including, as members, key department heads is one of the mechanisms that has worked well when it has been effectively constituted. However, this type of committee is usually not sufficient; successful PEMs have catalyzed department-level committees, interdisciplinary task forces to develop target population programs, patient education resource committees to organize resource people from each unit of the hospital, and so forth. Effective use of these committees, which in smaller institutions may appear as informal work groups, contributes to the overall need for broad support for patient education. (Details of the development and use of committees can be found in chapter 4.)

Policy and Procedure Support

A policy is a guide to action. It is an authoritative statement of what is or is not to be done. A statement of procedure usually accompanies a policy and defines how the tasks indicated in a policy are to be carried out. Written policies and procedures provide tools to (1) obtain agreement among staff about management of specific hospital activities; (2) define responsibilities of staff; (3) maintain consistency in implementation of specific hospital activities; (4) clarify relationships among departments; and (5) comply with requirements of accreditation bodies.[27]

Figure 1-3. Job Description for Patient Health Education Coordinator, VA Medical Center, Albuquerque (200 Beds)

As patient health education coordinator, the incumbent is administratively responsible for the implementation, coordination, and evaluation of all medical center-based patient health education activities. The incumbent will provide professional leadership, advice, guidance, and authoritative consultation to all services in matters relating to patient health education. The incumbent will be concerned with coordinating the patient health education program for direct care providers on an interdisciplinary basis.

The patient health coordinator will assume the following specific responsibilities and functions:

a. The coordinator develops goals and philosophy statements for the patient health education function, and establishes appropriate policies and procedures that govern the performance of such.

b. The incumbent makes diagnoses of organizational needs, identifies internal and external resources, and establishes priorities for health education programs based on identified needs and available resources.

c. The coordinator is responsible for centerwide program management including: preparing a budget, monitoring expenses, and analyzing costs of patient health education activities and programs; developing specific program goals, objectives, and content; ensuring the implementation, evaluation, and revision for each program; accurately tracking patient health education attendance and potential resources generated for the medical center.

d. The incumbent works with outside consultants as necessary to achieve project goals. Where appropriate, the coordinator participates in cooperative efforts with other VA facilities, on a national level, providing local and national leadership through professional memberships, community organizations and academic institutions to promote quality patient health education activities.

e. The coordinator consults with the associate chief of nursing for education and the nursing instructors, instructing their staff in the provision of patient health education.

f. On a local, regional, and national basis, the incumbent conducts educational programs for medical center staff who are responsible for patient health education programs, and provides consultation regarding problem-solving, program planning, evaluation, and research.

g. The coordinator provides technical guidance and direction in the selection of effective and appropriate educational/behavioral strategies, assessment and evaluation criteria, and documentation design.

h. The incumbent provides technical guidance and direction in the preparation, development, pretesting, and utilization of patient health education materials and audiovisual programs.

i. The coordinator chairs the medical center patient health education advisory committee and serves as an educational process consultant to subcommittees (convened to develop and implement specific programs). The coordinator represents patient health education at service chief and other medical center meetings.

j. The incumbent continually reviews and interprets outside research related to patient health education. He/she integrates these data into ongoing programs of quality assurance and future planning. The coordinator conducts and monitors research examining the impact of educational efforts, and assists with the development of quality review procedures and the development of quality assurance indicators pertinent to process mechanisms and patient outcomes. He/she analyzes evaluation data to provide feedback to all those involved in patient health education.

k. The coordinator functions as a preceptor and provides a training site for students and VA staff who have a special interest and/or academic preparation in health education.

l. The coordinator will be directly involved with the Salt Lake Regional Medical Education Center (SL RMEC) patient health education coordinator in program consultation, planning and implementation as appropriate for the Southwest Region and nationwide. In addition, a linkage with the national patient health education coordinator will be established and maintained. Involvement will include cooperative research, project development, and contributions of expertise, including faculty presentations. The incumbent will enhance networking and sharing through collaboration with the St. Louis Continuing Education Center (CEC) on national initiatives.

m. The incumbent participates in presenting papers at national patient health education programs, to promote a model for a patient health education program. Consultation services on issues of national concern to the field of health education are readily available.

n. The coordinator identifies opportunities for resource sharing to promote the mission of the medical center. Priority will be given to promoting cost effective approaches to deliver patient health education as a direct patient care activity.

o. The incumbent demonstrates expertise in identifying areas for sharing resources and successfully coordinates, prepares, and drafts a sharing agreement for review and approval by all concerned parties.

p. The coordinator is responsible for the direct supervision of a staff of volunteers, which supports the logistical functions of the ongoing patient health education programs as well as the operation of a centerwide distribution center for patient health education materials. Those logistical functions include maintaining a materials inventory, registering patients, reporting program attendance, and a variety of tasks necessary to assemble patient teaching manuals, handouts, and brochures.

Figure 1-3. (Continued)

q. The coordinator actively submits proposals for activation projects related to the patient health education program to meet the mission of the medical center. Such proposals include a patient health education learning center, spinal cord injury technology center, and other state of the art computer applications.

1. **Knowledge Required by the Position**
Skill in policy formulation for health education. Skill in determining the appropriate focus for health education. Skill in designated administrative activities. Skill in providing consultation to others. Skill in preparing others to perform health education related skills. Professional knowledge of the theories, principles, practices, and techniques of adult education. Skill in coordination and communication with senior level staff. Professional knowledge and skill to interpret research related to health education. Skill in facilitating communications. Knowledge and skill in planning for institutional, programs, and patient level activities.

2. **Supervisory Controls**
The patient health education coordinator is under the general supervision of the associate chief of staff for education (ACOS/E). With the approval of the ACOS/E, the coordinator attends to program management and staff development in an independent manner. Project assignments are initiated by the coordinator on the basis of organizational need.

3. **Guidelines**
Guidance is minimal, consisting of VA codes and regulations and past precedent or patient health education within the system. The coordinator practices a significant amount of professional discretion in the development and management of the patient health education function. Completed work is evaluated in terms of its overall effectiveness and its appropriateness in meeting the specific needs of the medical center, as well as regional and national VA training needs.

4. The 525-bed Veterans Administration Medical Center is referred to as the Regional Federal Medical Center in recognition of its landmark VA/DoD joint sharing agreement, whereby Kirtland Air Force Hospital is collocated with the VA facility. Both hospitals benefit from this arrangement and from their active affiliation with the University of New Mexico School of Medicine. The center is very involved in rural outreach efforts, as evidenced by the establishment of the Farmington, Artesia, and Raton community clinics.

   In addition, in 1989 there were approximately 197,742 outpatient visits per year. The center includes a spinal cord injury unit, nursing home care unit, long term and intermediate psychiatric facility, and a clinical services addition.

   The patient health education coordinator provides consultation and guidance to the center director, chief of staff, and service chiefs as well as direct care staff. The patient health education coordinator must frequently identify the origin of problems and assist the staff in developing an approach to meet the goals and objectives of the institution. This requires unusual modification of practices in applying educational principles and practices.

5. **Scope and Effect**
The mission of VA patient health education program is to promote the health of veteran beneficiaries through the provision of patient health education services, and to share program developments with the community at large. The purpose of the patient health education coordinator is to improve the coordination and quality of patient health education services in the medical center, in the community, and on a regional and national level within the VA system.

6. **Personal Contacts**
Personal contacts include face-to-face, telephonic, electronic, and written contacts with VA staff in the medical center, regionally, nationally, with health professionals in the community and on a collaborative basis with the Air Force.

7. **Purpose of Contacts**
The personal contacts involve exchange of information, consultation, continuing education and technical assistance.

8. **Physical Demands**
The work involves travel by automobile and air. The work includes some walking and carrying of light-to-medium weight items such as materials for continuing education or reports for meetings.

9. **Work Environment**
The work environment involves the normal risks and discomforts typical of an office, medical care setting, and travel.

Reprinted from the Department of Veterans Affairs, Albuquerque, New Mexico, 1989.

Figures 1-11 through 1-14 (pp. 28–32) offer samples of several policies and procedures and a process for developing and revising patient education materials. Although there is considerable disagreement about the number and type of policies and procedures that are needed as a base for successful implementation of a hospitalwide patient education program, the following categories of policy content should be considered:[28]

- Hospitalwide planning for patient education (Who is involved in planning and what is the planning process? What is the time cycle? How is the patient education plan integrated into the facility planning document?)
- Patient education program development and approval (Who is involved in target population program planning and development? What is the planning process? How is *program* defined? What is the facility review/approval process?)
- Delivery of patient education to patients (How is patient education delivered to the individual patient? Who provides this education and under what circumstances?)
- Patient education program review and evaluation (What mechanism/process reviews outcome data for the impact of patient education programs? How are patient education activities included in the hospital's quality management program?)
- Instructional materials—print and nonprint—for patient education (What selection criteria are used? Who is involved in the review process? What is the procedure for their purchase, storage, and distribution? Are the materials linked to program or activity objectives?)

Figure 1-4. Organizational Chart for Human Resources, El Camino Hospital, Mountain View

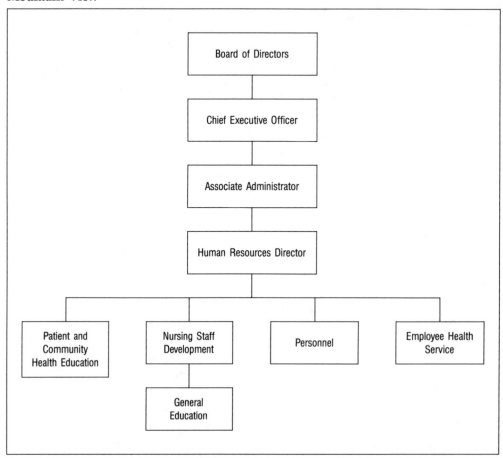

Reprinted, with permission, from El Camino Hospital, Mountain View, California, 1992.

- Coordination of patient education among departments and settings (Does the hospital have policies that facilitate coordination among departments and among settings? How is patient education coordinated with the discharge planning process?)
- Documentation of patient education in the medical record (Does the hospital have policies that facilitate all disciplines/departments to document patient education in the medical record? What should be documented? Where should documentation occur?)
- Budgeting and fiscal management of patient education (Does the facility have a policy that facilitates the budgeting process for patient education? Who is accountable for budget preparation? How is the budgeting process linked to the allocation process?)

Figure 1-5. Job Description for Manager, Patient and Community Health Education, El Camino Hospital, Mountain View (377 Beds)

Date	**Department**	**Position Title**
November, 1992	Patient and Community Health Education	Manager

Manage the following staff: Diabetes Educator, Enterostomal Therapy Nurses, Nutrition Educator, Parenteral Services Clinicians, Respiratory Nurse Counselor, Community Health Instructors, Support Group Facilitators, Secretaries.

Reports to: Human Resources Director

Job Summary:
Responsible for the management of planning, development, implementation, and evaluation of high-quality patient and community health education programs in order to provide a service to the patient and the community and promote positive community relations.

Responsibilities:
1. Identify patient and community health education programs through formal needs assessment.
2. Prioritize the development of patient education materials as indicated by needs assessment and implementation of patient and community programs.
3. Coordinate the development and implementation of patient and community health programs.
4. Provide departmental direction and support to personnel and programs under the auspices of patient education and community health education.
5. Coordinate the standardization of patient education tools for patient education in patient care departments.
6. Identify audit criteria to evaluate the effectiveness of patient and community health education.
7. Collaborate with public relations to promote community visibility of patient and community health education efforts.
8. Anticipate patient and community health education component in future ventures of the hospital.
9. Act as liaison with physicians and physicians' office staff regarding patient and community health education efforts.
10. Attend classes, workshops, and seminars for personal and professional growth.
11. Provide consultation to outside agencies on patient and community health education.
12. Facilitate research to validate patient and community health education strategies utilized for different patient groups.
13. Develop annual budget and review operating statements and staff expenses to determine adherence to budget.
14. Hire staff and complete annual performance appraisals.
15. Maintain contact with other community organizations for development of joint ventures, promotion of cooperation, and avoidance of duplication.
16. Serve as a member of hospital and medical staff committees.
17. Coordinate the development of documentation criteria for patient teaching efforts.
18. Act as internal resource concerning patient and community health materials and programs.
19. Review impact of existing patient and community health education efforts on a frequent basis with the use of user evaluations, quality assessment information, and cost/benefit analysis.

Reprinted, with permission, from El Camino Hospital, Mountain View, California, 1992.

Figure 1-6. Organizational Chart for Communications Department, St. Luke's Episcopal Hospital, Houston

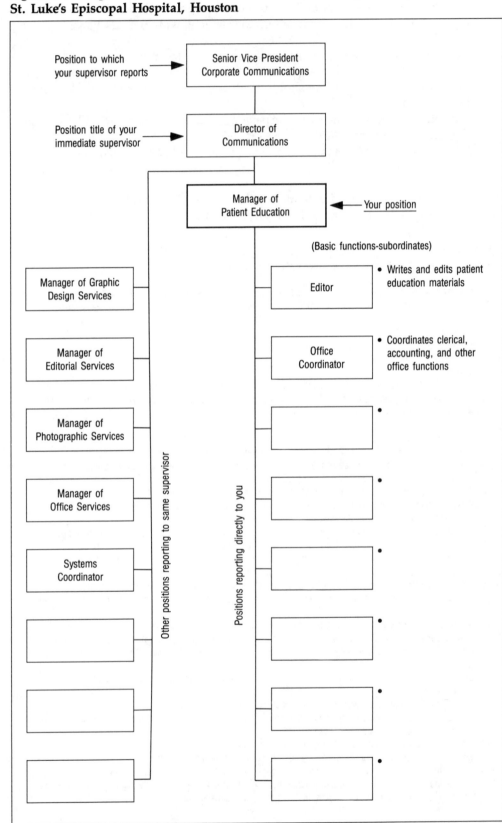

Figure 1-7. Job Description for Manager of Patient Education, St. Luke's Episcopal Hospital, Houston (785 Beds)

SECTION 1   HEADING

Position: Manager of Patient Education   Job Code: 1403

Incumbent: _____   Department: 40000

Reports to: _____   Payroll Section: 4010
                        (Name)
Director of Communications   Approvals: _____
                        (Title)   (Initials)   (Date)
Date: September 22, 1989   _____
                                                              (Initials)   (Date)

SECTION 2   BASIC FUNCTION

(Briefly describe the overall role of your job in the Hospital and the reasons for its existence.)

The basic function of my position is to coordinate the planning, implementation, promotion, and evaluation of patient education at St. Luke's Episcopal Hospital. This coordination involves chairing various task forces organized to produce printed and audiovisual patient education materials and working with the editor in the Office of Patient Education on the development of and revision to the text of any given project. I manage a support staff of one editor and an office coordinator.

SECTION 3   PRIMARY ACCOUNTABILITY

(Describe the specific responsibilities that you perform to accomplish the basic function of your job.)

1. Directs the planning, development, implementation, promotion, distribution, and evaluation of patient education printed and audiovisual materials by chairing task forces for specific projects and offering my technical assistance. In this coordinating role, I act as a liaison between our target audience (patients and family members) and the health care and administrative staff.
2. Manages the personnel activities within the Office of Patient Education, including completing performance evaluations, hiring new personnel, recommending promotions, carrying out disciplinary action, scheduling, assigning and approving work projects, and training staff in methods and procedures.
3. Manages the operational and financial activities of the office. This includes the planning of the annual budget, and responsibility for ensuring the department stays within the allotted budget for individual accounts and projects.
4. Serves as co-chair of the patient education subcommittee and directs the subcommittee's activities. In this capacity, I report to the members (physicians, directors of nursing, and additional department heads and administrative personnel) of the committee on the current status of various patient education projects. In addition, I review various requests from hospital staff with the subcommittee.
5. Reports quarterly to the medical education, research and publications committee, which is the parent committee to the patient education subcommittee. As done with the subcommittee, I review the activities that the office of patient education is involved in.
6. Directs office communication with other hospital departments, as well as with St. Luke's physicians in the Houston area.
7. Keeps patient education project clients informed of their project's status and projected dates of completion.
8. Coordinates the internal and external marketing of St. Luke's patient education materials, externally on a national basis.
9. Directs the planning and evaluation of patient education programming for the St. Luke's educational television channel, channel 4.
10. Plans and conducts staff inservices on the St. Luke's Patient Education Program.
11. Serves as cofacilitator of quarterly support–information program for cancer patients (*I Can Cope*) and similar programs for other patient populations upon request.

SECTION 4   SPECIAL REQUIREMENTS OR PROFICIENCY LEVELS

(Describe the education, experience, training and special licenses and accreditations required by the job.)

1. A master's degree in public health, preferably with class background in health education program planning, needs assessment, and evaluation development.
2. Four to five years of work experience in health education program planning and coordination.
3. An undergraduate degree and/or several years of experience in the area of communications, specifically relating to public speaking and writing experience.

(Continued on next page)

Figure 1-7. (Continued)

4. Computer skills with the minimum requirement being familiarity with word processing, database, spreadsheet, and basic DOS software.
5. Theoretical and practical (work) experience with marketing of health education materials.
6. Work experience with the production of printed education materials and/or videotapes, including interaction with graphic design and printing.
7. Knowledge of readability tests and principles, and experience with writing educational materials for the lay public.
8. Experience working and communicating with health care workers, physicians, and administrative personnel.
9. Troubleshooting skills used in solving problems in a highly political environment in an astute, respectable manner.

SECTION 5   DIMENSIONS

(Provide quantifiable measures of the scope of your position.)

Personnel:

	Direct Reports	Indirect Reports
	1 Exempt	0 Exempt
	1 Nonexempt	0 Nonexempt

Financial: Operating budget responsible for: $203,000.00
Patient education materials
budget (included in 203,000) : 80,000.00
Capital Expenditures (average) : 3,000.00

Money received from external marketing of patient education materials

Other Dimensions: Number of patient education booklets currently in production (to continue or increase in future): 27

These materials vary in length from one sheet of information to 45-page booklets.

I work with some 20 different hospital departments on these projects, most often with administrative or managerial personnel.

Patient education printed and audiovisual materials produced by this office impact over 31,000 patients annually.

Reprinted, with permission, from St. Luke's Episcopal Hospital, Houston, 1992.

- Personnel standards and performance appraisals (Does the hospital have a policy that facilitates the establishment of standards for all disciplines/departments in providing patient education? Are these standards used for performance appraisals for all disciplines/departments?)

System to Support the Acquisition, Development, and Distribution of Patient Education Materials

Fifteen years of reviewing patient education programs at various institutions across the country suggests very clearly the need for a centralized system, no matter how the actual patient education program is organized. Having a centralized system, however, does not mean that everything is done by one person or one department. However, it does mean that a hospitalwide process is designed that guides the development and review of in-house materials; the selection and acquisition of purchased or free materials; a distribution system that moves materials on a regular basis to locations accessible to clinicians who are providing one-on-one or group patient education; and a communication system that enables hospital staff to identify and access current materials. (For more information on systems for print and media, see chapters 16 and 17.)

Opportunities to Develop the Staff's Patient Education Skills

Most staff, no matter what their professional preparation, need continuing education in order to develop adequate skills to implement a variety of patient education activities.

Figure 1-8. Job Description for Coordinator, Patient Education, University of Nebraska Hospital, Omaha (290 Beds)

Position: Coordinator, Patient Education

Responsible to: Coordinator, Discharge Planning

Definition: A professional nurse who is responsible for the ongoing development, monitoring, maintenance, and coordination of the hospitalwide patient education program.

Qualifications:

A. Educational
   1. Graduate from a professional nursing education program: Associate degree, diploma, or baccalaureate.
   2. Bachelor of science degree required, masters degree preferred.
B. Professional and Personal
   1. Current license to practice nursing in Nebraska.
   2. Minimum of two years of experience in hospital nursing.
   3. Ability to communicate effectively, both in writing and orally.
   4. Ability to analyze situations, recognize problems, search out pertinent facts, and reach sound conclusions.
   5. Demonstrated competency in the organization and presentation of instructional programs.
   6. Knowledge of educational principles.
   7. Ability to effectively chair multidisciplinary committees.
   8. Demonstrated competency in leadership skills.
   9. Ability to work effectively with people.
   10. Knowledge of trends, practices, procedures, and requirements related to patient education.
   11. Knowledge of the patient education process.
   12. Optimum physical and emotional health.
   13. Professionalism in conduct and appearance.
   14. Membership and participation in professional and nursing organizations preferred.

Functions:

A. Development, maintenance, and coordination of patient education program
   1. Clarifies roles and responsibilities of disciplines involved in patient education.
   2. Coordinates patient education activities with medical staff, dietitians, physical therapists, respiratory therapists, pharmacists, and any other disciplines involved in patient education.
   3. Identifies conflicting patient education roles and goals and mediates solutions.
   4. Serves as chairperson of the patient education advisory committee, a multidisciplinary committee that (1) develops goals and philosophy statements that are consistent with University Hospital's mission statement and (2) reviews patient education materials.
   5. Serves as chairperson of the patient education contact nurse committee composed of inpatient and outpatient nursing representatives.
   6. Advises and participates on patient education committees for specific patient populations.
   7. Acts as a resource or consultant to individuals, groups, and departments institutionwide and seeks consultation with outside experts to achieve patient education goals.
   8. Identifies patient education needs through data collection and analysis.
   9. Develops and maintains patient education materials database through SYNAPSE, UNMC's health resource network available to regional physicians.
   10. Processes all orders and invoices for patient education materials.
   11. Maintains inventory of patient education materials.
   12. Assists employees in the development and review of teaching protocols and patient education materials.
   13. Provides technical guidance and direction in the development, implementation, and evaluation of patient education materials.
   14. Provides periodic evaluation of patient education efforts as necessary.
   15. Explores feasibility, implements, and manages a patient education skills laboratory.
B. Education and Development
   1. Conducts orientation session for new staff nurses on patient education.
   2. Assists nursing managers in identifying and providing needed ongoing education regarding patient education.
   3. Develops specific program goals, objectives, and content for educational programs on patient education.
   4. Maintains a resource library of patient education reference materials.
   5. Writes a column for the department of nursing's monthly newsletter, *The Communicator.*
C. Other
   1. Participates on nursing or hospital committees as requested.
   2. Relates to patients, families, and employees in a courteous and caring manner.
   3. Supports research activities within the department of nursing.
   4. Assists in other activities/special projects as assigned.

Although the majority of staff may feel that they can provide information to patients on a one-on-one basis, many will not know how to write a pamphlet at the fifth-grade reading level, teach a group of patients with chronic disease, evaluate the effectiveness of their teaching, document appropriately the process and effect of teaching, integrate media into their teaching, or organize a feasible teaching plan given severe time constraints. Sensitive assessment of continuing education needs and creative approaches to the design of educational events targeted to different levels and types of staff are important to increase the overall patient education skill level of staff. (Chapter 12 describes a variety of approaches to continuing education and staff in-service activities. Skill development also takes place when staff are involved in the planning of patient education programs and materials; see also chapter 4 on interdisciplinary involvement.)

□ Options in Choosing an Appropriate Coordinating and Management Structure

The economic pressures on hospitals, the changing utilization of service patterns, and the downsizing and other organizational changes currently facing many hospitals are having an impact on patient education management. PEM positions have become more vulnerable, as have other staff positions not seen as directly connected to patient care delivery. Yet the national picture is inconsistent with regard to current status of patient education positions.

Figure 1-9. Organizational Chart for Education Department, Dakota Hospital, Fargo

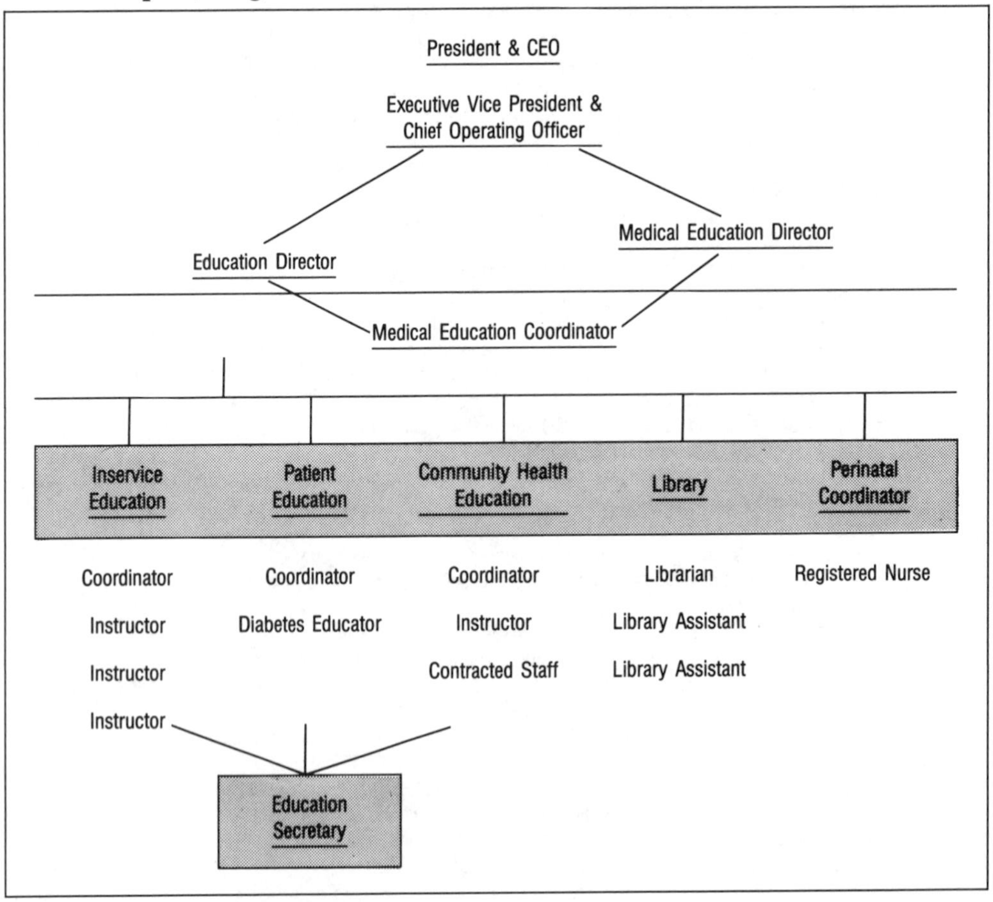

Reprinted, with permission, from Dakota Hospital, Fargo, North Dakota, 1991.

Figure 1-10. Job Description for Patient Education Coordinator, Dakota Hospital, Fargo (165 Beds)

Position: Patient Education Coordinator

Reports to: Director of Education

Position Description: This individual coordinates the planning, development, implementation, and evaluation of all patient education activities, and acts as a resource person to staff members.

This position requires graduation from an accredited school of nursing, current North Dakota licensure, and prior nursing experience. Advanced education and/or teaching or management experience is desirable.

Performance Standards:

Responsibility	Indicators	Relative Weight Percentage	Performance Point Value	Point Value
1. Quality:	Provides accessible and up-to-date reference of available patient education materials and programs through mechanisms of patient education inventory and directory.	_ 3	_____	____
	Keeps staff informed of program changes and new or revised materials.	_ 2	_____	____
	Evaluates patient education unit and house orientation monthly.	_ 1	_____	____
	Initiates problem-solving to enhance work efficiency.	_ 4	_____	____
	Provides annual staff education regarding diabetes care.	_ 1	_____	____
	Develops, maintains, and reviews policies and procedures for patient education annually.	_ 2	_____	____
	Adheres to hospital policies and procedures.	_ 1	_____	____
	Ensures that all JCAHO requirements are met.	_ 1	_____	____
	Suggests and implements quality improvement ideas.	_ 1	_____	____
	Revises materials and/or programs with accurate, updated information, current procedures and standards.	_ 5	_____	____
	Maintains diabetes certification.	_ 1	_____	____
	Evaluates content and patient satisfaction of patient education programs and materials annually by these methods: Patient verbal feedback and written evaluation. Consistent negative feedback from patients and staff implementing programs and materials constitutes reasonable cause for changes.	_ 2	_____	____
	Evaluates staff performance of patient education and documentation through these methods: Postdischarge chart audit for specific programs noting percentage who received teaching as documented. Unit-based QA committees: monitors documentation compliance on an intermittent basis.	_ 2		
	Patient education materials reflect current information and trends, accurate information, attractive format, a variety of educational approaches, and a readability scale consistent with 6–8th grade level.	_ 2	_____	____
	Maintains patient education materials in accessible, organized system.	_ 1	_____	____
	Bills education packets and material requests promptly and correctly according to program guidelines.	_ 2	_____	____
	Maintains original and historical files of all patient education programs and materials in an organized fashion or has access and knowledge of where to obtain them.	_ 2	_____	____

(Continued on next page)

25

Figure 1-10. (Continued)

Comments: _____   Subtotal

2. Productivity:	Establishes and achieves annual goals.	_ 2	_____ ___
	Attends and contributes on assigned committees.	_ 2	_____ ___
	Provides monthly patient education house orientation for all new employees.	_ 1	_____ ___
	Maintains, coordinates, evaluates, and revises patient education CCTV programming, equipment, and staff.	_ 4	_____ ___
	Submits end-of-month summary by the 15th of each month.	_ 1	_____ ___
	Prepares an accurate end-of-year report.	_ 1	_____ ___
	Acts as a resource person for all hospital departments for patient education-related requests.	_ 4	_____ ___
	Coordinates the development of new programs, protocols, and materials for all hospital departments with representation from appropriate departments.	_ 4	_____ ___
	Supervises prep center staff ensuring patient education excellence and focusing on friendly, courteous service.	_ 4	_____ ___
	Supervises, plans, and directs diabetes education programming according to ADA standards.	_ 2	_____ ___
	Assesses and instructs inpatient diabetic referrals according to ADA standards and outpatients in emergency situations.	_ 4	_____ ___
	Maintains and provides staff development for a core of patient education representatives whose function is to assist with unit patient education materials/program assessment, planning and development, and evaluation and revision.	_ 3	_____ ___
	Provides monthly calendar information for front desk, Ask-A-Nurse, monthly wellness ad, and quarterly Pulse.	_ 1	_____ ___

Comments: _____   Subtotal

3. Customer Service	Recognizes all staff members for program or material development.	_ 2	_____ ___
	Communicates with patient education representatives via newsletters, ad hoc meetings, or directly (verbally or by telephone).	_ 2	_____ ___
	Assesses and evaluates customer responses to patient education programs, service, attitudes, and content.	_ 2	_____ ___
	Provides patient education updates and consults in areas of expertise to outside agencies such as nursing homes, and home health agencies as requested and as time allows.	_ 1	_____ ___
	Represents Dakota Hospital in community activities related to health care by actively participating in community organizations and committees.	_ 2	_____ ___
	Sees that community classes and seminars are provided based on needs and potential for profit or break-even status.	_ 2	_____ ___
	Maintains and trains peer visitor program to provide patients with supportive services.	_ 2	_____ ___
	Manages, develops, markets, and facilitates support groups based on need, ensuring consumer involvement.	_ 3	_____ ___
	Collaboratively seeks solutions to work out problems.	_ 1	_____ ___

Figure 1-10.   (Continued)

	Displays an attitude that reflects high regard for teamwork, harmony, and cooperation.	_ 2	_____ ____
	Demonstrates support, respect, and kindness as an active attitude and behavior.	_ 2	_____ ____
	Appropriately addresses problems with and between departments.	_ 1	_____ ____
	Communicates positively and with sensitivity to patients and coworkers.	_ 2	_____ ____
Comments: _____		Subtotal	

4. Fiscal Responsibility	Prepares annual patient education budget (including prep center patient education component) in a timely and accurate manner.	_ 2	_____ ____
	Prepares a financial summary of all patient education seminars offered.	_ 1	_____ ____
	Assesses deviation between actual and budgeted costs monthly and annually.	_ 1	_____ ____
	Manages department purchases consistent with budget and justifies deviations.	_ 1	_____ ____
Comments: _____		Subtotal	

5. Other:	Maintains confidentiality.	_ 1	_____ ____
	Attends mandatory safety classes and observes all safety protocols.	_ 2	_____ ____
	Remains flexible to meet work demands.	_ 2	_____ ____
Comments: _____		Subtotal	

	Total Points	_____

Reprinted, with permission, from Dakota Hospital, Fargo, North Dakota, 1991.

Some hospitals have eliminated entire education departments in their need to cut expenses; others have eliminated individual positions such as the PEM and then divided the responsibilities of this position among other staff; still others have added additional responsibilities, including community health promotion, quality improvement, research, and/or staff development, to the PEM's job description. At the same time, there are examples of hospitals that have re-created the position of patient education manager, others where the PEM position has been the only education position to survive, and still others where additional patient education staff have been added, especially to manage expansion into ambulatory care areas.

For some hospitals these changes may result in at least the temporary demise of a coordinated patient education program. Others, however, appear to be developing a more organic approach to patient education coordination that utilizes many of the management structures that have been identified as essential to its success. Although new organizational arrangements are evolving, five options for overall coordination and management are described here along with potential advantages and disadvantages for each. These options will, of course, be more or less relevant to an individual hospital depending on bed size, patient population, patient care delivery system, extent of support for patient education, and available educational resources.[29]

Barbara E. Giloth, M.P.H., C.H.E.S.

Figure 1-11. Patient Health Education Policy and Procedure, VA Medical Center, Albuquerque

1. **Purpose:** To revise Medical Center Memorandum 9-22 and to define the policy, procedures, and responsibilities of the Patient Health Education (PHE) Program.

2. **Policy:** The Veterans Administration Department of Medicine and Surgery supports patient education as an integral part of delivering high quality cost effective patient care. Medical centers, through their professional staffs, are responsible for planning, coordination, and management of PHE and the delivery of PHE services throughout the facility.

3. **Definitions:**
   a. *Patient Health Education:* Any combination of activities designed to facilitate voluntary change in patient behavior toward good health. Activities typically focus on keeping patients informed about their health status, their rights, their treatment plans, and upon development of their self care skills.
   b. *Patient Health Education Program:* A written guide or set of planned interventions created in order to achieve specific health educational objectives for a group of individuals. The group may have a common health program (for example, Chronic Obstructive Pulmonary Disease, diabetes, hypertension), or utilize a common service (for example, surgical patients), or share common characteristics (for example, geriatric patients, Vietnam veterans).
   c. *Patient Health Education Activities:* Less formal patient teaching than occurs in full scale "programs." Materials may or may not be standardized; protocols or guides are generally not shared station-wide.

4. **Procedures:** All multidisciplinary patient education programs and activities will be coordinated through the Patient Health Education Coordinator and the Patient Health Education Advisory Committee in order to promote efficient use of resources, eliminate duplication of effort, and to ensure that all information given to patients is in agreement with approved program content as endorsed by the cognizant medical staff member(s).
   a. Planned Programs
      (1) Health care areas possessing high profiles for the development of planned patient health education programs will be identified by the Patient Health Education Coordinator in collaboration with Service Chiefs, Section Chiefs, and the PHE Advisory Committee. If indicated, multidisciplinary planning committees focused upon specific health problems or diseases will be established as authorized by the Patient Health Education Advisory Committee.
      (2) Planned patient health education programs will contain as a minimum:
         (a) Written educational content, approved by appropriate medical staff member(s).
         (b) A written delivery design.
         (c) An evaluation component including program and patient evaluation.
         (d) A standard documentation method, including reporting of outpatient teaching visits and/or family collateral teaching visits, as appropriate.
         (e) A staff training component.
         (f) Stated minimum resource requirements.
      (3) Following endorsement of the program by the Patient Health Education Advisory Committee, that program will be made available to those patients who have identified educational needs that can be met by the program.
      (4) The program will be reviewed thereafter on an annual basis.
   b. Patient Education Activities
      (1) Staff carrying out less formal patient education activities will be encouraged to upgrade such activities into planned programs if appropriate.
      (2) These activities will be documented, including reporting of outpatient teaching visits and/or family collateral teaching visits, as appropriate.

5. **Responsibility:** The Patient Health Education Advisory Committee will serve in an advisory capacity to the Patient Health Education Coordinator, and as a resource to the staff of the medical center. The committee will have overall responsibility for recommending policy, procedure and development of facilitywide patient education goals and plans, and will perform the following functions:
   a. Assist in identifying facility-wide patient education needs and establishing priorities.
   b. Select areas for patient education program development based on needs assessments and/or recommendation from the staff.
   c. Recommend proposed medical center policy and procedures regarding development of patient programs and activities.
   d. Appoint task forces of interested staff to develop and plan specific patient education programs.
   e. Advise task forces in developing educationally sound programs.
   f. Identify training and educational needs of staff related to patient education.

Figure 1-11. (Continued)

6. **Membership:**

   a. The Patient Health Education Advisory Committee is a multidisciplinary group comprised of the following:

   Patient Health Education Coordinator, Chairperson
   Associate Chief of Staff for Education, Ex-Officio Member

   Representatives from:

   Audiology and Speech Pathology Service
   Dietetics Service
   Nursing Service (2)
   Social Work Service
   Medical Service
   Geriatrics/Extended Care
   Dental Service

   Psychiatry Service
   Library Service
   Pharmacy Service
   Ambulatory Care Service
   Rehabilitation Medicine Service
   Spinal Cord Injury Service

   Consultants (Chief of Service or designee) from:

   Neurology Service
   Medical Media Production Service

   Surgical Service

   b. Members will be appointed by the chiefs of the represented services for a two year term or at the discretion of the service chief.

   c. Members will send an alternate from their service when unable to attend a committee meeting. The alternate will have the full power and authority to speak and/or vote for the absent member.

7. **Meetings:** The committee will meet monthly or more frequently at the call of the chairperson. Minutes will be prepared, including conclusions, recommendations, and actions taken by the committee.

8. References: M-8, Part IV, Chapter 4

9. Replacement: Memorandum 9-22, Patient Health Education Advisory Committee, dated March 6, 1984.

10. Automatic Recision Date: May, 1993.

Director

Reprinted from the Department of Veterans Affairs, Albuquerque, New Mexico, 1990.

Option 1: An Existing Department Coordinates the Program

Under this option, a department is designated to coordinate patient education, most likely the hospitalwide education department or nursing education department. Patient education coordination and management responsibilities are split among the department's staff, many of whom are likely to have staff education as their primary focus. There is likely to be a hospitalwide patient education committee that sets policy for the hospitalwide patient education activities. If the department director and committee chair are interested in patient education, and if the committee chair is powerful and well respected within the organization, this management model has a good chance of being successful. The integration of patient education into the job descriptions of a variety of departmental staff can increase the likelihood that activities will be implemented.

Option 2: A Committee Coordinates the Program

Another option is to designate a committee to coordinate patient education. Members of the committee should come from a variety of disciplines and have varying levels of experience with patient education program development. The Veterans Administration, for example, has had a great deal of experience with this option since a 1986 national Patient Health Education Program policy mandated the establishment of an administrative structure for patient education.[30] Although approximately 15 percent of 171 VA medical centers now have a full-time coordinator for the patient education function,[31] the majority implement a variety of programs with a multidisciplinary patient education committee at the helm.

Figure 1-12. Policy and Procedure Manual, Patient Education Materials, The Ohio State University Hospitals, Columbus

Number __03-13__

Effective Date __July 10, 1984__

Revision Date __May 20, 1992__

Prepared by: Patient Education Coordinator, Educational Services/Development

Authorized by: _____
                        Executive Director

Policy

Patient education materials are intended to communicate patient self-care health instructions and information. The materials may be written, visual, or audiovisual and distributed by the hospital and medical staff members. Hospital and medical staff members are required to develop/revise patient education materials in consultation with the Patient Education Coordinator, Department of Educational Services and Development.

All patient education materials developed by staff members are the property of The Ohio State University Hospitals. These materials are distributed to the Hospital's departments and outpatient facilities for use with patients and their families by the Department of Educational Services and Development.

Responsibilities

1. The Patient Education Coordinator is responsible for the following: (a) to assist hospital and medical staff in all aspects of preparing materials; (b) to plan, coordinate and promote patient education materials; and (c) to format and print the patient education materials on Patient Education Paper according to the standards established by the Hospitals Department of Communications and Public Relations and the Health Education Advisory Committee.
2. Hospital departments are responsible for ensuring that the information contained in the materials is current, complete, accurate, and meets Hospital's standards.

Procedure

1. *Development/revision, approval, and distribution of Patient Education Materials prepared by OSUH staff members:* When a hospital or medical staff member desires to develop/revise and distribute patient education materials with The Ohio State University Hospitals, Clinics, and outreach facilities, that individual must complete the "Request to Develop or Revise Patient Education Materials" (form available from the Department of Educational Services and Development).

   Once completed, the form should be sent to the Patient Education Coordinator for appropriate disposition (See figure 1-13: Process for Developing/Revising Patient Education Materials).

   A Patient Education Resource Manual, containing detailed information on the development/revision, approval, and distribution process and references to help in developing materials is available to all departments and nursing units. Nursing units are to obtain this Manual from the Division of Nursing, Chair of the Patient Education Committee. All other departments are to obtain this Manual from the Patient Education Coordinator.
2. *Internal Distribution of Patient Education Materials:* All patient education materials will be listed in the "Inventory List and Order Form" (available through Educational Services and Development). The cost of Patient Education materials to departments is for the printing, only. The Hospital's Department of Communication and Public Relations will be responsible for the cost of the Patient Education Paper.
3. *Approval of Patient Educational Materials prepared by Outside Agencies:* Any Hospitals department wishing to distribute materials published by outside agencies (that is, voluntary agencies—Heart Association, Cancer Society, Lung Association, manufacturers, pharmaceutical companies, vendors, other hospitals) should contact the Patient Education Coordinator in order to coordinate the need for such materials.
4. *External sale/distribution of Patient Education Materials:* Selected patient education materials are available for sale to non-Ohio State University health services providers upon request to the Department of Educational Services and Development.

   In order to be cost effective, maintain quality and protect external sales income, patient education materials *may not* be reproduced in any manner to any individual without written permission of the Patient Education Coordinator. Funds generated from the sale of these materials will be allocated though the patient Education Coordinator for use in furthering or enhancing patient education activities throughout the organization.
5. *Requests for Patient Education Funds:* Hospital departments may submit written requests for the use of patient education funds to the Patient Education Coordinator. Requests may include the following: the purchase of commercially made patient education materials or staff education resources on patient education; support for staff to attend conferences on patient education outside the Hospitals; and monies for patient education research activities.

Questions concerning this policy should be directed to the Patient Education Coordinator in the Department of Educational Services and Development.

Figure 1-13. Process for Developing/Revising Patient Education Materials, The Ohio State University Hospitals, Columbus

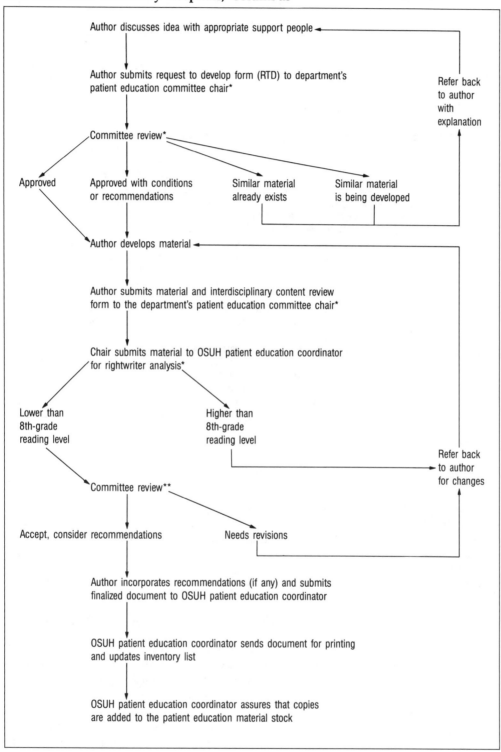

Reprinted, with permission, from The Ohio State University Hospitals, Columbus, 1992.

*If the department does not have a patient education committee, the forms are sent to and reviewed by the patient education coordinator and their department's health education advisory committee's representative.

**The material is reviewed by the patient education coordinator, the health education advisory committee's department representative, and a third person from the department chosen by this representative if no department patient education committee exists.

Figure 1-14. Division of Nursing Policy and Procedures at The Ohio State University Hospitals, Columbus

	Number __A-12__
	Effective Date __10/85__
	Revision Date __8/90__
	Approved by: _____

Title: Patient Education, Registered Nurse's Role and Responsibilities

Policy Statements:
1. *Patient education* is an individualized teaching–learning experience. The overall responsibility for coordinating the teaching–learning experience lies with the registered nurse.
   a. The registered nurse may delegate aspects of patient education to other members of the interdisciplinary team or other ancillary nursing personnel.
   b. The registered nurse will include the patient/family and/or significant other as an active partner in the teaching–learning experience.
2. The registered nurse will provide all patients and families the opportunity to acquire knowledge, skills, and attitudes regarding their health status. The RN will coordinate resources to assist the patient/family in achieving the educational goals.
3. The patient education process includes assessment, planning, implementation, evaluation, and revision. This process begins upon admission and continues through discharge.
4. Patient education materials developed by the Division of Nursing at OSUH undergo a review process to assure quality and accuracy of content (refer to patient education resource manual for process detail).
   a. The individual nursing unit may obtain these materials by completing a patient education materials order form and submitting it to the chairperson of the patient education committee.
5. All aspects of the patient education process, including the patient/family response to teaching, must be documented in the nursing record.
6. Patient education materials developed outside OSUH need to be reviewed by the patient education committee prior to distribution.

Reprinted, with permission, from The Ohio State University Hospitals, Columbus, 1992.

This option is applicable to a wide variety of organizational structures, but its success is dependent on an effective committee chair and dedicated members. A hospital with a number of departments that have already made philosophical and personnel commitments to patient education could select this option and realize important accomplishments. Because of the lack of a specifically designated manager, however, many activities can fall through the cracks if no one is charged with clear responsibility for follow-up.

Option 3: A Separate New Department Coordinates the Program

A third option is to establish a separate department of patient education. In general, this department not only has management responsibility for coordinating patient education activities within the institution, but it also has responsibility for implementing specific patient education programs. It may also have the responsibility for community health education. Often such a department runs prenatal classes, the diabetes education program, cardiac rehabilitation, and/or ostomy education. Such a department may hire full-time instructors or a range of part-time staff or contractors to deliver specific patient education services.

This model appears very effective where the director of the department can balance the activities related to hospitalwide management with the need to offer specific patient education services. Often such a department offers a variety of community education programs and may reach out through grants and other resources to encompass a range of community-based programs. Although such a department can establish specific revenue streams for some of its activities, it is not likely to be able to cover even its direct costs, making it vulnerable to budget cuts.

Option 4: A Patient Education Manager within a Clinical Department Coordinates the Program

In this option, a PEM position is created within a clinical department, usually nursing. Because of the broad range of nursing activities, such a manager may have broad impact within the hospital. Often the incumbent may have discharge planning or staff development responsibilities, which can complement and strengthen the patient education role. Because such a position usually reports to nursing, there are less likely to be turf issues related to implementing the role; the PEM will have increased access to all of the nursing units as well as the ear of nursing leadership. However, there may be turf issues that surface between nursing and other hospital departments. Depending on whether the department is focused on nursing care alone or the broader provision of patient care services, this position may be able to staff a multidisciplinary patient education committee, or it may be limited to nursing committees such as a unit-based nursing patient education resource committee. The major risk for such a position is that it becomes too involved in nursing concerns, thus being less sensitive to the multidisciplinary issues that continue to dominate the patient education field. Another risk is that multiple responsibilities will make it difficult for the position to implement the patient education role effectively. This, however, may be a risk under any of the options because of the tendency for such positions to be balancing multiple roles.

Option 5: A Patient Education Manager within a Nonclinical Department Coordinates the Program

The last option is to establish a PEM position within a nonclinical department, such as the department of human resources or the department of education. Such a position is likely to be free from some of the territorial constraints that may exist if the PEM is in one clinical department; however, the position also risks isolation if the coordinating department is not well connected to clinical services. Usually such a position is able to effectively use a variety of hospitalwide committees and target population task forces to address a wide range of patient education needs. It may also be able to more easily develop the critical mass of staff with an interest in education than a position that is tied to a specific discipline. Depending on the job requirements, the position may not be filled by an incumbent who has a clinical background in addition to educational skills. This may be viewed as an advantage or disadvantage in planning target population programs.

☐ Considerations in Making the Choice

Many hospitals have asked, ". . . but what is the best way to organize patient education?" There is no easy answer to this question. (Chapter 2 discusses the process of internally assessing the status of patient education activities within the institution.) The decision on how to develop a coordinating mechanism for this function relates to many issues, including the following:

- Bed size and already-existing hospital services
- Interest level in patient education by executive staff and individual departments
- Already-existing patient education activities, especially committee structures and policies

- Already-existing hospitalwide education and training resources
- Patient care delivery processes, including team development
- Importance of other complementary innovations such as patient-centered care initiatives, total quality management, and so forth
- Availability of specialized services such as the medical library, health promotion, the community health information center, and centers for excellence

Whatever the structure, the ultimate aim of patient education management is to enable health care providers to work more effectively with patients and their families so that they are prepared to cope with their diagnoses and manage their conditions over time. To accomplish this facilitating role, PEMs (and those with the function but not the title) must address changing the hospital environment to promote more effective patient involvement, making the discharge preparation process more efficient and effective, enhancing the continuity of education services among delivery sites, increasing clinical staff's access to a variety of teaching tools, defining and addressing quality and productivity concerns related to the provision of patient education, and better defining the role that hospitals can play in the provision of effective consumer education.

Although more qualitative and quantitative research examining the impact of hospital-wide and target population management structures and processes on the extent, efficiency, and effectiveness of patient education interventions at the case level will provide critically needed information about the management requirements, such research is not likely to be forthcoming. Those senior managers and others with an interest in patient education should look creatively at their institutions to identify a variety of ways to increase and improve the coordination and management of this important function.

☐ Conclusion

Evidence from the past 15 years points to the importance of developing management structures to support hospitalwide patient education program development. The complexity of the patient education function, the broad involvement of staff throughout the institution, and the challenges of helping patients and families implement difficult behavior changes require hospitalwide policy and procedures, interdepartmental communication processes, and a mechanism to coordinate program development if these objectives are to be achieved. Hospitals have a wide latitude to develop their management structures given bed size, degree of vertical and horizontal integration, their own staff resources, and the patient populations they serve. The challenge is to fashion structures that will work and then assess their impact on the effective provision of patient education services.

References and Notes

1. Bartlett, E. E. Historical glimpses of patient education in the United States. *Patient Education and Counseling* 8(2):135–49, June 1986.

2. *Implementing Patient Education in the Hospital.* Chicago: American Hospital Association, 1979 (out of print).

3. Deeds, S. G., Hebert, B. J., and Wolle, J. M., editors. A model for patient education programming. Special project report, Public Health Education Section, American Public Health Association, 1979.

4. American Hospital Association. *Hospital Inpatient Education: Survey Findings and Analyses, 1975.* Atlanta: Centers for Disease Control, 1977.

5. American Hospital Association. *Hospital Inpatient Education: Survey Findings and Analyses, 1978.* Atlanta: Centers for Disease Control, 1980.

6. American Hospital Association. Special Survey on Selected Hospital Topics for 1981, unpublished data.

7. American Hospital Association. *Hospital-Based Health Promotion Programs: Report and Analyses of the 1984 Survey.* Chicago: AHA, 1985.

8. Final Report—Census of Hospital-Based Health Promotion and Patient Education Programs. Chicago: American Hospital Association, 1988 (unpublished).

9. American Hospital Association. *Annual Survey of Hospitals, 1986–90.* Chicago: AHA, 1991.

10. AHA/ASHET Patient Education Liaison Program. Patient education management and job descriptions: survey and resource document. American Hospital Association, 1990 (unpublished).

11. Stanton, M. P. Patient education in the hospital health-care setting. *Patient Education and Counseling* 5(1):14–22, 1983.

12. Office of Academic Affairs. *Patient Health Education Profile in VA Medical Centers.* Washington, DC: Veterans Administration, 1987.

13. Giloth, B. What makes patient education effective? *Promoting Health* 4(4):6–8, July–Aug. 1983.

14. Kernaghan, S. G. Responding to the prospective pricing challenge: 1984 patient education leaders point the way. Supplement to *Promoting Health,* Nov.–Dec. 1984.

15. AHA/ASHET Patient Education Liaison Program.

16. Hospital-Based Health Promotion Programs, 1985.

17. Office of Academic Affairs.

18. Kernaghan, S. G., and Giloth, B. E. *Tracking the Impact of Health Promotion on Organizations: A Key to Program Survival.* Chicago: American Hospital Publishing, 1988 (out of print).

19. Office of Academic Affairs.

20. Palma, L., and DuShaw, M. Joint study looks at quality of patient education programs. *Michigan Hospitals* 18(1):10–11, Jan. 1982.

21. National standards and review criteria for diabetes patient education programs. *The Diabetes Educator* 12(3):286–91, summer 1986.

22. National Standards Steering Committee (NDAB). National standards for diabetes patient education programs; pilot study results and implementation plan. *The Diabetes Educator* 12(3):292–96, summer 1986.

23. Redman, B. K., Levine, D., and Howard, D. Organization resources in support of patient education programs: relationship to reported delivery of instruction. *Patient Education and Counseling* 9(2):177–97, Apr. 1987.

24. Lorenz, R. A., Pickert, J. W., Enns, S. J., and Hanson, S. L. Impact of organizational interventions on the delivery of patient education in a diabetes clinic. *Patient Education and Counseling* 8(2):115–23, June 1986.

25. Adapted from: *Implementing Patient Education in the Hospital.* Chicago: American Hospital Association, 1979, pp. 13–14 (out of print).

26. VA Patient Health Education Program, Office of Academic Affairs. Facilitator's guide. In: *Patient Health Education: Building Medical Center Commitment.* Washington, DC: Veterans Administration, 1988.

27. This material has been adapted from *Implementing Patient Education in the Hospital,* p. 111.

28. This list of categories was adapted from correspondence to Barbara Giloth from Nan Stout, then national coordinator for patient education, Veterans Administration, L. Nan Stout, Sept. 3, 1985.

29. The documentation of patient education management structures is very limited. See, for example, Kernaghan, S. G. *Responding to the Prospective Pricing Challenge: 1984 Patient Education Leaders Point the Way* and Facility Management Case Studies/Target Population Case Studies in VA Patient Health Education Program, Office of Academic Affairs. *Patient Health Education: Building Medical Center Commitment* Section 6, pp. 1–42; Section 7, pp. 1–46, 1988.

30. Stout, L. N. Veterans Administration patient health education policy statement. *Patient Education and Counseling* 10(3):301–4, Dec. 1987.

31. Personal communication with Rose Mary Monaco Pries, national coordinator for patient education, Veterans Administration, St. Louis, 1992.

Chapter 2

Performing Strategic Planning in Patient Education

Patricia A. Mathews, M.A., F.H.C.E., R.N.

☐ Objectives

The reader will be able to:

- Define strategic planning and describe its benefits in planning patient education programs
- List the key elements of the strategic planning process
- Describe the components of the patient education strategic planning model and how they can be used in developing programs

☐ Strategic Planning in Patient Education

Before planning specific patient education programs, patient education managers (PEMs) should adopt a strategic planning approach that will ensure that their program goals tie in to those of the institution at large. *Strategic planning* involves transferring into action a vision or a point of view of what something should be by first setting goals and then describing the means for achieving them. When used to plan a patient education program, strategic planning clarifies the program's vision and outlines its direction for a specific long-term period (usually three to five years).

In this era of rapid change in the health care environment, sound strategic planning is the responsibility not only of senior managers, but also of department managers such as patient education managers. (For example, see the article by Beckham,[1] which describes the mind-set for strategic planning.) All managers need to be involved in moving the hospital forward to meet new challenges and in looking beyond the traditional needs of their own areas of responsibility to participate in a process of continuous improvement that depends on teamwork across hospital lines.[2] Although this book refers to one individual—the patient education manager—as the person primarily responsible for patient education activities, it is recognized that strategic planning for patient education may also be done by a committee composed of individuals from various departments assuming responsibility for different phases of the planning process.

Patricia A. Mathews, M.A., F.H.C.E., R.N.

Advantages of Using a Strategic Planning Approach

The advantages of using a strategic planning approach when planning patient education programs include the following:

- *Programs can be designed to fit into the overall hospital plan.* By identifying the hospital's goals and assessing the patients' educational needs, the PEM has the opportunity to determine how the patient education program will fit into key hospital strategies and can develop programs to specifically address the goals of those strategies.
- *Focus on long-term goals and hospitalwide needs can be maintained.* Strategic planning can result in a strong patient education program that helps meet the long-term needs of patients and their families, as well as of the hospital. This is because strategic planning is proactive rather than reactive, and reflects a commitment to achieving long-term goals rather than short-term solutions to immediate problems.[3] This approach also encourages a broad view of patient education needs and discourages responding only to special interests within the hospital.
- *Support and visibility for patient education programs within the hospital are provided.* Because the patient education manager must work effectively with various members of the hospital team during the planning process, a strategic planning approach helps to ensure cooperation and support from top management as well as other departments essential to the success of a new patient education program. This also increases the visibility of patient education throughout the organization.
- *Data necessary to justify the resources needed to implement a patient education program are provided.* These data may be reflected either in the centralized budget or as part of the budgets of those departments involved in the patient education program, depending on the hospital's system. The chances of obtaining needed funding and other resources are greater for strategically planned programs. When making a case for additional resources for programming, PEMs report greater success if the process has answered the decision maker's questions. One case specifically cited in the literature is Seattle VAMC, where strategic planning resulted in funding.[4]
- *Data needed to persuade others of the benefits of patient education are provided.* Strategic planning can result in useful qualitative and quantitative data that illustrate the need for, and the impact of, patient education programs. Throughout the strategic planning process, the patient education manager collects data that can be communicated to other members of the planning team and thus makes the potential benefits of patient education known to others throughout the hospital. Such data are also useful in getting additional programs approved if they illustrate the success of previous patient education efforts.
- *The hospital's quality improvement efforts are enhanced.* Well-planned patient education programs can contribute to the quality of patient care. There are many definitions of quality: Some define *quality* as "zero defects," others as "conformance to customer requirements." Leebov and Ersoz use a definition that has specific application in health care. They define *quality* as doing the right things right consistently to ensure the best possible clinical outcomes for patients, satisfaction for all of the hospital's many customers, retention of talented staff, and sound financial performance.[5] Planned and coordinated patient education services can contribute to this definition of quality in many important ways. According to the AHA management advisory on patient education services, well-planned patient education can enhance efficient use of hospital services and increase physician support, staff satisfaction, patient satisfaction with hospital services, and community support for the hospital.[6] Gorman and Ludemann also point out that patient satisfaction is being accepted as one legitimate indicator of quality of care.[7]

In short, strategic planning can be used to ensure the quality of the patient education program and ensure that it helps meet the goals of the institution at large.

Key Elements of a Strategic Planning Approach

There are a number of key elements in the strategic planning approach to patient education. They include the following:

- A clear definition of the program's business or mission, especially with regard to hospitalwide goals
- A vision statement for the specific program
- External and internal assessments of markets and their needs
- An action plan for program development

Definition of the Program's Business or Mission

The PEM should define the mission of the hospitalwide patient education program. The program's mission should complement the hospital's mission and goals, but not necessarily duplicate them. The mission statement says, "This is what we are, this is what we are here for, and this is what we believe in and want to be known for." The following is an example of a mission statement for a patient education program:

> The Anywhere Hospital patient education program exists to ensure that every individual receives the appropriate educational experiences needed to assist in coping with changes related to illness, and to provide an environment for learning, formulating, and reinforcing goal-directed health behavior.

Vision Statement

In developing a strategic plan, it is helpful to take a long-term perspective and create a *vision* of what the patient education program should be within a specified period of time. Patient education program development needs to consider at least the next two to three years.

The following is an example of a vision statement for a patient education program:

> By 1994, the General Hospital Patient Education Program will provide patient education to all hospital inpatients and to outpatients seen in the two ambulatory care clinics. In addition, the new patient education program for pediatric patients will be expanded to become the most comprehensive and innovative of its kind. In light of the hospital's mission to serve the elderly in the community, a community-based geriatric patient education program will be completely in place by 1994.

This vision statement describes a long-term view of the patient education program overall, and provides specific goals for various aspects of the program.

The vision statement should also focus on the contribution that patient education activities can make to the success of the goals of the entire organization, rather than just those of the patient education department. By using strategic planning as a basis for planning patient education activities, the PEM can select goals that are consistent with the hospital's mission and that will strengthen the position of the patient education department throughout the hospital. For example, the sample vision statement described how a potential element of the geriatric program would support the hospital's mission in the community.

External and Internal Market Assessments

The next step involves collecting data on the markets in the overall industry environment (external assessment) and the specific hospital environment (internal assessment) in which patient education will take place. This market research will determine how a proposed patient education program will be affected by national and local trends in technology, education, government regulation, economics, and other areas, and how the program will fit with such hospitalwide concerns as the types of programs needed, the funds available, the objectives of other departments, the types of patients most likely to be readmitted, and so forth. (External and internal assessments are described in greater detail in the section of this chapter on the patient education strategic planning model.)

Action Plan for Program Development

Action planning begins with the development of strategies and incorporates the development of patient education management objectives and the planning of specific programs. (These elements are discussed in detail in connection with the patient education strategic planning model.)

Strategic Planning and the Business Plan

A process that is intertwined with strategic planning is the development of a business plan. A *business plan* clearly defines the specific means used to achieve the goals of the strategic plan and outlines strategies for operational issues such as financing, staffing, and marketing. It is prepared in conjunction with specific project initiatives or program proposals—such as a new patient education program—and provides an orderly plan for their development and operation. For example, the business plan for a new patient education program should outline specific financial and marketing goals and identify specific steps for implementing the program.

The strategic planning process *should not be separated* from the business planning process.[8] The strategic plan and the business plan must share goals, should be in agreement with the goals of the hospital's strategic plan, and should indicate how the program can strengthen the overall organization.

Too often, patient education managers fail to recognize the importance or even the existence of a hospital's strategic plan and are not able to plan programs that will enhance and complement the hospital's goals. This may be because the hospital's strategic plan is not formalized or fully distributed throughout the hospital, but is known only to top management. However, planning and developing patient education programs in this type of information vacuum can result in fragmented programming that does not meet the needs of all patients, poorly planned programs that fail, or program proposals that do not relate to the organization's goals and thus do not receive the approval or support needed to proceed.

Patient education managers who recognize the importance of linking their own planning to the plans of the hospital can devise well-coordinated and effective programs. If PEMs are aware of the hospital's goals, they can coordinate the overall approach to a given goal and thus avoid fragmentation and poor planning. For example, if a PEM knows that providing senior services is an organizational goal that affects several departments, he or she may realize that several programs may need to be developed and co-ordinated and may check with all involved parties when planning programs.

☐ The Patient Education Strategic Planning Model

Thus far, this chapter has defined the strategic planning process, identified some of the benefits of and key elements in using strategic planning to develop patient education programs, and discussed how strategic planning and business planning should be linked. This section describes the major steps in a patient education strategic planning model that begins with assessing trends and concludes with conducting an evaluation to determine whether the programs developed have been effective in accomplishing their goals. The patient education strategic planning model (figure 2-1) helps the patient education manager to proceed through the strategic planning process in an organized manner, identify patient education program needs, and prioritize program objectives and goals. Using

Figure 2-1. A Patient Education Strategic Planning Model

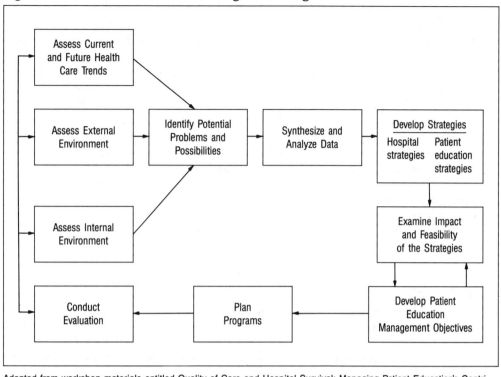

Adapted from workshop materials entitled Quality of Care and Hospital Survival: Managing Patient Education's Contribution, American Hospital Association, 1986.

this model, the PEM can ensure a firm link between the hospital's goals and those of the patient education program.

This strategic planning model was developed by Cornett, Giloth, Mathews, and Ruzicki, and has been used by the author of this chapter in actual patient education practice. In planning an AHA conference, these patient education professionals conducted a literature search to see if there was a strategic planning model specifically for patient education and found that one did not exist. They felt that a model was needed to help managers begin to use planning to align organizational goals. After developing the model, they presented it in 1986 at the AHA series of conferences titled Quality of Care and Hospital Survival: Managing Patient Education's Contribution, which was held in Philadelphia, St. Louis, and San Francisco.

The patient education strategic planning model incorporates several approaches that differ slightly from traditional strategic planning. First, the development of the action plan in traditional strategic planning corresponds with the development of strategies, patient education management objectives, and program planning phases of the patient education model. The development of a business plan is not part of the patient education model, but would be incorporated by using information gathered in the impact and feasibility phase of the model. Because patient education exists as part of many hospital programs, it is difficult to utilize a traditional business plan and make it meaningful in this setting.

Successful use of the strategic planning model for patient education first requires that key personnel within the organization be identified and given an active role in the process. From the very beginning, in addition to the patient education manager, strategic planning for patient education should involve those key health care professionals who have a role in educating patients. This is because patient education must be integrated into the overall plan of patient care, and it will be provided by a variety of care givers

41

including nurses, physicians, and other clinical staff such as dietitians, pharmacists, physical therapists, and social workers. Involving representatives from these different disciplines in the strategic planning process helps ensure that they will (1) provide valuable input during the planning stages and (2) be fully involved and supportive of the program once it is implemented.

One way to involve staff other than the PEM is to organize a committee for the strategic planning process, with various individuals assuming responsibility for specific phases of the process. If a patient education committee does exist, it may already include the appropriate individuals. If not, in addition to the PEM, participants could include a nursing director; the director of education; key physicians; representatives of hospital departments such as pharmacy, food service, social service, and physical therapy; and others involved in patient education, such as the wellness director, discharge planners, volunteers, and the outpatient manager. Position titles, politics, and degree of involvement will vary from hospital to hospital. (See chapter 4 for more information on building effective committees.)

The following sections present the key steps in the patient education strategic planning model.

Step 1. Assess Current and Future Health Care Trends

The first step in the patient education strategic planning model includes identifying and assessing both general health care trends and trends that are more specific to patient education.

General health care trends that are key to the planning and implementation of any health care service include the following:[9]

- Increased competition for patients among providers
- Increase in the number and types of outpatient services with a corresponding decrease in need for inpatient acute care beds
- Increased acuity of hospitalized patients
- Increased emphasis placed on the costs of service
- Increased scrutiny of patient outcomes
- The growing aging population and its impact on health care
- The growth in managed care
- Changes in reimbursement
- Increased demand and opportunity for alternative delivery systems (for example, outpatient clinics, birthing centers, and women's centers)
- The growing consumer interest and involvement in health and health care

Although these trends may vary in the level of impact they will have on planning according to hospital size and location, they are examples of the kinds of information that should be considered by the PEM when doing this assessment. For example, the increased acuity of hospitalized patients has been an important trend that affects how PEMs approach their jobs. In the past, most patient education could take place in the inpatient setting. Patients stayed in the hospital until they were better able to participate in the programs needed to ensure safe discharge. Now, inpatients are more acutely ill, requiring that the PEM utilize a variety of different approaches. For example, family education has taken on new importance, and careful coordination with community agencies and development of outpatient education and/or support groups has consumed more of the PEMs' and the care givers' resources.

The patient education manager can obtain information about general health care trends by reading health care journals and hospital association newsletters, especially those read by top managers (such as *Healthcare Forum*, *Hospitals*, and *Modern Healthcare*), by reading the health care sections of newspapers, and by attending meetings at which health care trends are discussed. If attending meetings is difficult, reading their proceedings can help identify trends. Having discussions with hospital top management can also help the PEM learn about important health care trends.

When assessing health care trends, it is also important to focus on the impact of current and future trends that specifically affect patient education. Some of these trends include:

- Increased emphasis on discharge planning
- Increases in prevention and wellness services for patients
- Integration of patient education into most hospital services and product lines
- The changing role of the patient education manager

The last trend deserves further explanation. Patient education managers are becoming more multifocused and are less likely to have positions or titles that reflect only inpatient education. Commonly, the PEM position includes discharge planning, outpatient education, community health education, staff development, quality assurance, and other related activities.[10] Although multiple roles can be an advantage in planning because the PEM has a wider scope of knowledge, they can also cause time constraints that make strategic planning more difficult.

The trends specific to patient education are discussed at regional and national patient education conferences and at local patient education groups. In addition, journals related to patient education, such as *Patient Education and Counseling, Journal of Healthcare Education and Training, American Journal of Nursing,* and *Nursing '92,* are good sources for tracking patient education trends.

In addition to gathering information on general health care and patient-education-related trends, PEMs should pay particular attention to patient education research and its impact on patient outcomes. Today's increased emphasis on cost-effectiveness demands that the PEM be prepared to use research and evaluation data to justify existing patient education programs and to develop new ones. In addition, the increasing acuity levels of inpatients requires that program design take into consideration the continuity of patient education through the inpatient, outpatient, and home care phases of patient care. Fortunately, the amount of research available on patient education in these phases of care is increasing. (See chapter 14 for information on using the research base to improve program design, chapter 15 for self-efficacy theory in patient education, and the section in chapter 16 on CCTV research and patient education.)

Step 2. Assess the External Environment

Assessing the external environment, which includes the national environment, the community environment, the external market beyond the hospital, and other agencies and professional groups, is the next step in the patient education strategic planning model (table 2-1). This phase of planning involves collecting external data that may influence patient education planning. Assessing the external environment requires examining the broad environmental context in which the organization operates, and this information forms the basis for key planning assumptions later in the strategic planning process. Knowledge of the external environment also allows the PEM to make realistic assumptions regarding events or trends and their potential impact on the organization and, more specifically, on patient education.

Analysis of the external environment includes examining both national and local trends that are more specific to patient education than those examined for the overall health care environment. National trends, such as technological advances and political and regulatory developments, can be gleaned from various newsletters and journals. It may also be helpful to communicate with the peer review organization representative in the hospital. This individual can provide information on regulatory developments that could affect patient education. For example, as inpatient lengths of stay become shorter, the PEM needs to be more aware of national regulatory trends that could affect the type of educational programming that patients need. The PEM also needs to be aware of financing regulations regarding outpatient programs, because more patients need to utilize them and may not have the money to pay fee for service.

Technological changes, such as continued growth in noninvasive treatments, certainly will affect the variety of educational approaches used in the outpatient setting. The PEM may need to coordinate with physician offices or staff of freestanding hospital-run centers to ensure that patients receive information about procedures. PEMs can provide office staff with materials and resources for use in educating patients. Pamphlets and video-

Table 2-1. Assessment of the External Environment

National Trends	How to Gather Data
1. What political and regulatory developments are occurring that will affect patient education?	Newsletters from regulatory agencies PRO requirements JCAHO requirements, read journals
2. What technological advancements may affect patient education?	Read journals
3. What educational trends affect patient education (for example, greater consumer expectations of health care services, credentialing health educators, and so on)?	Read journals, newsletters

Local Trends	How to Gather Data
1. What local voluntary agencies are involved or have an interest in patient education?	Call local representative of major organizations (for example, Visiting Nurses Association [VNA], Bureau of Veterans Affairs, American Cancer Society [ACS], health department, YMCA, American Heart Association, and so forth). Contact specialty patient educators (for example, cardiac rehabilitation, oncology, diabetes, and so forth).
2. What patient education activities are performed by community agencies?	Interview or survey person responsible for patient education activities in these agencies. Identify agencies through discharge planning process.
3. What feedback system is set up between the hospital and community agencies?	Interview or survey person responsible for activities in these patient education agencies.
4. What patient education activities are being conducted by other area hospitals?	Advertisement/newspaper coverage Informal discussions, interview representatives
5. What professional groups in the area have major interests in patient/health education?	Interview representatives. Monitor attendance at conferences.
6. What potential markets and clients are available?	Epidemiologic data Interview health care providers and sample of potential target population.
7. What population, social, and economic trends are occurring in the community that could affect patient education?	Newspapers Government reports Interview community leaders, organizations.
8. What utilization/service demand trends, including consumer perceptions in terms of quality, service, and price, influence patient education efforts?	Community surveys
9. What health care delivery trends are occurring in the community?	State hospital association newsletters Read newspapers, journals.

tapes are the most common educational approaches, but computer-assisted instruction is becoming more frequent. Also, as more physicians' offices make equipment and procedures available, patients may be diverted from the hospital setting, requiring careful coordination to ensure that patients receive education when they need it.

The PEM also needs to focus on the health care delivery trends occurring in the community. Assessment of patient education activities conducted by other hospitals can avoid duplication of programs. It is important that the PEM be aware of other types of providers in the community and the educational programming they offer. Networking with other providers can be a means of identifying local health care trends, and can also serve to help establish cooperative programming.

Table 2-1 provides additional external assessment questions and suggests ways to gather data. For example, in response to the first question under "Local Trends," suggested ways to gather data on local voluntary agencies involved in or having an interest in patient education include calling representatives of major organizations such as the American Cancer Society (ACS) or the American Heart Association and contacting area specialty patient educators to determine which agencies they work closely with. Establishing joint projects with these agencies rather than duplicating efforts may be the best way to provide specific patient education programs.

Step 3. Assess the Internal Environment

The next step in the strategic planning model involves assessing the internal organizational environment that affects patient education. In this step, data are collected to identify the activities, needs, and resources of the organization.

Assessing the internal environment (the hospital itself) actually involves getting to know the organization's culture and can be valuable in determining the role of patient education hospitalwide. Figure 2-2 contains questions to ask to assess the organization's internal environment.[11] The answers to such questions as "What are the most important things that your organization wants to accomplish in the next three years?" or "What are your organization's greatest internal problems?" may not be easily available. In many organizations, such information is a closely guarded secret. Suggested ways to gather these data include meeting individually with different administrators to discuss forecasting and future trends, and networking with key people in the organization to informally discuss concerns.

The internal assessment may involve some "digging" on the part of the PEM, but the information derived from it is vital to the planning process. During this phase, gathering information from members of the patient education committee or, if no such committee exists, networking with other department managers can often be helpful. Interviews with key individuals in the hospital can help the PEM to focus on important internal issues for the organization. Reviewing the hospital's existing mission statement, goals, objectives, and policy statements is also helpful during this phase.

During the internal assessment, a review of the organization's strategic plan can provide useful information. If top management and board members have participated in a strategic planning process, answers to questions such as "What are the most important things your organization wants to accomplish in the next three years?" and questions involving the positive and negative forces affecting organizational goals, internal problems, and opportunities will usually have been addressed in the strategic plan.

The internal assessment should also focus on assessing hospital departments, their resources, goals, job descriptions, and performance standards as they relate to patient education. Next, reviewing patient data reveals key information on the most common diagnoses, average lengths of stay, reasons for readmission, and mechanisms for patient education in the preadmission and outpatient areas (see table 2-2, p. 47). This information is helpful when developing strategies for new programs. Finally, documentation forms used in patient education activities need to be reviewed to find out how well and how

Figure 2-2. Assessment of the Internal Environment

Questions to Ask:

1. What is the most fundamental purpose of your organization (mission statement)?
2. How did your organization come into existence?
3. What are the most important things your organization wants to accomplish in the next three years?
4. What are the most positive and the most negative environmental forces impacting your organization?
5. What are your organization's greatest internal problems?
6. Where are the best opportunities for your organization?
7. How is the government helpful and harmful in relationship to the delivery of health care?
8. What are the major issues facing your organization this year?
9. What are your top ten organizational values?

How to Gather Data:

1. Participate in key management meetings. Read minutes of meetings you did not attend.
2. Review hospital's mission statement, policy statements, philosophy, goals/objectives, strategic plan (if available).
3. Review departmental goals and objectives.
4. Meet individually with administrators to discuss forecasting and future trends for organization.
5. Analyze patient statistics (admissions, average length of stay [ALOS], number of surgeries, outpatient visits, and so forth).
6. Listen to the "grapevine."
7. Talk to planners.
8. Network with key people in the organization (nursing, medicine, chief financial officer [CFO], and so forth).
9. Analyze quality assurance (QA) data and risk management information.
10. Examine top 20 admissions.

The questions to ask are reprinted, with permission, from L. Kaiser. Organizational mindset: ten ways to alter your world view. *Healthcare Forum* 29(1):50–53, Jan.–Feb. 1986.

consistently patient education efforts are being documented. Discharge summaries, care plans, flow sheets, and audit tools can be reviewed to assess the current status of documentation. Quality assurance professionals and unit-based staff can assist the PEM in collecting these internal data. This approach involves other members of the health care team who have expertise in data collection.

An internal assessment for patient education strategic planning would be incomplete without assessing current patient education data. Table 2-2 poses questions and tells how to gather data for an internal assessment of patient education. The assessment should begin with a review of current programs, teaching materials, and participating staff. The PEM needs to find out whether programs have written goals, policies, teaching plans, appropriate interdisciplinary involvement, documentation, and evaluation methods. A review of written materials coupled with interviews with those conducting the programs can be utilized to assess the completeness of existing programs.

The internal assessment of patient education is critical to effective planning for a variety of reasons. First, knowing what patient education activities already exist within the hospital helps the PEM to avoid duplication and conflicts. For example, in one East Coast hospital two department heads unknowingly submitted a bid to conduct the same patient education program for a local industry. One department won the contract, and the other department head was surprised to find out that there was a competing program within the organization! A thorough internal assessment is the best way to avoid such problems.

Step 4. Identify Potential Problems and Possibilities

After collecting data in the assessment phases, the patient education manager should next identify potential problems in the planning process in both the internal and external environments and begin to identify possibilities for successful patient education interventions to address them.

Table 2-2. Assessment of the Internal Environment of Patient Education

Questions to Ask	How to Gather Data
1. What are the current patient education programs, materials, and participating staff?	Use surveys and/or interview department directors, and have informal staff meetings concerning current and needed patient education programs.
2. What organizational characteristics (structures) of the hospital will support or hinder patient education program development?	Review policies and procedures that affect patient education. Brainstorm with patient education advisory committee.
3. What resources are available for patient education? • Funds budgeted • Media equipment • Auxiliary • Current use of media and materials for patient education	Obtain examples from media department, library, education department. Preview materials. Survey and/or interview staff currently doing patient teaching.
4. Which departments have goals that relate to patient education?	Review department goals, interview appropriate managers.
5. Are patient education roles and responsibilities included in job descriptions, performance standards, performance evaluations?	Review job descriptions and performance evaluation criteria of staff in departments.
6. What are the top 20 common diagnoses of patients admitted to the hospital?	Medical records DRG data
7. What are the average lengths of stay and ages of patients with these diagnoses?	Patient statistics report Medical records
8. What problems have patients identified on patient questionnaires?	Review results of patient opinion satisfaction questionnaires.
9. For what reasons are patients being readmitted?	Review data from UR, medical records, morbidity statistics.
10. What information is currently given to patients in the preadmission phase? When, by whom, and in what format?	Interview or survey admissions department, public relations, outpatient services, referral agencies, emergency room, physician offices.
11. What patient data base is collected, and could this information be useful in determining patient education needs?	Review data base forms.
12. What patient education is included in discharge summaries?	Chart audits Quality monitoring indicators
13. What patient education criteria are included in audit tools?	Quality monitoring indicators
14. Do standard care plans include patient education components?	Review standard care plans.
15. How are patient education outcomes and activities documented?	Review documentation procedures.
16. Has there been interdisciplinary involvement in patient education planning and implementation?	Audit charts of specific patient population.
17. How complete are existing patient education programs for specific populations? • Written program purpose and goals • Written policies, procedures for smooth running of the program • Teaching plans • Interdisciplinary involvement • Staff orientation procedures to the program • Coordinating mechanisms • Documentation and communication procedures • Evaluation methods for patient/family outcomes and program effectiveness	Review written program materials such as standard teaching guidelines, evaluation tools, handouts, and so forth. Interview staff responsible for program and providers who participate in it. Observe actual teaching activities. Chart audits to determine if all components of patient education are included.

Figure 2-3 gives several examples of questions to ask to identify potential problems and possibilities. Answering these questions allows the PEM to organize the data in such a way that trends are easily identified. For example, the external data may assist in identifying needs not currently being met by community agencies, and may also identify potential sources of support and collaboration with these agencies.

Internal organizational data may help the PEM identify new educational services that may be needed, the sources of support and opposition to patient education, and the priorities of key decision makers. Having this information provides more objective data on patient education needs and can help justify new program development.

Although the PEM may believe that the internal patient education environment is easily assessed daily on an informal basis, formalized use of assessment questions and subsequent analysis often provides surprises. For example, interviews with staff and patients may provide information about strengths and weaknesses of current education programming that are not readily apparent. Later in the process, decisions can be made regarding revising or eliminating current programs.

The last question in table 2-2 can be asked to help identify program strengths and weaknesses. For example, one of the weaknesses often identified is the lack of multidisciplinary involvement in a program. Other personnel may need to be involved to make the program better, or when the disciplines are involved, duplication may be discovered. One of the strengths often identified is strong medical staff support, always essential for a sound program.

Figure 2-3. Identification of Potential Problems and Possibilities

A. External Environment (community/national)

1. What national trends seem most applicable to our situation?
2. What key events are happening in the community that can provide opportunities or create potential problems for patient education?
3. What patient education needs are not being met in the community?
4. Where are the major sources of support for patient education within the community and nation?
5. What are the top priorities for health care in the community that may be affected by patient education programming?

B. Internal Environment (hospital)

1. What appear to be the programmatic priorities for key decision makers?
2. What are the major current and future problems facing the organization that might be affected by patient education programming?
3. Where are the major sources of support for patient education within the hospital? Is there opposition to organized patient education planning?
4. Which patient education programs, services, products, and ideas support current organizational goals?
5. What do the hospital's key decision makers believe is the business of patient education in terms of services performed?
6. What organizational mechanisms are in place for extending patient education services into the preadmission and postdischarge periods of health care delivery?
7. What new health services is the organization investigating that should have a patient education component?

C. Internal Patient Education Environment

1. What is the level of functioning (strengths/weaknesses) of patient education in the system as compared to the standards?
2. What opportunities and problems are identified from an analysis of the patient education activities data base?
3. What patient education activities would staff like to develop and/or change? How would they change them?
4. What educational activities do patients and their families want?
5. Which patient education services could generate revenue?

To facilitate the identification of problems and possibilities, organizations may want to consider a patient education planning retreat. As described by Cordell, such a retreat is a way to ensure that adequate time is allotted for this step in the strategic planning model for patient education. A 7½-hour retreat focusing on patient education was held for The Seattle Veterans Administration Medical Center (VAMC) group, which consisted of 9 out of 12 Patient Education Committee members representing the disciplines of nursing, library, social work, dental, psychology, surgery, medicine, and education. This commitment of time and participation was essential to meeting the organization's strategic planning goals. The use of the group process, with adequate time for brainstorming and networking, supported both the needs of the participants and the overall planning process.[12]

Step 5. Synthesize and Analyze Data

After collecting data to identify potential problems in the internal and external environments and ways to address them, the PEM can begin to synthesize and analyze the data. This type of analysis requires searching for patterns in the data gathered, making sense of them, coming up with conclusions or interpretations of them, and comparing them with patterns in an ideal scenario. As the following two examples show, the conclusions drawn from the data gathered can lead to useful changes in patient education programs.

In one hospital it became clear during the strategic planning process that although there were ample educational programs for patients, the programs' goals were not well understood by top management or even most department heads. The PEM took an objective look at the data and determined that several programs were the "pet" projects of energetic individuals; realistic goals had never been established for these programs, nor had their effectiveness ever been evaluated. As a result, the PEM worked with staff to reorganize one program and build in an evaluation mechanism, and discontinued another program, freeing up resources for existing well-developed programs.

In another example, at the Seattle VAMC the strategic planning process helped participants focus on patient needs for programs in chronic obstructive pulmonary disease, diabetes, and smoking cessation.[13] After patient education needs were identified, they were prioritized. This enabled patient education committee members to deal with the high priorities for patient education programs first, as well as to gain an overall perspective of the needs of the organization. Development of the patient education program plan was based on the priority needs coupled with the resources available (staff time, facility space, and money).

This step of the strategic planning process can also help the PEM identify program efforts by other organizations, by either addressing ways to develop programs for unmet community needs or coordinating plans with an existing program in the community rather than duplicating it. For example, during the strategic planning process one PEM became aware of an excellent prenatal exercise program offered by a local Young Women's Christian Association and was able to link prospective parents with the program through the hospital. This increased the reputation and visibility of both organizations while conserving the time that the hospital would have needed to develop its own program. Using the expertise of the planning/marketing professionals on the hospital staff is often helpful.

Step 6. Develop Strategies

Prior to this phase of planning, the PEM should have identified several overall hospital strategies and goals and now be ready to develop a broad course of action for designing a hospitalwide patient education program to help achieve those goals. The value of this step is that it allows the PEM to align patient education strategy with hospital strategies. This step is really a two-part process. First, hospitalwide strategies should be clearly defined and written down. Next, the PEM should list any patient education strategies that would support clearly identified organizational goals. Table 2-3 shows several hospital-wide strategies and the specific patient education strategies that would support them. For example, if a hospital strategy is to develop new outpatient services, among the patient education strategies to be considered might be preadmission education programs, disease-specific classes/services (such as an ostomy workshop), risk reduction programs, and services related to new markets (such as women's services). The PEM would then choose one strategy to work on. If preadmission is of prime importance to the hospital, the PEM might focus on possible programs in this area. Next, the PEM would examine the impact and feasibility of this strategy. Some of the patient education strategies may eventually become action items in the hospitalwide strategic plan, focusing general attention on the importance of patient education within the overall organization.

Step 7. Examine Impact and Feasibility of the Strategies

Once the strategies have been identified, the PEM needs to develop criteria to help prioritize them according to how they will improve the future position of the hospital and whether they are feasible to implement. Figure 2-4 lists questions to assist the PEM in

Table 2-3. Samples of Coordinated Hospital and Patient Education Strategies

Hospital Strategy	Patient Education Strategy
Develop new outpatient services.	Develop preadmission programs.
	Develop an outpatient ostomy clinic.
	Develop a women's program.
Reduce the risk of unplanned readmissions.	Develop a risk reduction program.
	Develop a patient self-management program.
	Increase emphasis on discharge planning.
	Increase postdischarge educational support services.
	Increase family involvement and training.
Improve efficiency of inpatient care delivery.	Streamline inpatient teaching.
	Use nonprint material (for example, videos) to convey repetitive information.
	Support patient teaching with print materials (pamphlets, instruction sheets, and so forth) when patients need to refer to information often.
	Provide staff development so major barriers to staff teaching can be overcome.

Figure 2-4. Questions to Examine the Impact and Feasibility of a Patient Education Strategy

1. Why was this patient education strategy chosen?
2. Is the strategy congruent with management policies, philosophy, preference, priorities, and politics?
3. What is the extent of potential future impact?
4. What are the legal issues?
5. What interdepartmental and/or interdisciplinary collaboration is necessary? What problems might exist?
6. Does the strategy have market strength and attractiveness?
7. How will budgetary limitations affect further development of the program?
8. What risks (consequences) are acceptable should components of the strategy fail?

assessing each strategy. The PEM should describe the strategy and determine why it was chosen. Legal issues, the extent of interdepartmental collaboration required, and any risks of the strategy should all be identified during this step of the strategic planning process. A risk might involve alienation of a key support person; for example, a physician who thinks that ostomy education should be done in the surgeon's office or who favors a local supplier could undermine the program and cause its collapse. In addition, turf issues commonly surface during this step and should be dealt with before trying to implement a multidisciplinary patient education program. Retreats or other opportunities to help key players get to know and trust each other may be used if improved cooperation is needed.

Time spent examining the impact and feasibility of strategies can save both dollars and effort later in the strategic planning process. This is especially true if it can be determined at this stage that the proposed strategy is too costly, poses legal risks, or lacks essential support from key players.

Step 8. Develop Patient Education Management Objectives

Once the impact and feasibility of a strategy have been assessed, the PEM could brainstorm ideas with hospital staff or committee members. For example, ideas related to preadmission programs could include general preadmission surgical classes for adults, coordinated preadmission activities with physicians' offices or HMOs, preadmission classes for specific target groups, or the incorporation of educational protocol into existing preadmission testing visits.

After a list has been generated, the PEM should select several ideas that have potential for success and develop patient education management objectives for them. This step outlines specific action steps that will lead to plan accomplishment. For example, for the strategy of preadmission programs, the PEM has generated patient education ideas to support the goal and is now ready to define a patient education management objective that relates to this strategy. In this scenario, a possible patient education management objective is to develop a preadmission education program for total hip replacement surgical patients by October 1993. Other possible objectives are to develop, in conjunction with the office staff of Dr. Cornea, a preadmission program for cataract surgical patients by July 1993, and to develop a pediatric puppet show orientation by December 1993.

Once developed, the impact and feasibility of each management objective should be evaluated using a set of questions similar to those used to examine the strategy (see figure 2-5). Questions relating to cost, staffing facilities, and equipment needed, in addition to the fit of the new objective into the existing structure, all need to be addressed at this point. Proceeding with program planning prior to taking this step may result in

Figure 2-5. Questions to Examine the Impact and Feasibility of a Patient Education Management Objective

1. What are the possible patient education management objectives that relate to the patient education strategy?
2. How will the management objectives fit into my existing patient education structure?
3. What human resources in terms of time, type and numbers of staff, and training needs will be necessary? Who is to be involved? Focus on the pro and con positions, and map critical linkages.
4. What material resources (such as print, video teaching materials) and financial resources are required and available?
5. What facilities/equipment are needed and available?
6. What are the legal issues for the patient education management objective?
7. What interdepartmental/interdisciplinary collaboration is necessary? What problems might exist?
8. What is the extent of potential future impact?
9. Does the patient education management objective have market strength and attractiveness?
10. What risks (consequences) are acceptable should components of the management objective fail?

lack of funding and/or cooperation from essential allies within the hospital and other areas involved.

Step 9. Plan Programs

Having completed the preceding steps, the PEM should now prioritize the management objectives according to their feasibility at the present time. This will help the PEM choose one objective that will provide the basis of a program that truly supports the organization's goals. Assuming that the management objective chosen is to develop a preadmission education program for total hip replacement surgical patients by October 1993, moving from the objective to the program consists of the following steps:

1. Identify target population.
   - Research the number and types of patients coming to the hospital for this type of surgery. This includes admission patterns, special needs, age, sex, and physical abilities. (See chapter 13 for more information on target population programs.)
2. Develop program objectives.
   - These are outcome objectives of the proposed program and are not the same as the management objective. They should cover what the learner should be able to do at the conclusion of the program. For example, an objective for this program might be to demonstrate that patients would be able to walk with crutches correctly and effectively.
3. Identify barriers to instruction.
   - These might include illiteracy, pediatric patients who cannot understand, or bedfast patients who are unable to meet all the outcome objectives.
4. Determine performance criteria.
   - For each objective these will determine when, how often, or how well the learner needs to perform. Does the crutch walking need to be demonstrated before surgery? Does the crutch walking need to be for 100 yards without stopping? Must it be done every day?
5. Select instructional methods.
   - This includes the choice of individual versus group instruction; use of print and audiovisual media; use of pre- or posttesting; and use of demonstration, lecture, role-playing, and other instructional methods. (See chapter 13 for information on planning programs for target populations, chapter 16 for use of CCTV and other technologies, and chapter 17 for the use of print materials.)
6. Develop lesson plans.
   - In this step, the PEM lists each performance objective, the content included, the method and teaching aid used to teach, and the means of evaluating the patient's attainment of the objective (observation, paper and pencil test, and so on).
7. Decide on a method to document that patient education took place (see chapter 9).
   - Methods can include flow sheets, narrative notes, and computer entry.
8. Develop a budget/business plan.
   - Projection of start-up costs and ongoing direct and indirect expenses for a new program is a critical part of the planning process. If appropriate, specific and realistic income projections should also be made based on assumptions about institutional goals and market strength that have been identified earlier in the planning process. These estimates will enable the manager to identify and resolve potential shortfalls before the program is implemented. (See chapter 7 for information on identifying resources for patient education.)
9. Develop an evaluation mechanism.
   - This is different from the learner evaluation described in the lesson plan, and implies evaluation of the total program. If evaluating process, questions could

include: How many patients enrolled in the program? How many completed the program? What percent of the medical staff referred patients? If evaluating program outcome, questions might include: What percentage of patients who completed the program were able to perform to the standards of the program?

The program planning step is probably familiar to PEMs. It is the step that many early program managers viewed as the entire planning process. In the strategic planning model, this step, although no less important, is now tied in with a sound planning process.

Step 10. Conduct Evaluation

After the patient education program is planned and implemented, it must be evaluated. Evaluation uses methods to determine whether the original program objectives are being met. The time at which evaluation takes place should be determined at the start of the program. For some programs it may be appropriate to conduct evaluation after one year; for others, after two to three months. Evaluation data and feedback are essential to determine whether the strategic planning process has had the desired result and impact. Ruzicki outlines an excellent program evaluation process, which is described in the following paragraphs.[14]

The purpose of evaluation is to come up with data to be used in decision making. Evidence or data are information that will show what is actually happening with regard to the specific evaluation question—in the form of acts, words, numbers, or other proof (a picture of what exists). Preestablished criteria are standards that depict the ideal situation and are often found in program objectives. The technique used refers to ways used to collect evidence.

When doing evaluation, the PEM simply gathers evidence about the existing situation to answer a specific question and compares the evidence to preestablished criteria. For example, if the PEM is interested in finding out whether patients who must self-administer insulin by injection are able to do so upon discharge (question), he or she must find evidence through observation, medical record audit, or some other mechanism to compare to the established criteria for the program (for example, 100 percent of patients will have the necessary injection skills upon discharge).

Many PEMs are frightened by the notion of evaluation, thinking that it implies rigid, formal research techniques; however, most program evaluation can be conducted by anyone familiar with the program. It is helpful if the process for evaluating the program is determined before implementation and if evaluation is a routine part of the program. Evaluation can help the PEM spot problems and deal with them before they grow. Evaluation also helps identify program trends and continually ensure program quality.

Evaluation needs to be conducted at two levels, the program level and the hospital level. Evaluation conducted at the program level can focus on outcomes such as how well the program met its objectives for the patient, or in terms of other identified criteria, such as the number of people who attended the program, or the level of patient or physician satisfaction. Whole programs or parts of programs can be evaluated. PEMs may look at specific procedural or structural elements of the patient education program, such as the registration process for a preadmission program.

To evaluate programs from an organizational level, as implied in the evaluation step of figure 2-1, requires revisiting the hospital's strategic plan to determine whether the program was implemented according to the management objective and whether it actually affected the organization in the way it was intended to. The PEM may find that although a program is effective in some ways, it does not actually have the desired impact on the hospital. Attaining the desired impact may not require dropping the program, but it will certainly require reexamination of the program's design.

As a result of using this evaluation process at one hospital, several patient education programs were redesigned and at least one was eliminated. In addition, new methods to keep key individuals informed of patient education programming and evaluation data were designed. These included monthly reports, presentations at department manager meetings, and inclusion of patient education program activities in hospital publications.

☐ Conclusion

Patient education managers have responsibilities that cross departmental lines and therefore are in a unique position to effect change. The planning process described in this chapter can be one of the elements of a strong patient education effort, one that looks not only at strategies for meeting the needs of individual patients but also at a much larger picture—the goals of the hospital.

Strategic planning for patient education is a process that, at first inspection, may seem overwhelming to the PEM. However, once familiar with the steps and techniques, the process is easily and effectively used in a hospital setting. When patient education managers and/or committees embrace strategic planning as a mind-set for change, they begin to actively seek out ideas, concepts, and innovations, and look for ways to contribute to the overall mission of the hospital.

References

1. Beckham, J. D. Strategic thinking and the road to relevance. *Health Care Forum* 34(6):37–47, Nov.–Dec. 1991.

2. Leebov, W., and Scott, G. *Health Care Managers in Transition: Shifting Roles and Changing Organizations.* San Francisco: Jossey-Bass, 1990, p. 5.

3. Bartlett, E. E. Preparing for strategic planning. *Patient Education and Counseling* 11(1):1–2, Feb. 1988.

4. Cordell, B., Linnell, K., and Price, J. Strategic planning in patient education: a key element of successful management. *Patient Education and Counseling* 11(1):69, Feb. 1988.

5. Leebov, W., and Ersoz, C. J. *The Health Care Manager's Guide to Continuous Quality Improvement.* Chicago: American Hospital Publishing, 1991, pp. 4–7.

6. American Hospital Association. *Management Advisory, Patient Education Services.* Chicago: AHA, 1990, p. 1.

7. Gorman, A., and Ludemann, M. A. Comparing satisfaction levels of inpatients and outpatients with a diabetes teaching program. *Patient Education and Counseling* 12(2):121–29, Oct. 1988.

8. Abendshien, J. *A Guide to the Board's Role in Strategic Business Planning.* Chicago: American Hospital Publishing, 1988, pp. 1–2 (out of print).

9. American Hospital Association. *Hospital Inpatient Education: Survey Findings and Analysis.* Atlanta: Centers for Disease Control, 1980.

10. Giloth, B. Managing patient education in U.S. hospitals. *Patient Education and Counseling* 15(2):101–11, Apr. 1990.

11. Kaiser, L. Organizational mindset: ten ways to alter your world view. *Healthcare Forum* 29(1):50–53, Jan.–Feb. 1986.

12. Cordell and others, pp. 65–73.

13. Cordell and others.

14. Ruzicki, D. Evaluation: it's what you do with what you've got that counts. *Promoting Health* 6(5):6–9, Sept.–Oct. 1985.

Chapter 3

Creating an Educational Environment in a Hospital Setting

Laura Gilpin, M.F.A., R.N.

□ Objectives

The reader will be able to:

- Identify the elements of an educational environment within a hospital
- Discuss the role of hospital staff members as teachers of patients and families
- Identify the architectural and design elements that support an educational environment
- Understand the role of access to information in encouraging patient and family involvement
- List educational materials that reinforce an educational environment

□ Illness as an Educational Opportunity

For many patients hospitalization is an unfamiliar and unexpected experience. Because of the apprehension that generally accompanies a serious illness or accident, hospitalization is rarely recognized as a potential opportunity for learning and growth. Yet hospitalization provides a situation in which the patient is surrounded by experts (physicians, nurses, pharmacists, nutritionists, and other professionals) who are knowledgeable in a vast array of health and medical areas.

Hospitals are well established as teaching institutions for medical students, interns, nursing students, and various others who require technical knowledge and practical skills. However, patients are rarely regarded as fellow students; instead, they are seen as the passive recipients of the knowledge and skills acquired by others.

Because of the decreased length of most hospital stays, patients and their families are now frequently required to perform many technical skills that used to be strictly the domain of trained professionals. In addition, many consumers are finding that they need to be more knowledgeable about health care issues because the complexity of medical care and treatment options is requiring that they make informed decisions about their care. Thus it is important to create an environment within the hospital that encourages patient learning.

Laura Gilpin, M.F.A., R.N.

Components of an Educational Environment

To meet the changing needs of consumers, hospitals must become teaching centers and community resources, not only treating illnesses but also promoting independence, well-being, and health. One of the components of an educational environment that this shift requires is a change in attitude on the part of all hospital staff. Fortunately, an attitude of openness costs nothing. Even if no additional nursing time is allotted, even if no resources or materials are provided, patients and family members can be encouraged to ask questions and participate in their own care.

Unfortunately, attitudes are difficult to change. The entire medical establishment, it seems, has developed around an atmosphere of withholding information, creating passive, or at least submissive, patients. Many nurses remember being taught never to reveal the patient's vital signs. In many hospitals today, the medical record still remains a closely guarded secret, available to most hospital personnel but withheld from the patient. But the complex health care establishment is changing: Consumers are better informed; physicians and nurses are more open about giving information; and hospitals, fearing litigation, are providing patients with more opportunities to make choices regarding treatment options.

Another component of an educational environment is the free exchange of information. Questions by patients and families are encouraged, including those that may be unrelated to the patient's current medical diagnosis. A patient hospitalized with cholecystitis may be more concerned about a parent's recent diagnosis of Alzheimer's or a child's diagnosis of anorexia nervosa. In an environment that truly supports education, patients and families are provided with ample health and medical information and staff have access to a wide range of resources.

One of the most valuable sources of information for many patients is the medical record. Whether the patient reads it daily or never looks at it, an open medical record policy is a powerful symbol of the patient's right to know and encourages patients to become actively involved in all aspects of their care.

In an educational environment patients are not only provided with access to information, they are also empowered and encouraged to make use of their knowledge by participating in decisions regarding their care. An educational environment includes respect for patients' choices, even when their decisions are not those the health care professionals would have made.

Patients are also given the option of not learning and not actively participating in making their own health care decisions. The specific needs and interests of all patients are respected even if their need is to be passive. However, it is possible that simply being exposed to an atmosphere of open communication and free access to information will cause patients to begin to shift their traditional attitude of dependence.

To create an environment that supports an attitude of openness and education, all aspects of patient care must be addressed. It is not enough to hire a patient education manager (PEM) whose role is to carry out an entire education program in isolation. Nor is it effective to simply provide a rack of educational pamphlets and expect patients to become knowledgeable and actively involved on their own. To be truly effective, an atmosphere of education must pervade all aspects of a patient's hospital stay. A bath, a dressing change, a meal, or watching a funny movie can all be opportunities for learning.

Nurses play a vital role in sustaining an attitude of openness and communicating it to patients. Adequate training and ongoing support for nursing are essential, as is providing resources for answering a wide range of questions.

Physician involvement also is critical in encouraging patients to participate in decisions regarding their care. Physicians are also vital links in sustaining the patient's involvement in his or her own care after discharge.

In an educational environment, the patient's family members and close friends are also encouraged to actively participate in the patient's care and to practice the skills they may need when caring for the patient at home.

Nutritional information is another essential component in educating patients and families about health maintenance and possible long-range illness prevention. Hospital dietitians as well as staff from other departments, such as physical therapy, pharmacy, and social services, can provide valuable educational resources throughout the hospital.

The architectural design of the hospital must also reflect the educational focus of patient care. A library and a lounge can provide access to educational materials and interactions. A unit designed with a kitchen can facilitate teaching patients and families about nutrition.

To truly become an educational institution, hospitals must also become community resources by providing ongoing opportunities to learn about health and illness. Consumer health libraries (see chapter 19), classes, and support groups can help establish hospitals as valuable sources of information within the community.

If patients and their families have learned how to learn, are aware of what resources are available, and know how to make use of their knowledge by participating in decisions regarding their care, the process of education can continue long after the patient has left the hospital.

Examples of Educational Environments

Educational environments are as individual as the patients who occupy them. There is no magic formula for creating an environment that supports patient education. Each unit and each hospital will be different, depending on the needs of specific patient populations and the availability of staff and resources to meet those needs.

Many hospital settings incorporate various aspects of an educational environment. Some oncology units and rehabilitation facilities have emphasized patient education and family involvement for many years. It is somewhat more difficult, however, to find examples of hospital settings where education and active participation permeate all aspects of the patient's care. Fortunately, there are several examples that can serve as models for other health care facilities moving toward increasing patient and family involvement.

The Cooperative Care Unit

Probably the oldest and best-known educational environment in the United States is the Cooperative Care Unit at New York University Medical Center in New York City. Open since 1979, this unit provides care for 104 acute care patients and their care partners (usually a family member who assists with patient care). The Cooperative Care Unit provides a homelike setting for patients who meet acute care criteria, but are ambulatory or mobile enough to go to centralized locations for meals, education, and clinical needs. They must also be medically stable enough not to require close monitoring or significant supervision by professional nursing staff. For example, an AIDS patient might be admitted for a diagnostic workup and to be started on IV medication that could then be administered at home. Each patient must have a family member or friend available to serve as a care partner to stay overnight, provide assistance with personal needs, and communicate critical information about the patient's health status to the professional staff.

Comprehensive education is provided for patients and their care partners at an education center staffed by nurse educators, social workers, nutritionists, a pharmacist, and a recreation therapist. Patients administer their own medications and a nutritionist is available in the dining room at mealtimes to work with patients on dietary choices.

The Cooperative Care Model has demonstrated that many patients who would have otherwise been hospitalized in a traditional setting can retain much of their independence and autonomy and still receive the necessary medical treatment at a substantially reduced cost. In addition to creating a more pleasant, homelike atmosphere, the Cooperative Care Unit provides an environment in which patients and their care partners can learn and practice the skills they will need when the patient goes home.

The Day Hospital at Memorial Sloan–Kettering Cancer Center
Another innovative unit is the Day Hospital at Memorial Sloan–Kettering Cancer Center in New York City. Because of the intensity of some cancer treatments, such as high-dose chemotherapy, oncology patients are frequently hospitalized so that they can be closely monitored during and after treatment. For patients who have a family member who can monitor them after they go home, the Day Hospital provides an alternative to hospitalization.

Patients receive their treatment in a carefully supervised setting while family members are provided with education and training on any ongoing care the patient may need at home. Staff are available around the clock to answer questions if problems arise later. If patients at the Day Hospital have difficulty tolerating their treatment or require more acute care than a family member can provide, they may be admitted to an inpatient unit at Memorial Hospital. For most patients the Day Hospital offers an alternative to the disruption of frequent hospitalizations.

Planetree Model Units
Planetree is a not-for-profit consumer health care organization founded in 1978 to assist hospitals interested in providing humanistic patient care. One of this organization's most important aspects is its provision of patient education and access to information.

The Planetree Model is a comprehensive approach, focusing not only on patient education but also on changes in nursing, family involvement, nutrition, arts, massage, and architectural design. The patient is always at the center of humanistic care. In the Planetree Model, the nurse plays a key role in creating a nurturing environment in which patients are free to choose any, all, or none of the options available. Illness is seen in the context of the patient's life experience and for some patients may be an opportunity for growth and learning. (See figure 3-1 for a conceptual model of Planetree.) The goal of these changes has been to transform the way patients experience hospitals: from being impersonal and intimidating institutions to becoming nurturing, healing, and educational environments.

The first Planetree Model Unit, a 13-bed medical–surgical unit, opened in 1985 at California Pacific Medical Center (then Pacific Presbyterian Medical Center) in San Francisco. This pilot project, initially funded by grant support and evaluated by the University of Washington, incorporated a variety of changes to create a healing, nurturing environment in which medical–surgical patients and their families are encouraged to participate fully in their care. Results of the four-year evaluation have shown that patient, nurse, and physician satisfaction are significantly higher compared to other medical-surgical units in the hospital.

The second Planetree Unit, a 25-bed medical–surgical unit, has been in operation since 1989 at San Jose Medical Center in San Jose, California. Additional Planetree Units are under development in Oregon, New York City, and Central California. Mid-Columbia Medical Center in The Dalles, Oregon, is the first institution to implement the Planetree Model hospitalwide.

Medical criteria for admission to the Planetree Units is the same as for any other medical-surgical unit. Patients are not screened or preselected and do not have to have a family member available to assist with care. Any patient may be admitted provided he or she has a medical or surgical diagnosis and a physician who supports the Planetree concept of access to information, including the open medical record. Over 200 physicians at each hospital admit patients to the Planetree Units.

Patients on the Planetree Units and their families are free to participate in as many or as few of the programs as they like. They are provided with a variety of educational resources, including fact sheets, in-depth research packets, nutritional counseling, and a self-medication program. Unrestricted visiting hours and the availability of overnight stays encourage family members to take an active role in caring for the patient. A massage program and an arts program offering soothing music or funny movies encourage patients to learn about relaxation and stress reduction.

Figure 3-1. Conceptual Model of Planetree

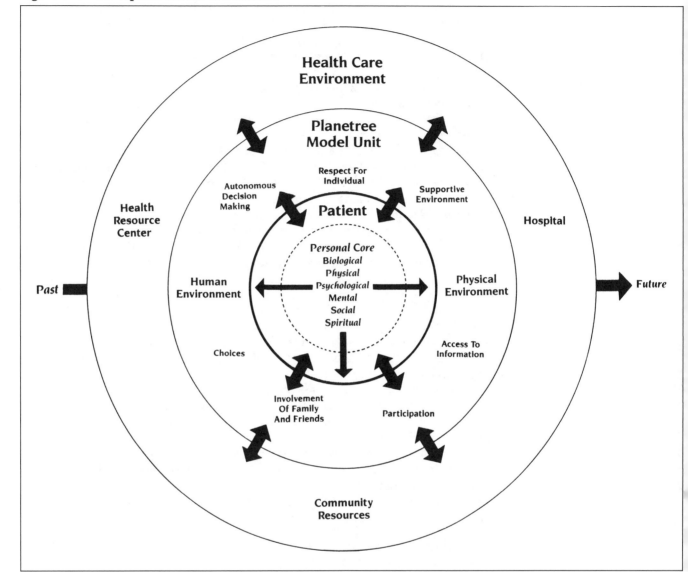

Because the Planetree Model can be adapted to any patient population, it is the one that will be referred to in this chapter. Although there are variations in the implementation of Planetree concepts at the five model sites, the goal at each hospital has been to create a healing and educational environment for patients and their families.

Obstacles in Creating an Educational Environment and Some Ways to Overcome Them

Implementing a comprehensive educational program on any unit or in any hospital involves overcoming a number of obstacles and barriers. Whereas some of these obstacles are very real, others are only illusions. Unfortunately, the invisible obstacles are far more difficult to overcome. Policies are tangible and can be changed and rewritten; however, illusions are pervasive and persistent. Most successful education programs such as Planetree and the Cooperative Care Unit exist despite the illusions and may eventually help to dispel them.

One of the most significant barriers to patient education is the myth that patients do not want the information or that they would misuse it if they were given it. "A little knowledge is a terrible thing" is a phrase frequently heard among hospital staff when discussing patient education. There is also a common belief that younger patients might want information but elderly patients either would be overwhelmed by the information or would not know what to do with it. Another illusion is that if patients wanted information they would simply ask for it. In focus groups that Planetree conducts with patients and family members at numerous hospitals nationwide, many people report that they are too intimidated to ask, do not want their physicians to think they are dumb, or feel that nurses are too busy to respond. Yet a lack of questions is often perceived by hospital staff as evidence of a lack of interest on the part of patients and families.

Many health care professionals also have a subtle fear of the empowered patient. Nurses are often afraid they will be asked difficult questions. Physicians frequently believe patients will refuse medications, treatments, or diagnostic tests or will question the practitioner's medical judgment. Another common fear is that patients will be upset by reading their medical records or will be more likely to initiate litigation.

However, studies support the experience at Planetree Units that knowledgeable patients are not more likely to ignore their doctors' advice, nor are they more likely to file lawsuits.[1] On the contrary, a lack of information rather than too much information is often cited by angry patients as a contributing factor in their decision to sue.[2-4]

In addition to the challenge of changing the beliefs and attitudes of some health care providers, implementing an education program in any hospital setting also presents many barriers in that patients are usually acutely ill and families are often anxious or in a state of crisis. Some patients, particularly the elderly, either have no family or their family members are themselves ill and unable to participate in the patient's care. Low literacy levels and language barriers also are common problems.

Medical–surgical patients also present a challenge in the variety of diagnoses seen. Formalized teaching plans are difficult to develop to meet the needs of such a broad range of patients. Flexibility and a personalized approach to patient teaching are essential so that the needs and interests of patients and families can be identified early, and useful resources made available. A variety of resources, such as fact sheets, audio- and video-tapes, and foreign language materials need to be easily accessible.

Another barrier is the enormity of the task of implementing an educational program hospitalwide. There are certain advantages to creating an educational environment on only one unit to start with. Yet, there are also a number of disadvantages, one of which is the significant lack of economy of scale. Although decentralization is very effective in bringing decisions regarding education as well as actual implementation to the unit level, the expense of developing resources to be used only on a single unit is unnecessary. However, once materials have been found to be useful, they can be distributed hospitalwide.

Another obstacle is the tremendous confusion over who should be responsible for patient teaching. Recent studies show that most patients want their physician to be their primary educator.[5] On the other hand, nurses believe that patients see them as the primary educator.[6] Physicians were significantly less likely than nurses to believe nurses should have primary responsibility for educating patients.[7] Multidisciplinary committees can be useful in clarifying the roles of all health care professionals. Changing patient perceptions of who can provide information seems to occur over time as they receive education from a variety of sources.

Another area of resistance in creating an educational environment is the issue of cost. Many aspects of a comprehensive program can require substantial budgetary increases, including the cost of nurses' wages if they are to spend more time teaching, the additional salary if a patient education manager is hired, the cost of buying or developing extensive patient education materials, or the expense of establishing a community-based health library. Providing patient education can cost more than maintaining current ways of doing things, and there is certainly ample justification for the need to increase patient education budgets. But there are also many aspects of patient education that do not have to add significantly to a hospital or unit budget.

One of the least expensive aspects of an education program is the open medical record. The patient's medical record is a valuable document filled with relevant information. It is very useful in helping patients ask questions and begin a dialogue with their physicians.[8] Answering a patient's specific questions is no more time-consuming than answering vague questions, yet far more useful information can be conveyed. Implementing the open medical record policy on only one unit can help to overcome the physicians' initial anxiety about patients reading their medical records.

Patient education programs also offer the potential of significant cost savings by decreasing length of stay, avoiding rehospitalization, and preventing complications.[9,10] Unfortunately, these areas are often difficult to document. Increased patient satisfaction in a competitive market and a potential decrease in patient litigation cases by providing adequate information and patient involvement may help offset cost considerations.

The possibility of reallocating existing funds may be helpful in justifying patient education expenses. A community-based health library, such as the Planetree Health Resource Center, provides valuable public relations and marketing opportunities. Media coverage of community outreach events may be less expensive than purchasing advertising space. Sometimes local businesses and foundations can be found to form a consortium of funding sources to support various community and hospital-based education programs.

Creating an environment that is supportive of patient education requires the cooperation and approval of the medical staff, administration, nursing department, and other departments. Most resistance seems to result from a lack of information regarding the value of patient education or the fear that implementation will be too difficult. A step-by-step approach to address both these issues seems to be the most effective.

☐ The Human Environment

One of the most vital aspects of humanistic care is the relationship that forms between patients and those who provide their care. Although patient education materials are essential tools, they are not a substitute for human interaction. This is not to say that teaching requires lengthy one-on-one sessions between patients and staff; however, such interactions do set the tone for the sharing of information and encourage patient questions and involvement.

Although patients should be encouraged to seek information independently, most initially require the assistance of a knowledgeable staff member who can explore their needs and interests and determine how best to meet them. The staff are vital in creating an atmosphere conducive to patient education. Most of the material in the following sections focuses on how various staff members can serve as teachers. The role of patients and families as teachers and the importance of administrative support for patient education are also covered.

Nurses as Teachers

In many educational environments nurses are the primary educators of patients and their families. This is not meant to diminish the role of physicians as educators; certainly some information can come only from the patient's physician. But nurses have a distinct advantage in that they are accessible to patients 24 hours a day, 7 days a week. "Teachable moments" can occur at any hour of the day or night, whenever a patient or family member has a question or needs information.

Nurses are also frequently perceived by patients to be somewhat less intimidating than physicians, so nurses may be more likely to be asked questions, particularly questions that are unrelated to the patient's current diagnosis. The disadvantages of having nurses responsible for patient education include a lack of time allocated for patient teaching, inadequate resources to provide adequate information, and the fact that patient education is often not seen as a priority by administration or other nurses.

In a setting supporting education, reallocation of the nurses' time with a priority on advocacy and education is a primary goal. Adequate and easily accessible resources such as fact sheets, audio- and videotapes, and in-depth information packets on topics not within the nurses' range of knowledge help to make better use of the nurses' time. A patient education manager can be a useful resource for nurses in providing patient education and in overseeing the development and maintenance of educational materials. If the role of this position is to coordinate patient education throughout the hospital or on several units, this person's salary does not add significantly to the overall budget.

Accountability and Continuity of Care

One of the most critical issues in implementing an educational environment is that of nursing accountability to ensure that every patient has someone who is responsible for coordinating his or her care throughout the entire hospital stay. In many hospitals there is a serious lack of continuity of care: Nurses care for different patients each day, so patients find it difficult to establish a rapport with any one nurse. Nurses are accountable only for the patients they are caring for on a given day. No one is accountable for the patient's teaching needs over the entire stay in the hospital or on a particular unit.

Another related problem is that no one is responsible for patient teaching, although the nurse who discharges the patient is ultimately responsible for documenting that the patient went home adequately prepared. As a result, much of the information given to patients is presented on the last day of admission, often when the patient is excited or anxious about going home and the family is busy making necessary arrangements. It is not uncommon for information about the patient's medications to be given during the last hour, sometimes even during the last 20 minutes, of the patient's stay.

To address the issues of lack of continuity of care and accountability, some educational environments such as Planetree have implemented *primary nursing* as the most effective means of providing an individualized, humanistic approach to patient care. This system of nursing ensures that each patient has one nurse who is responsible for coordinating his or her care throughout the entire hospital stay. Although case management, which may encompass a patient's entire episode of illness across all settings, may also be effective in providing a high level of continuity, primary nursing has an advantage over case management in that the primary nurse delivers more of the patient's routine care, offering many spontaneous opportunities for teaching throughout the day.

Although other nurses will care for the patient, the primary nurse develops the plan of care, with the patient's input, and communicates the plan to the other nurses. Due to the broad scope and comprehensive nature of nursing care, the primary nurse becomes the central figure in encouraging patients to take an active role in their care. He or she is also responsible for coordinating patient teaching and providing information where appropriate. Other nurses may assist with the teaching according to the primary nurse's plan.

Whenever possible in elective admissions, the primary nurse makes a home visit before the patient is admitted. This is an ideal time to provide information and begin preoperative and postoperative teaching, because patients are often more relaxed in familiar surroundings. The same nurse then follows the patient throughout the hospital stay on the unit and follows up with a telephone call after the patient is discharged.

Discharge Planning

Because the primary nurse is responsible for coordinating the patient's care throughout the hospital stay, discharge planning can begin as soon as the patient is admitted. The primary nurse may also be responsible for noting the patient's estimated length of stay, based on the appropriate diagnostic-related group (DRG). To facilitate open communication, a care-planning conference involving the attending physician, the primary nurse, and the patient (as well as the family, if possible) is set up by the nurse within 24 hours of admission to jointly discuss the patient's treatment, care, and discharge needs. This helps the patient and family anticipate the kind of training that will be necessary before he or she goes home.

A social worker or hospital discharge planner knowledgeable in community resources often assists the primary nurse. After a patient's discharge, a home health nurse or hospice nurse can contact the primary nurse for better continuity of teaching needs. The primary nurse also calls the patient following discharge to provide any additional information. (Chapter 8 provides more information on discharge planning.)

Training

Many nurses are trained in patient education while in nursing school. Because the nursing process of assessing, planning, implementing, and evaluating is familiar to most nurses, its use is facilitated in patient teaching. What is often lacking, however, is a sense of enjoyment about learning and teaching. Learning is frequently perceived as work or punishment rather than an enjoyable, natural process innate to all human beings. Teaching is often perceived as a task rather than a human interaction.

Effective training programs elicit an understanding of the different ways people learn. Experiential exercises are sometimes helpful in reestablishing a sense of enjoyment and natural curiosity in learning. Various teaching theories can be presented, including Martin Gardner's multiple intelligences[11] and the Myers–Briggs personality types.[12,13] These approaches stress different learning styles and the need for flexible teaching styles. Practical approaches to patient teaching can be adapted from David Werner and Bill Bower's book, *Helping Health Workers Learn.*[14] Other valuable resources include the work of Judith Waring Rorden[15] and Barbara Klug Redman.[16]

It is also vital to sensitize staff to the patient's perspective of illness and hospitalization and to emphasize the empowerment aspects of learning as well as the importance of open information exchange.

Ongoing Support and Training

To maintain the vision that patient education is a priority despite the numerous other demands of nursing, periodic meetings and in-services need to be scheduled throughout the year. These meetings can take the form of potluck dinners or other informal gatherings where nurses can discuss a variety of issues, including patient education. Educational in-services on patient care can be provided, usually at no cost, by hospital staff such as social workers; respiratory, physical, and occupational therapists; pharmacists; and chaplains. Physicians are valuable resources in teaching staff specific skills such as dressing changes required for new surgical procedures. These skills can then be taught to patients and family members by the nurses.

Physicians as Teachers

The word *doctor* comes from the Latin word *doctore,* meaning "to teach." Patients look to physicians for information, particularly regarding their own medical needs. Although some physicians enjoy the interactions involved in teaching, many are concerned about the time required to answer numerous questions. Some physicians may worry that patients will make unwise decisions if they have access to information.

By providing patients with information and encouraging them to participate in decisions regarding their own care, patients are better able to become partners with their physicians in maintaining their health. This partnership requires trust: the patient's trust in the physician as well as the physician's trust that the patient is capable of taking on this new responsibility. In this new relationship the physician becomes an educator and advisor.

Education for physicians may help them in assuming these new roles. Some physicians inadvertently undermine the patient's attempts to get involved, subtly reinforcing passive behavior. Physicians often rely heavily on their armament of medications, routinely prescribing sedatives instead of providing information about stress reduction or prescribing antihypertensives without discussing diet, exercise, or life-style changes, all of which involve trusting the patient's ability and interest in becoming actively involved in his or her care.

Many physicians feel caught between the patient's demand for more personalized service and the hospital's demand to keep the cost of care within strict reimbursement limits. It is essential to find ways that physicians can provide information to patients that do not require an unreasonable commitment of time. Encouraging nurses and pharmacists to take more responsibility for patient teaching helps to ensure that the physician's time is spent answering questions specific to the patient's needs. It is also helpful to provide physicians with a range of resources, such as consumer health libraries, so that patients or family members can be encouraged to obtain information on their own whenever possible.

Pharmacists as Teachers

Pharmacists can be a valuable resource for patients and their families by educating them about their medications. They are usually the experts best able to provide information about medications, particularly in terms of food–drug interactions and the drug–drug interactions that can occur when medications are combined inappropriately.

Where internship programs are available, pharmacy students also can be valuable resources. The students can develop their teaching skills and, at the same time, augment existing teaching staff. For example, pharmacy students can assist nurses with the teaching phase of a self-medication program that requires one-on-one instruction on each medication that the patient is taking.

In some hospitals pharmacists are routinely involved in discharge medication teaching. Unfortunately, much of this teaching is done on the last day of hospitalization when there is little opportunity for follow-up questions. Incorporating pharmacists and pharmacy students into the overall teaching plan from the time of admission can help to ensure that patients and their families receive vital medication information.

In addition to the information that pharmacists can provide while patients are in the hospital, it is helpful to teach consumers that pharmacists are also valuable resources in the community. Questions about medications can often be answered by patients' local pharmacists when having prescriptions filled.

Nutritionists as Teachers

If hospitals are to become educational resources for patients and families, nutrition is an important aspect of teaching people about good health. Many major illnesses today, such as heart disease, cancer, stroke, hypertension, and diabetes, may be preventable through good nutritional habits. Although many people may be aware of the importance of nutrition, learning how to incorporate good nutritional habits into their daily routine is often difficult. Hospitalization can provide the unique experience of bringing the patient or family in contact with a nutritionist who can assist in personalizing a healthy nutritional plan.

Nutritionists also are vital in helping to prevent malnutrition, which is often prevalent in hospitals.[17] Many medical tests and procedures require that patients refrain from eating for a certain number of hours. Other patients are heavily sedated or may be too nauseated to eat. Teaching patients how to maintain adequate nutrition even while they are hospitalized may be essential in providing high-quality care and helping to prevent complications.

In an educational environment a nutritionist sees all patients at least once while they are on the unit. Nutritional information can then be provided to meet their specific interests and needs. Classes on various topics can be organized for small groups of patients or families with similar interests. A kitchen on the unit enables the nutritionist to provide cooking demonstrations for patients and families.

Social Workers as Teachers

In many hospitals social workers see only select groups of patients, such as those with cancer or AIDS. Many other illnesses, such as emphysema or heart disease, can be just as debilitating and devastating, but these patients frequently are not provided with the support or expertise of a clinical social worker.

Social workers can teach families how to find the support and resources in the community that they will need to care for the patient at home. Information can also be provided about support groups and other resources to meet the patient's and family's emotional needs.

Other Hospital Staff as Teachers

In addition to providing essential services to patients, physical therapists as well as respiratory and occupational therapists can become valuable educational resources. Although many already see themselves in this role, other staff often fail to recognize the value of these professionals as teachers. Better coordination among all staff might result in more efficient use of all the hospital's resources. For example, in addition to helping patients walk, physical therapists can provide instruction on how to prevent falls at home.

Chaplains also can be seen as teachers by helping patients and families learn new coping skills and understand what spiritual resources are available to them in the community. Arts coordinators, massage coordinators, and recreational therapists can provide instruction in relaxation training that can be used in both the hospital and the home.

Medical Librarians as Teachers

Although most hospitals have medical libraries available to the staff, these resources are rarely available to patients or their families. Some hospitals occasionally provide medical information for those who are not employees, but because these libraries are usually not staffed to accommodate these requests, this service frequently is not made known to the general public. The information in medical libraries is usually highly technical, although some libraries also contain nursing literature that general consumers may more easily understand.

Linking the hospital with a consumer health library, such as the Planetree Health Resource Center, or a public library that has an emphasis on health can provide a valuable service to patients and families. These libraries offer access to information on a wide range of health and medical topics, support groups, and coping skills. The ability to offer computer searches of the latest medical literature can also be helpful. A librarian, library researcher, or other liaison is a vital link in providing material to those who are hospitalized.

Patients and Families as Teachers

Although the hospital is filled with a wide variety of well-trained professionals, sometimes the best teachers are patients and families who have shared similar experiences. Creating opportunities for interaction between patients and among families can provide educational resources that few health care professionals can offer.

For example, a patient who has had an ostomy for many years is able to offer emotional support and practical suggestions to a patient for whom an ostomy is new. In some hospitals this opportunity might be lost unless the patients happened to be roommates. Many patients value the opportunity to share their experiences with others who are in similar situations.

Family members and significant others can also exchange information on how to cope with a difficult situation or provide suggestions on how to manage home care. Families can also create informal support groups to help each other cope with the realities of hospital life or the anxieties of preparing to care for the patient at home. An event such as a movie night or a group meal can serve as a catalyst to bring patients or families together who otherwise might not meet.

The Importance of Administrative Support

Expanding the role of every health care professional in the hospital to include a focus on patient teaching requires commitment and support at all levels of the administration. The chief executive officer (CEO), vice-president of patient care, and nurse manager must all agree on the importance and value of patient education if it is truly to be seen as a priority in patient care. All too often, patient education is said to be a priority but is not adequately supported to be successful. Decentralization, although useful in bringing the decisions regarding patient education to the unit level, can place the entire responsibility for developing and implementing a teaching program on those who do not have adequate training or time.

Implementing policy changes such as the open medical record or a self-medication program often requires the support and involvement of other departments. Having broad administrative support is important in obtaining the cooperation of others. (See chapter 5 for more on the importance of the administration's support.)

Financial support is also vital both in the actual implementation of a patient education program and as a powerful symbol of the value the hospital places on informing patients. Hiring a patient education manager, although adding a salary, is helpful in developing and implementing an education program and provides tangible evidence to all staff that patient education is a priority.

☐ The Physical Environment

Two aspects of the physical environment that affect patient education are its architecture and its access to various kinds of information and education. A well-designed hospital not only creates a comfortable, homelike environment, it also provides the physical structure that will support and augment the delivery of patient-centered care. The education of patients and families is not a separate, isolated event: It is incorporated into all aspects of the patient's care and therefore needs to be reflected in all areas of the architectural and interior design of the hospital. An environment that limits patient independence, restricts family interaction, and impedes staff flexibility cannot at the same time encourage patient participation, family involvement, or staff responsiveness.

For many patients and their families, the traditional hospital environment is unfamiliar, frightening, and often dominated by intimidating medical equipment. Illness itself is often accompanied by fear and anxiety, and an inhospitable environment may only intensify the negative experience. All environments influence behavior either positively or negatively. A well-designed hospital space enables and encourages certain interactions to occur that can enhance the learning and teaching opportunities for patients, families, and staff.

Architecture That Empowers

The ideal way to create a physical environment that supports education is to design the hospital from the ground up with an emphasis on active involvement of patients and families. Unfortunately, few new hospitals are being built and many of those that are, are replicating the traditional institutional designs of the past. Fortunately, many substantial changes can be made by renovating and remodeling existing facilities. Hospitals that are old enough to require renovation or that need to reconfigure existing space are finding that the design of an educational environment need not cost significantly more than the reconstruction of the traditional hospital design. Even small cosmetic changes can contribute to an atmosphere that fosters education.

An educational environment is one in which patients and their families sense they are valued, respected, and encouraged to actively participate in all aspects of care. This attitude is communicated in every element of the design, from the most significant considerations of space allocation to the most subtle details of imagery, symbols, and metaphors. For example, the high counter at most nurses' stations can create a symbolic as well as a real barrier that separates staff from patients and families. Removing this barrier encourages positive interaction and communicates that patients and families are valued and equal participants on the health care team. The absence of this barrier also provides patients with easy access, both real and symbolic, to their medical records. The addition of round cafe tables can encourage discussions between patients and staff. (See photographs of Planetree Units in San Francisco and San Jose in figures 3-2 and 3-3.)

An empowering environment by design encourages the patient's independence. Chairs are easy to get in and out of. Handrails are positioned to encourage mobility. Patients are given control over their environment by being able to adjust the temperature, the lighting, and privacy in their rooms, ideally using controls they can access from their beds without assistance.

Figure 3-2. Nurses' Station: View toward On-Unit Library at the Planetree Unit, San Jose Medical Center

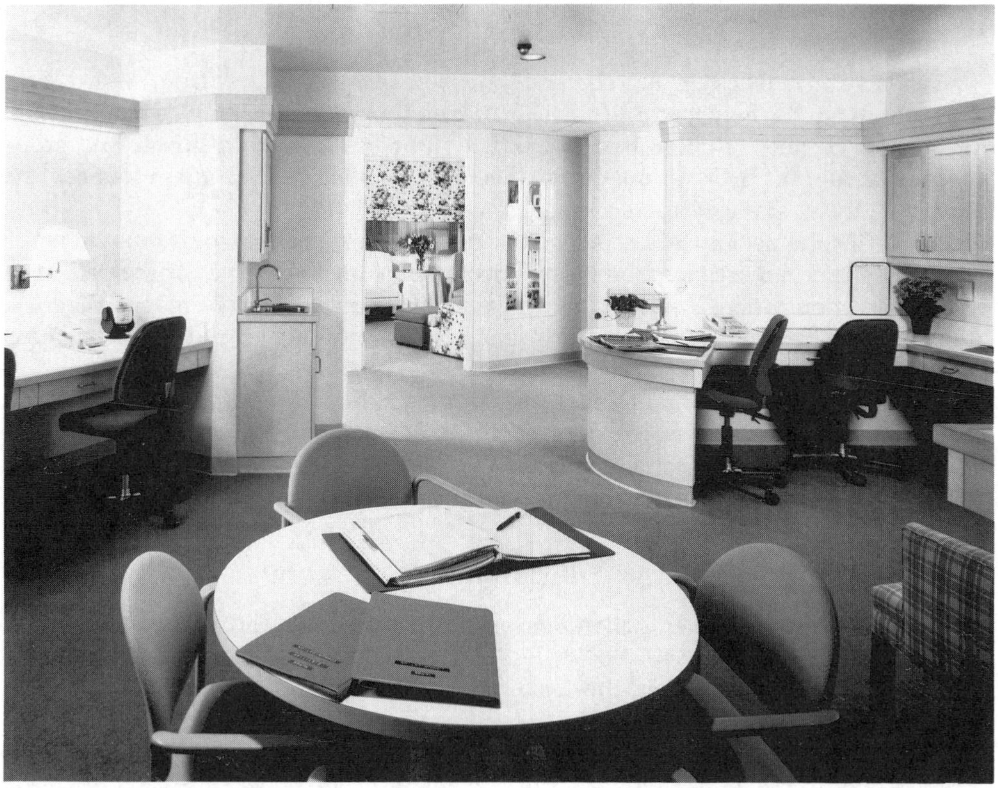

Photograph by Donna Kempner, San Francisco, copyright ©1991. Used with permission.

Figure 3-3. Nurses' Station: View toward Library/Lounge at the Planetree Unit, California Pacific Medical Center, San Francisco

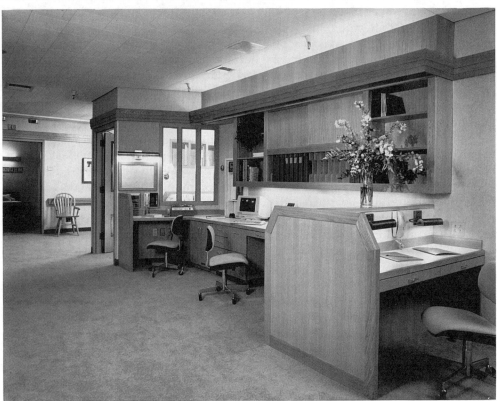

Photograph by Christopher Irion, San Francisco, copyright ©1991. Used with permission.

Patients and families are also offered a variety of spaces to choose from. Varied social spaces, from busy activity rooms to quiet libraries and cozy lounges, provide many options for differing degrees of interaction and activity. Families have both private and group spaces that support their various needs in stressful situations. Seating in lounges and activity rooms is arranged to encourage conversation.

Family involvement is also encouraged by providing a kitchen on some units, in which family members can prepare food brought from home for themselves or the patient. A care partner room where families can stay overnight encourages involvement at all times. A homelike ambiance helps convey the message that patients are viewed within the larger context of the family.

An educational environment must also empower the staff and provide a nurturing space for those who work there. An uncluttered, quiet environment seems to be soothing for staff as well as for patients and families. A staff lounge, away from the sounds and stresses of the unit, offers care givers an opportunity to care for themselves.

Access to Information and Education

An essential element of the educational environment is the availability of numerous educational resources and materials. Books, fact sheets, and medical record access not only provide a range of information, they also visually communicate the attitude that questions are encouraged.

A library on the Planetree Unit for patients and families provides the most obvious access to information. Books and magazines offer information on various diagnoses, medical tests and procedures, and medications. Patient education materials such as fact sheets and nutritional information are also available to browse through. The library is furnished with comfortable chairs and adjustable reading lights. Although it was designed to be a quiet reading area, windows facing the nurses' workstation maintain visual contact with the patients.

A kitchen on the unit is vital in creating a home atmosphere. In addition to functioning as a unique learning laboratory where nutritionists can give cooking demonstrations for patients and families, the kitchen serves as an important social space where families can gather, forming spontaneous support groups.

The patient lounge or activity room also is an important social space, bringing patients and families together who otherwise might not meet. Informal classes and support groups can be held in this type of space if it is big enough.

Ideally, every area is imbued with the sense that every opportunity can be an educational one. Even the arts and massage, although primarily entertaining and relaxing, can educate patients and families about the role of relaxation. Providing a variety of spaces with flexible functions helps ensure that all patients and families will be able to have the most meaningful and educational experience possible.

☐ Resources for Patients, Families, and Staff

The next section briefly mentions various patient education resources, such as written and audiovisual materials, the patient's medical record, self-medication programs, and the care partner program. (See chapter 17 for further details on print materials and chapter 16 for technological options.)

Patient Education Materials

Patient education materials are an integral part of an educational environment, providing patients and their families with consumer health care information. These materials need to be easily accessible to patients, families, and staff at all times. Whenever possible, patients are provided with materials they can take home and refer to later.

Fact Sheets
In an educational environment fact sheets can provide basic information on a broad range of topics, including common diagnoses, tests, and procedures and medications, as well as home care, self-care, and health promotion. These materials are presented as much as possible from the patient's perspective, based on what consumers want to know rather than solely on what health care professionals want them to know.

The goal of the fact sheets is not only to explain medical topics in simple terms but also to help consumers learn the language of medical terminology so that they can better understand what is being said to them in the hospital and can communicate more effectively with nurses, physicians, and other staff. For example, stroke patients probably hear the term *cerebral vascular accident* or *CVA* and need to understand what it means.

Ideally, fact sheets provide basic medical information in language that is empowering and nonthreatening. Commands (for example, "Do this") or words such as *must* and *should* are to be avoided. The term *physician's orders* can be rephrased as *physician's advice*. Explanations are provided whenever possible. It is helpful if fact sheets are available in a variety of languages that meet the needs of the specific patient population. However useful they may be, fact sheets cannot be relied on to be the sole source of information because some people are unable to read due to literacy problems or visual impairment.

Audiotapes and Videotapes
In the age of television, audio- and videotapes are very useful, especially in providing information to people with low literacy levels or to those who are not comfortable with written

information. For many people the visual format of videos is a familiar method of acquiring information. Audiotapes are particularly useful for the visually impaired, although difficulty in operating tape players is sometimes a drawback.

High-quality videotapes at reasonable prices are sometimes difficult to find. Some hospitals with large audiovisual departments are able to produce their own tapes.

Closed-circuit television also is effective in making videotapes available. Unfortunately, many patients are unaware that this service is available and nurses are not always knowledgeable about when certain programs are shown. (For more on closed-circuit television, see chapter 16.)

Books and Journals

A small library of books, magazines, and journals for patient and family use is a valuable asset in creating an educational environment. In addition to providing valuable information, books available on health topics symbolically encourage patients and families to acquire knowledge about their care. Books can cover a wide range of health and medical topics, including basic information on common illnesses, diagnostic tests, various treatments, and medications. Health magazines and journals provide timely information on consumer health issues. A book cart pertaining to health topics can be taken by volunteers from room to room throughout the hospital.

In-Depth Information

For those patients or family members who would like information beyond the scope of fact sheets or dealing with topics not covered by fact sheets, in-depth research packets are a valuable resource. On Planetree Units research packets consist of information gathered from the Planetree Health Resource Centers, which are freestanding medical libraries for the lay public. In both San Francisco and San Jose, the resource centers are across the street from the hospitals and thus are easily accessible. In San Jose, the PEM first talks with the patient or family member who has requested the packet to assess his or her interests or needs. The PEM then gathers the appropriate information from articles and books in the resource center with the assistance of the librarian. If necessary, a computer search is provided. At the San Francisco Planetree Unit, nurses fill out request forms outlining the patients' or families' interests. A staff research assistant at the resource center prepares the information packet and serves as a liaison to the unit. If a computer search brings up a useful article that is not available at either the resource center or the hospital's medical library, the article can be sought from other university libraries.

In addition to up-to-date information, research packets may also include listings of support groups, agencies, and resources in the community. At the patient's request, information about complementary therapies such as visualization or massage may also be included.

Whenever possible, packets are delivered to patients while they are still in the hospital. If patients need the information immediately to help them make an informed decision on treatment options, packets can be rushed to them, usually within 24 hours of their request.

The Patient's Medical Record as an Educational Resource

One of the most valuable learning resources available is the patient's own medical record. Encouraging a patient to read his or her own medical record helps to create an environment of trust and openness, often initiating dialogue between patients and staff. Reading the medical record often elicits questions from the patient, which, when answered and supported, encourages more questions. The open medical record also helps patients understand the process of diagnosis and the selection of various treatment options.

In educational environments patients are encouraged to read their medical records, but are never required or pushed to do so. Generally, the patients who choose not to read their medical record are those for whom the experience could create anxiety. To protect confidentiality, only the patient has access to his or her medical record. If the patient would like a family member to have access to the medical record, he or she signs a form that releases information to the designated person.

The open medical record is also a valuable asset in risk management. Patients have prevented numerous errors from occurring by noticing that important information, such as allergies, was missing from the record or by pointing out discrepancies in medication orders.

The Self-Medication Program

A self-medication program provides an opportunity for patients to begin taking responsibility for their own care while they are in the hospital and have access to a variety of resources. Any patient who is mentally alert and interested in learning about his or her medications is encouraged, but not required, to participate in this program. Pharmacy students at the San Francisco Planetree Unit assist the nurses with the teaching phases of the self-medication program.

Various protocols for self-medication programs are available. Planetree developed a three-stage protocol that begins with patients learning the names, dosages, side effects, and proper use of their medications. Patients are later responsible for asking the nurse for the medication at the appropriate time and eventually keep an eight-hour supply of the medication at the bedside to be fully responsible for its appropriate administration. A physician's order is required to initiate the self-medication program.

For patients who have been taking medications for years, a self-medication program reinforces their ability to manage their own medications rather than disempowering them by taking their medications away. For patients who are going home with new, unfamiliar medications, a self-medication program enables nurses and pharmacists to serve as educational resources, helping to spot problems before they occur. The program helps to identify those patients who may have difficulty with compliance.

The Care Partner Program

In the care partner program the patient's family members or close friends are encouraged to participate in his or her education, physical care, and emotional support. Sometimes one specific person is designated the patient's care partner, the one who becomes most actively involved in the patient's care, with others providing a smaller support role. A care partner is often the person who continues to care for the patient after he or she goes home. The care partner program provides in-depth training in a supportive, supervised environment to teach whatever skills are needed. These skills may be as simple as helping the patient bathe or as complex as suctioning a patient on a ventilator.

A care partner agreement is a verbal or written plan agreed on by the patient, the primary nurse, and the care partner. It is specific enough to meet the patient's needs, but flexible enough to accommodate the care partner's varying levels of interest and involvement. Based on the agreement, the primary nurse develops an educational plan that meets the needs of both the patient and the care partner.

Volunteer care partners are useful for patients who do not have families. Although they may not be as involved in the physical care of the patient as a family member, they can make the hospital stay friendlier and help coordinate the patient's care at home.

☐ Ways to Inform Patients and Families of the Resources Available

Regardless of how many resources are available, they are of no use if patients and families are unaware of them. When patients are admitted to the Planetree Units, they are provided with folders, called patient information kits, that outline the resources that are available. The folder includes a copy of *How to Make the Most of Your Stay* (see figure 3-4), as well as a membership to the Planetree Health Resource Center. In addition, nurses provide orientation tours for patients and families to familiarize them with the resources on the unit.

Patients also need to be aware of resources outside the hospital—those the community can provide. When a patient is discharged from the hospital, a social worker, a discharge planner, or the primary nurse usually initiates contact with a community agency, such as home health or hospice, if necessary. For many patients the person who assesses their discharge needs is their only link to resources in the community. Once the patient has left the hospital, it may be very difficult for patients and their families to know what services and information are available to them. If hospitals are indeed educational resources for communities, the access to information must extend beyond hospitalization.

Planetree Health Resource Centers are open to the public at no cost, providing a range of current health and medical information as well as listings of national and local services and support groups. All patients on the Planetree Units are given free one-year memberships to their local Planetree Health Resource Center. The membership includes borrowing privileges for books, audio- and videotapes, and discounts on the Planetree class series.

The Planetree Health Resource Center model was developed to provide consumers with access to a range of information so that they can make informed decisions regarding their health and participate more fully in their care. A unique classification system was developed for the library's books, journals, and clipping files that is designed to be user-friendly. Consumers with no medical knowledge or special expertise can easily access the information. The Planetree Health Resource Center at San Jose Medical Center also includes a large collection of materials in Spanish and Vietnamese.

If consumers are unable to visit the Planetree Health Resource Center, the research staff can, for a fee, provide consumers with the same in-depth research packets that are available to patients and families on the Planetree Units. At no cost, the resource center staff will provide consumers with information by telephone about community agencies and support groups.

Education is an ongoing process. Regardless of whether consumers are interested in wellness, health maintenance, coping with an acute illness, or learning how to live with a chronic disease, access to information is vital if they are to make informed decisions about their lives.

□ The Hospital of the Future

Hospitals need not wait until the future to become educational resources for patients and their families. The information age has already arrived. Consumers are already demanding, often through litigation, to be included in the medical decisions that powerfully affect their lives. Years ago, only the most innovative hospitals supported such once-strange and radical concepts as the birthing movement and home hospice care; but today, these changes are successfully integrated into mainstream health care.

One can only guess at what tomorrow's health care system will look like. Significant changes are likely to occur in the areas of reimbursement and access to insurance. The rationing of care is also a likely possibility. What will probably not change is the tightness of budgets or the availability of money for anything but the most essential aspects of care. But the changes that do take place will probably be those considered most essential. Preventing illness will start to take precedence over expensive treatments. Home care and ambulatory care will continue to grow. Diminishing resources will require better collaboration among the resources that are left.

Figure 3-4. How to Make the Most of Your Stay

How to Make
The Most of Your Stay

PLANETREE
MODEL HOSPITAL
UNIT AT PACIFIC
PRESBYTERIAN
MEDICAL CENTER

Welcome
to Planetree

Welcome to the Planetree Model Unit at Pacific Presbyterian Medical Center (PPMC). The Planetree Unit is an innovative medical-surgical unit designed to provide you with the latest in medical technology in a healing, nurturing environment. At Planetree, we believe peaceful, comfortable surroundings, warm and supportive caregivers, and access to health information and education can help you get well faster and stay well longer. During your hospital stay, the Planetree staff encourages you and your family to become actively involved in every aspect of your care. While the degree of participation is entirely up to you, the Planetree staff will work to support you at every level.

The Physical Environment

There are a number of differences between our unit and other hospital environments you may have seen. The Planetree Unit is designed to be homey and comfortable. We hope you will enjoy the comfortable furnishings, artwork, and soothing colors. To make your room more familiar and cozy, we encourage you to bring special belongings from home such as photographs or a favorite pillow *(Please leave your valuable possessions at home so they will not be lost)*. Near your room you will find:

The Planetree Lounge
The Lounge is a place for you and your family and friends to relax, read, share a meal, or watch a movie. Within the Planetree Lounge you will find a library of health care books and fact sheets, as well as fiction, poetry, audio-cassettes and videos.

The Planetree Kitchen
We encourage you and your family to prepare meals in the Planetree Kitchen located right next to the Lounge. You may bring favorite foods from home or enjoy the healthy snack foods provided by Planetree. *Please help us by labelling all food kept in the Planetree Kitchen with your name and the date.*

The Planetree
Health Care Team

Planetree believes that you, the patient, are the most important part of the health care team. As a member of the health care team, we encourage you to participate in decisions regarding your care. In doing so, you and your family will be working with the other important members of your health care team, including your doctor, your primary nurse and the Planetree nutritionist.

Your Doctor

In addition to diagnosing and treating your medical condition, your doctor is a valuable resource for learning how to take care of yourself. You and your family are encouraged to talk directly with your doctor, ask questions about your health concerns, and participate in your care.

Your Primary Nurse

At Planetree we provide you with a caring and knowledgeable nursing staff. During your stay you will have a primary nurse who will coordinate your care, provide support, be an advocate for you, and help you learn about your health.

The Planetree Nutritionist

Nutrition is an important part of the healing process and staying healthy in the future. Being able to enjoy favorite foods while in the hospital can help you to feel more at home. During your stay, the Planetree Nutritionist is available to answer any dietary questions you may have, assist you in learning how to meet your nutritional needs, and help you make use of the hospital menu to choose enjoyable and nutritious foods.

Learning About
Your Health

During your stay at Planetree we encourage you to learn more about your health and become actively involved in your care. We have created many educational opportunities on the Planetree Unit, ranging from books and fact sheets in the Planetree Lounge to the availability of a caring and knowledgeable staff. You may read about additional resources on the back side of this page.

(Continued on next page)

Figure 3-4. (Continued)

Your Medical Chart

We encourage you to read your own medical chart and ask your nurse or doctor to answer any questions you may have. You may write about your own experiences and observations in the section of your chart called "Patient's Progress Notes". Your chart is available at the nurses' station or you may ask your nurse or doctor to bring it to you.

The Patient Health Information Packet

We encourage you to request a free Patient Health Information Packet from the Planetree Health Information Service during your stay on the Unit. Your **free** Patient Health Information Packet will contain materials from the current health and medical literature. Your packet will be sent to you in the hospital or shortly after you return home. A Packet Request Form is included in your Patient Information Kit, or you may ask your primary nurse to assist you in requesting a packet.

The Self-Medication Program

This program can help you learn about your medications and how to take them during your hospital stay. The program will also enable you to become more knowledgeable and confident about taking your medications when you return home.

Your Family, Friends and Care Partner

Hospitals are sometimes intimidating places and visits from your family and friends can help you feel less isolated. Visiting hours on the Planetree Unit are unrestricted and children may visit provided they are in good health. You are also encouraged to involve family members or friends in your care and choose a "care partner" who will work closely with you and your primary nurse in providing your care. Your care partner may spend the night in the Lounge or in your room when a space is available.

Helping You Relax: Massage Program

A soothing massage may help you relax and feel better. During your stay on the Planetree Unit your primary nurse can arrange for you to receive a massage from a Planetree volunteer certified massage therapist. There is no charge for massage.

Planetree and the Arts

Planetree believes that the arts can play an important role in the healing process. Music, comedy, poetry, storytelling, film and the visual arts are all available on the Planetree Unit, and can provide a relaxing diversion for you and your family. Audio-cassette players are available and the Planetree Lounge features a wide selection of music on cassettes. A VCR and a collection of movies are available in the Planetree Lounge, or a portable VCR is available so that you may watch a movie in your room. The Planetree Lounge also has a variety of books, magazines and art supplies for your use. The Planetree Arts Coordinator is available to help you take advantage of the Arts Program on the Unit.

The Planetree Health Resource Center

The Planetree Health Resource Center is located across the street from the hospital at 2040 Webster Street. The Center is a health and medical library for the layperson that is free and open to the public. We encourage you to visit our Center where you will find a wide selection of health and medical books, a clipping file of current medical information, a health bookstore, and many other health resources. Included with your Patient Information Kit is a form which offers you a free one year library card at the Center. For more information please call the Planetree Health Resource Center at 415-923-3680.

We Welcome Your Suggestions!

We hope you find your stay on the Planetree Unit to be comfortable and supportive. We welcome your ideas and suggestions for improving the Planetree Unit. For more information about Planetree please feel free to ask your primary nurse, or call our office at 415-923-3696.

A special thanks fo The Henry J. Kaiser Family foundation, The San Francisco Foundation and the J.M. Foundation for their generous support to fund the development of the Planetree Model Hospital Project at Pacific Presbyterian Medical Center

Planetree wishes to acknowledge Pacific Presbyterian Medical Center for their dedication to providing the best medical care available within an environment that is both innovative and humanistic.

Although technology is likely to reign supreme well into the next century, patient education will probably make significant inroads into the delivery of hospital care. Giving consumers the knowledge and skills to manage their own health is practical, economically sound, and, most important, it is what consumers are asking for.

□ Conclusion

Creating an educational environment in a hospital setting requires an atmosphere in which information is freely given to patients and their families and in which questions are encouraged, including health questions that may not pertain to the patient's current diagnosis. To create an environment supportive of patient education, all aspects of patient care must be addressed, including training of nurses and other staff members, involvement of the patient's family or friends, addressing nutritional concerns, and, when possible, the redesign of hospital architecture. Access to various educational materials, including the patient's own medical record, and resources in the community is also vital. Patients may choose to make use of their knowledge by assisting in making decisions on the course of their treatment and participating in their own care. The hospital must expand its role to not only treating illnesses but also promoting independence, well-being, and health.

References

1. Kinnaird, L. With hospitals' malpractice risk rising, patient education offers positive response. *Promoting Health* (American Hospital Association) 7(4):6–8, July–Aug. 1986.

2. MacStravic, R. S. Therapeutic pampering. *Hospitals & Health Science* 31(3):59–69, May–June 1986.

3. May, M. The malpractice malady. *The Social & Health Review* 4:71-75, Nov. 1986.

4. Sommers, P. Malpractice risk & patient relations. *Legal Aspects of Medical Malpractice* 13(10):1–8, Oct. 1985.

5. Tilley, J., Gregor, F., and Thiessen, V. The nurse's role in patient education: incongruent perceptions among nurses and patients. *Journal of Advanced Nursing* 12(3):291–301, May 1987.

6. Tilley and others.

7. Caffarella, R. The nurse's role in hospital based patient education programs for adults. *The Journal of Continuing Education in Nursing* 16(6):222–23, 1984.

8. Stevens, D., Stagg, R., and Mackay, I. What happens when hospitalized patients see their own records. *Annals of Internal Medicine* 86(4):474–77, Apr. 1977.

9. Webber, G. Patient education: a review of the issues. *Medical Care* 28(11):1089–1103, Nov. 1990.

10. Green, L. The potential of health education includes cost effectiveness. *Hospitals* 50:57-61, May 1, 1976.

11. Gardner, M. *Frames of Mind: The Theory of Multiple Intelligences.* New York City: Basic Books, 1983.

12. Myers, I. B. *Gifts Differing.* Palo Alto, CA: Consulting Psychologists Press, 1980.

13. Lawrence, G. *People Types and Tiger Stripes: A Practical Guide to Learning Styles.* 2nd ed. Gainesville, FL: Center for Applications of Psychological Types, 1983.

14. Werner, D., and Bower, B. *Helping Health Workers Learn.* Palo Alto, CA: Hesperian Foundation, 1982.

15. Rorden, J. W. *Nurses as Health Teachers: A Practical Guide.* Philadelphia: Saunders, 1987.

16. Redman, B. K. *The Process of Patient Education.* 6th ed. St. Louis: Mosby, 1988.

17. Teitelman, R. Skeletons in the closet. *Forbes*, Apr. 9, 1984, pp. 156–57.

Chapter 4

Building Effective Committee Structures and Interdisciplinary Collaboration

Sandra J. Cornett, Ph.D., R.N.

☐ Objectives

The reader will be able to:

- Describe the importance of interdisciplinary collaboration in patient education
- Determine whether preexisting committees have or can assume patient education functions
- Describe three types of committee structures for patient education
- Describe the characteristics and functions of interdisciplinary care delivery teams
- Describe the role of the patient education manager on patient education committees
- Identify barriers to interdisciplinary team collaboration and strategies to enhance collaboration

☐ Importance of Interdisciplinary Collaboration in Patient Education

To be effective, patient education efforts need a tremendous amount of coordination among individuals from many hospital departments. Responsibility for facilitating team development and coordinating programs often falls to the patient education manager (PEM). Therefore, to plan and implement effective patient education, the PEM must have team-building skills and be able to identify and utilize mechanisms that will ensure interdisciplinary involvement and collaboration. In most hospitals these mechanisms include committees, task forces, ad hoc groups, and care delivery teams, all with membership from a variety of departments. This chapter first defines what is meant by an interdisciplinary approach and discusses why it is so important in patient education efforts, and then describes various committee structures and functions.

There are many definitions of *interdisciplinary teamwork*, but the essential element in all of them is that it is the work of a group of individuals with specialized roles who collaborate or coordinate the services provided to a patient or group of patients. This group perceives and believes in collective action; therefore, there is a tendency to act in a unified manner.

Why is interdisciplinary collaboration essential in patient education? There are several important benefits for patients, care givers and other staff members, committee members, and even the PEM. First and foremost, the patient is a dynamic, interactive, and integrated whole, and thus his or her individual problems are interrelated and cannot be adequately treated in isolation by one health care professional. Similarly, problems brought up by the patient's family also must be considered with the patient in mind. In fact, most patients learning how to live with a chronic illness need family members and significant others to assist them. Using different health care professionals to educate a patient about the various aspects of his or her illness maximizes expertise to better meet the complex needs of the whole individual and his or her family. One person cannot be an expert in all phases of a patient's care.

There are many benefits for care givers and other staff members involved in patient education when a collaborative approach is used. More than any other aspect of health care, patient education is the responsibility of almost every health professional in the hospital. This generic responsibility for patient education across all disciplines is supported by each profession's practice act and by JCAHO standards for patient and family education. A well-planned approach to educational efforts can reduce uncertainty about what role each staff member plays in patient education.

When a variety of professionals provide services to patients, there is an increased need to clarify lines of communication and authority within the organization. Interdisciplinary collaboration offers a way to more efficiently plan programs and deliver care by organizing ways to exchange relevant information and reduce duplication of effort. Such collaboration may also very well serve to reduce costs. As committee members share tasks and solve problems together, accountability and productivity increase. When group decision making and accountability for coordinated activities occur, there is less likelihood that patients' problems are overlooked or ignored; therefore, improved quality and continuity of care result.

Team members themselves enjoy additional benefits when interdisciplinary collaboration occurs. For example, their morale often improves, and stress often decreases when members share frustrations and successes. Members grow professionally in an environment where trust and respect flourish and where relationships between disciplines are important.

For the PEM personally, committees and task forces may also function as support groups, particularly if the PEM's role is new in the hospital. Committee members can provide valuable insights into how individual hospital departments work and can identify effective ways to gain support, not only for patient education in general but also for the PEM's role. They can also introduce the PEM to professionals in their own departments, which helps legitimize the PEM's efforts with the staff.

☐ Committee Structures and Teams

To meet the ongoing challenge of getting those involved in patient education to coordinate their activities, PEMs should consider several kinds of committee structures. Given the variety of hospital settings, patient education committees are organized in different ways, with different titles, membership, and functions. They may be new committees having only patient education responsibilities, or they may be integrated into existing committees that have assumed one or more patient education functions. Three general types of committees can be distinguished—those at the hospitalwide level, the departmental level, and the specific patient population levels of patient education programming.

The Hospitalwide Patient Education Committee

A hospitalwide patient education committee may vary for a particular setting, depending on several factors. These include the size of the hospital, the format and number of already-established patient education activities, whether the hospital management sees patient education as a priority, and how much time the PEM actually has to perform the role of leader.

Deciding on Committee Functions

Hospitalwide patient education committee functions are usually phased in gradually. The committee gives priority to those functions that meet the organization's most pressing needs at a certain period of time. Depending on the hospital's structure and size, some of these functions may be done by other committees within the organization that have ties to patient education.

Functions that require expertise in the care and education of specific patient populations should be done by department-level patient education committees or by interdisciplinary teams that develop and implement specific patient population education programs. For example, whereas the hospitalwide committee sets the standards, policies, and procedures for the development and review of patient education materials, department-level patient education committees review them.

Functions of the hospitalwide committee may include:

- Gaining support for patient education and the role of the PEM from the hospital's top management. This can be accomplished by:
  - Using formal and informal lines of communication to inform departmental staff of the committee's activities
  - Supporting a systematic, comprehensive, coordinated approach to patient education programming
  - Obtaining information from the various departments on patient education issues and needs that are best attended to hospitalwide (for example, problems with materials distribution and staff training needs in patient education)
- Communicating patient education issues between the departments and the organization
- Developing a strategic plan for patient education that translates the hospital's plan into patient education management objectives (see chapter 2)
- Developing and recommending policies, procedures, and standards, and coordinating mechanisms for keeping patient education activities needing a hospitalwide approach centralized (for example, distributing materials) and keeping activities, such as developing materials, that are done best by the departments and interdisciplinary teams, decentralized
- Assessing hospitalwide patient education needs, identifying priorities, and recommending allocation of resources for patient education
- Developing and implementing a standardized process for planning, and implementing specific patient population education programs that include an interdisciplinary team approach
- Reviewing and approving patient education programs for specific patient populations
- Monitoring and evaluating the effectiveness and quality of patient education activities from a hospitalwide perspective
- Developing and recommending criteria and strategies for program monitoring and evaluation of patient education activities at the departmental level
- Consulting with departments on patient education activities and with interdisciplinary teams on planning and implementing specific patient population programs
- Providing learning opportunities for all levels of staff to increase knowledge and skills in providing patient education and developing and managing programs
- Recognizing staff and interdisciplinary teams for excellence in patient education

Forming a New Committee versus Using an Existing One

Once hospitalwide patient education committee functions have been defined, the decision needs to be made to either form a new committee or integrate patient education into a previously existing committee. Existing committees where patient education may be integrated include patient care, education, quality assurance, or discharge planning. In some settings, integrating the hospitalwide functions into an already-existing committee that has administration's strong support may result in greater visibility, credibility, and coordination of activities. This approach may help keep patient education efforts from being duplicated, and, in addition, resources may be used more efficiently and effectively. On the other hand, a new committee may be needed if patient education is to be given the emphasis needed to change practices.

The following questions can be used to help evaluate whether an existing committee can assume hospitalwide patient education functions:[1]

- Has the committee been given legitimate hospitalwide authority from administration to effect interdepartmental change?
- Does the membership represent those departments that are necessary to provide input on patient education?
- Is there expertise on the existing committee to fulfill patient education functions?
- Is the committee small enough (8 to 10 members) or does it have a subcommittee mechanism to accomplish specific tasks for committee review?
- Do members have a genuine commitment (for example, participate in patient education activities or act as role models for patient education) to patient education?
- Will patient education functions be a priority for members, or will previously established objectives take precedence over patient education concerns?
- Does the committee meet often enough to carry out patient education functions?

In addition to using the proposed hospitalwide patient education committee functions and the preceding questions, the following tasks can help further determine whether a new committee should be formed:[2]

1. Identify all or most of the existing committees as either hospitalwide committees or specific departmental committees. Find out who the members and chair of each are. Determine whether the members serve on a variety of committees.
2. Learn about each committee's charges, functions, and tasks. Determine which existing committees might have an interest in patient education functions.
3. Talk with the chair of each selected committee to find out more about the committee's focus and whether it would be possible to incorporate patient education responsibilities.
4. Solicit opinions from other managers and staff on the formation of a new patient education committee or the incorporation of patient education functions into a current committee.
5. Identify people who have said they would like to serve on a patient education committee or who have expertise and unique talents for patient education. Identify ways these people may be involved in patient education without forming a committee.

Deciding on Committee Membership

If either the membership or the objectives of an already-existing committee do not coincide with or cannot be adapted to the identified patient education needs and functions, the formation of a new committee becomes necessary. Who should be on the committee then becomes an important question. Members chosen for the hospitalwide committee should be at least in a first-line management position in their department, such as nurse manager, department supervisor, or assistant director. By virtue of their managerial position, these individuals have responsibility and authority to make key decisions within their department that can affect patient education activities. Members of the hospitalwide committee have a managerial position within the hospital hierarchy that ensures access both to their staff who teach patients and to top-level administrators. In this way, they serve as a link between the staff and managers in specific departments and the hospitalwide patient education committee, resulting in better communication. Committee appointments should be made by top-level administration, which further legitimizes decisions made by the committee and facilitates implementation of those decisions.

A number of tasks need to be done to help the PEM determine which individuals should serve on, and which should be represented on, the hospitalwide patient education committee.[3]

1. The PEM should first list all the departments and professions that could potentially have an impact on patient education. Usually those departments with professionals who provide direct care to patients and their families are included, as well as some personnel from other areas related to patient education, such as quality assurance, continuity of care (discharge planning), patient relations, communications, marketing, administration, education and staff development, library, auxiliary, chaplaincy, medical records, finance, admitting, and outpatient services. Depending on the hospital and the objectives and functions outlined for the committee, different departments and professionals will need to be included. Many times, a core group is appointed and other departments are included on an ad hoc basis as the goals of the committee change.
2. The PEM should then write down next to each department or profession which person(s) he or she wants on the committee and why each should be appointed. Reasons may include the following:
   - Interest in and knowledge of patient education
   - Member of a department that should be represented
   - Ability to gain support from staff and key management
   - Formal leader appointed by management
   - Informal leader who is listened to by staff and provides a good role model in patient education
   - Good representative of the profession
   - Reputation for meeting commitments
3. The names and reasons for recommended participation should then be reviewed. Are there people who could better be involved on an ad hoc basis? Are there people who have special problems working together? The hospitalwide committee should be limited to 15 to 20 members; otherwise, it will become unmanageable even with subcommittee mechanisms.

Once the committee membership is decided, the next step is to plan how the committee should be formed. Should a chair be named before convening the committee, or should the committee choose its own chair? Should the PEM become the chair, or should a key manager in the organization be appointed?

Planning the First Meeting

To get a patient education committee off to a good start, it is important that the PEM (and others, if necessary) spend time planning the first meeting. Although all committee meetings take some degree of planning, the first one often sets the tone and stage for future success. A poorly planned first meeting can alienate members and foster unwillingness to participate in future activities.

How much preparation is needed and who does it depends on the particular situation. The PEM will play a primary role if he or she is the chair, or a supporting, consultative role if someone else is appointed chair. The following list will help with the preparation:[4]

1. A general plan should be outlined showing how the committee is to function (see figure 4-1). (Information and decisions with regard to tasks 1 and 2 in figure 4-1

need to be made before the meeting, with input from the committee during the first and subsequent meetings.)

2. To maximize attendance, it is important to find out what times during the day committee members are most available. That information will determine the time and date of the first meeting.

3. A letter should be sent expressing appreciation for each committee member's willingness to participate. This letter should also identify the information committee members need to have before coming to the meeting. The following list provides some guidelines to consider:

- An overview of committee responsibilities, objectives, and membership should be provided.

- Some indication of the potential member's commitment to the group should be given, for example, the amount of time required for meetings and other responsibilities. This may give the member a better chance to decide whether to participate or to ask for another department member to be appointed.

Figure 4-1. Management Tasks to Ensure Effective Functioning of a New Patient Education Committee

Tasks	Questions/Examples
1. Clarify committee responsibilities, schedule, and member roles	• What is the charge of the committee? • What are specific duties or objectives? • Why has each member been selected? • What deadlines exist (for example, reports, administrative meeting review, budget planning period)? • How frequently will the committee meet? • How much time is needed in committee meetings or for outside work?
2. Establish operating procedures	• What are standard operating procedures for scheduling meetings, assigning work to members, developing a work plan, establishing subcommittees? • Who will document committee actions and decisions, and how will that be done? • What are the reporting mechanisms between the committee and appropriate management? • How, when, and by whom will the work of the committee be evaluated? • What will be the relationship between the PEM and the committee chair?
3. Provide background information and materials	• For the hospitalwide committee, resources could include the hospital patient education-related policy statements; materials that support planned, documented patient education; examples of program materials used by other hospitals for coordinating a hospitalwide program. • Standards for designing and implementing programs for specific patient populations including defining goals, objectives, content, materials, methods, evaluation, cost, and operational procedures. • Outlines of specific patient population programs from other hospitals; examples of materials used for the specific population; pamphlets, brochures; procedures used elsewhere; resource lists.
4. Provide resource persons to the committee	• Staff who are exceptional at program planning or working with groups. • Staff who have already completed similar tasks at the hospital or elsewhere, for example, chairing a patient education committee, developing administrative support, writing policy statements, developing a specific patient population program, teaching patients and staff.

Adapted from E. A. Lee, J. Garvey, G. Finnegan, and B. Giloth. *Implementing Patient Education in the Hospital.* Chicago: American Hospital Association, 1979, table 4-1, pp. 68–69 (out of print).

- Background information on patient education should be provided, such as JCAHO standards, policies, and procedures; material on patients' rights; AHA management directives; professional statements; and so on.
- Tasks to be completed before coming to the first meeting should be described, such as a review of the materials, completion of a self-assessment about patient education values and beliefs, completion of a departmental assessment, and so forth.
- Personal contact should be arranged with each appointed member to answer questions and discuss any concerns initiated by the material he or she received. A short memo sent out just before the meeting will serve to remind participants of the location, date, and time.

Departmental Patient Education Committees

In some hospitals, particularly large ones, departmental committees are formed to help coordinate activities and meet the patient education standards for that patient care area. Participation on departmental committees provides staff with an opportunity for professional growth and senior-level staff with an opportunity to model positive behaviors. Committee membership can also assist staff in meeting criteria for promotion to other positions within the department. Departmental patient education committee members become a cadre of resource people for other staff.

It is important that a mechanism be developed that allows interfacing between the hospitalwide committee and the departmental patient education committees. For example, minutes of patient education committee meetings can be copied and sent to the PEM. Also, the chair of a departmental committee could sit on the hospitalwide committee or the PEM could serve as a member of the department-level committee.

The criteria used to help decide whether an existing committee within the department can assume the patient education functions for that area or whether a new committee needs to be established are the same as those mentioned in the previous section on the hospitalwide patient education committee. The range of functions often varies for departmental patient education committees, depending on the resources available and the focus that committee members want to take.

Deciding on Committee Functions

The functions of this type of committee may include:

- Implementing decisions, policies and procedures, standards, and so on set by the hospitalwide committee
- Assessing departmental needs and concerns about patient education
- Communicating these needs, concerns, accomplishments, and ongoing and new activities in patient education to the hospitalwide committee
- Communicating hospitalwide activities to appropriate staff within the department
- Reviewing and approving programs and materials developed by the staff according to hospital standards
- Monitoring and evaluating departmental patient education activities using a quality improvement process and program evaluation techniques to determine patient education effectiveness and efficiency at this level
- Providing resource people and support to the staff for patient education efforts
- Providing staff development activities on patient education (see chapter 12 for more on staff development)

Deciding on Committee Membership

Membership on departmental committees is intradisciplinary, that is, comprising only one profession, and represents the various groups or areas within a department. For example, a nursing department's patient education committee may have representation from each major inpatient clinical area (medical–surgical, critical care, woman and infant, neurorehab, and so on), as well as outpatient clinics and the emergency department. Nurses from all levels of the hierarchy are usually represented (staff nurse, clinical nurse specialist, assistant nurse manager, nurse manager, director). In addition, nurses from other areas of the hospital, who do not report to the department of nursing but are doing patient education, may be asked to serve so coordination of efforts is increased. Half the membership rotates off the committee every year, so tenure is for two years and there is continuity.

The Specific Patient Population Program Planning Committee

Whereas the hospitalwide committee and departmental committees can effectively handle policy, procedural, and standards issues having a hospitalwide or departmental impact, another type of committee is usually needed to develop programs for specific patient populations. Often this type of committee or task force is formed on an ad hoc basis. Once a given program assigned to a specific program planning committee is functioning, the committee takes on an advisory role. This is not to say, however, that some members of this type of committee are not involved in implementing the program.

In some hospitals a subcommittee of the hospitalwide committee or some other interdisciplinary patient care committee may assume responsibility for planning a specific patient population program. A process similar to the one described in the hospitalwide committee section of this chapter should be followed by the PEM to decide whether to form a new committee and to identify its functions and membership. In general, it is usually necessary to have some kind of new group because of the detail and expertise involved in planning and implementing a specific patient population program.

Deciding on Committee Functions

Specific patient population program planning committee functions may include:

- Obtaining necessary administrative authorization and support
- Conducting an assessment of the patient population to be served
- Determining organizational support and resources
- Establishing the program's purpose and goals
- Writing standard teaching plans and protocols, including expected outcomes (objectives), content, and methodology, to meet the educational needs of the specific population
- Developing and/or reviewing appropriate print and audiovisual materials
- Defining the roles and responsibilities of the interdisciplinary team members who will implement the program
- Designing and implementing staff training programs associated with the program
- Disseminating information on the program
- Evaluating the program's impact on patient knowledge, behavior, and health status as well as on the organization
- Providing advice and review on an ongoing basis to an already-established program

During the course of establishing specific program planning committees, member roles and committee responsibilities need to be defined. Also, operating procedures such as subcommittee work; the meeting schedule; reporting mechanisms; work plans describing who will do the work when and how it will be evaluated; and the relationship between the chair of the ad hoc committee and the PEM all need to be negotiated. Figure 4-2 provides an example of guidelines developed to help this type of committee function effectively and efficiently.

Deciding on Committee Membership

Specific patient population program planning committees are usually composed of five to eight interdisciplinary health care professionals who serve a specific patient population. The different disciplines chosen to be represented on this type of committee depend on the patient population being served and whether the hospital employs staff from a particular profession. For example, the core group of interdisciplinary team members for a cardiac rehabilitation program usually includes a physician, a nurse, a dietitian, a physical therapist, an occupational therapist, and a social worker. A pharmacist, an exercise physiologist, a psychologist, a chaplain, or a health educator may also be included, if available.

The following questions should be considered when developing a list of potential members to serve on a specific patient population program committee:[5]

Figure 4-2. Specific Patient Population Program Planning Committees

Functions of the Chair:

The chair will be picked by the members of the group. The chair will be the primary contact person for the patient education manager. Functions are as follows:

1. Start and end the meetings on time.
2. Facilitate discussion of agenda items and get input from every member.
   a. Restate decision by the group for clarification and summary.
   b. End meetings with a restatement of decisions, assignments, and deadlines.
3. Monitor the committee's progress relative to the objectives and the process used to accomplish the objectives.
4. Assign minutes of the meeting to be taken and distribute to members along with agenda prior to the next meeting.
5. Set meeting dates determined by a consensus of members.
6. Develop written agenda and send out a meeting reminder.
7. Evaluate and improve meeting agendas.
8. Convey progress reports to the appropriate administrative personnel, including the patient education manager, if not present at the meetings.

Role of the Patient Education Manager:

1. Discuss standards for developing a structured specific patient population program. Ensure that guidelines for developing programs are used, specified procedures are standardized, and ideas and resources are shared by groups.
2. Provide input into guideline development, as needed, and review materials produced by the committee.
3. Work with the chair to manage meetings more effectively, if needed. Provide input to the committee on how to reach objectives and solve problems that may be decreasing the effectiveness of the group.

Schedule:

How often the committee meets will be determined by its members. The decision should be based on the amount of work to be done and the deadlines set by the members. Most committees meet every two to three weeks during the planning phase.

Assignments:

1. Some tasks will have to be assigned to individuals on the committee to get the work done within a reasonable length of time. Committee members are responsible for completing their assignments within the agreed-upon time. They are also responsible for sharing their efforts with staff and managers in their departments to get their input.
2. Subcommittee mechanism:
   - Subcommittees or task groups may need to be formed periodically to assume tasks that are identified as needed by the committee members.
   - Subcommittee membership will be on a voluntary basis.
   - Deadlines for completion of the tasks will be set by the total group membership.
   - The subcommittee will disband after the assignment results have been reviewed and accepted by the total committee.

- Who has the expertise to help determine content and methods for the selected patient population?
- Who has patient care responsibilities for the patient population?
- Who is already involved in functioning programs for this population?
- Who can sell the program to peers?
- Are there disciplines not involved in teaching these patients that could serve as valuable resources during the planning phase?
- Should representatives of both outpatient and community services be included?
- Should the patients' and their families' point of view be represented by a person who has experienced the health care problems targeted in the program?
- Are there staff who have had previous experience in developing and implementing a specific patient population education program?

☐ Interdisciplinary Care Delivery Teams

In most instances, members of the interdisciplinary ad hoc committee that developed the guidelines for structuring a specific patient population education program will implement and evaluate the program. During the final stages of program development, committee members provide in-services to other interdisciplinary staff who care for that patient population and therefore will be involved in various aspects of the program.

The PEM is usually involved in helping the ad hoc program committee plan and provide these in-services. Coordination of the interdisciplinary care delivery team who is doing the patient education, however, is not done by the PEM. Coordination activities are delineated in the guidelines and are discussed with all team members during the in-services. The person responsible for coordinating the care delivery team is usually a member of the planning committee or a staff member appointed by management.

An interdisciplinary care delivery team is composed of individuals with varied specialized training who coordinate their activities to provide services to a group of patients or clients. For a team to exist, there must be more than the presence of a variety of providers; each provider must function as a subunit of the whole in a collaborative relationship.

Effective patient education at the case management level requires interdisciplinary staff to engage in a series of task-related activities. These tasks are divided into those carried out by individual team members and those performed by the interdisciplinary care delivery team as a whole. Thus the work of staff involved in the management of a patient's care is coordinated through team conferences and other activities. Figure 4-3, modified from a model developed by A. J. Ducanis and A. K. Golin,[6] shows how five team task activities correspond to the processes used in delivering patient care and education.

The PEM can help facilitate interdisciplinary care delivery team activities by ensuring that resources, materials, and procedures are in place that help the members complete their tasks. For example, a tool to assess a patient's and family's learning needs and readiness to learn will help team members collect essential data as a basis for teaching.

☐ Role of the Patient Education Manager on Patient Education Committees

The role of the PEM on the various patient education committees is defined by many of the organizational variables already discussed—whether the committee is new or already established, the specific committee functions, committee membership, the number of staff available, and the expertise of staff in the educational program planning process. Five overlapping functions may be assumed by the PEM at different times and with different committees: convener, committee chair, facilitator, advisor, and coordinator.[7] They are discussed in the following sections.

Convener

Because the PEM is likely to be the person who initiates establishing a committee, he or she may be responsible for determining committee functions, choosing members, and planning the first meeting. Some PEMs organize the first meeting's agenda to include the election of a chair.

Committee Chair

Although chairing a committee is a potential role for PEMs, it is one that should be carefully thought through and taken for a specific reason. On the hospitalwide level, the PEM may want to be the chair. He or she may be the only one who comes from a "neutral" point, has an overall perspective for patient education, can gain some visibility for the function, or has enough time to assume the position's responsibilities. On the other hand, the PEM may want to have a person more influential with physicians and department directors to chair the committee while he or she plays a supportive role. In some hospitals interdisciplinary committees are traditionally chaired by physicians. In an effort to involve committee members, some PEMs rotate the role of chair, with each member assuming responsibility for a limited period.

Figure 4-3. Individual and Team Activities for Delivering Patient Education

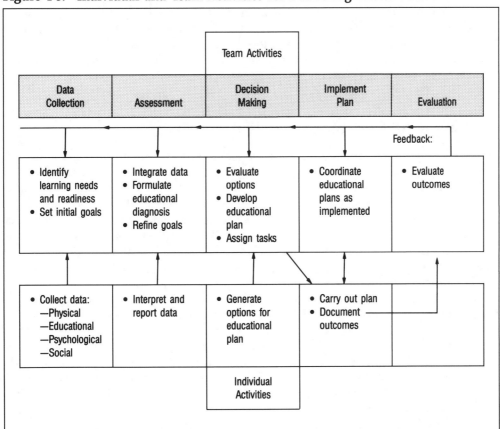

Modified from A. J. Ducanis and A. K. Golin. *The Interdisciplinary Health Care Team: A Handbook.* Germantown, Maryland: Aspen Systems Corp., 1979, pp. 106–8.

For departmental patient education committees and specific patient population program committees, the PEM is usually too removed from actual program operations to accept responsibility for being chair. Another reason why PEMs might decline such duties is that ownership for activities at this level needs to remain with the staff expected to implement committee actions.

Facilitator

The facilitator role makes good use of the PEM's management, communication, and team-building skills. The PEM needs to work with the chair of the various committees to manage meetings effectively, provide input into the team process, and solve problems that appear to be inhibiting group effectiveness.

Advisor

When numerous committees and groups are in the various stages of planning and implementing different programs and initiatives, the PEM may need to serve in an advisory role, acting as a consultant to the members. Much of the activity for this role can take place outside the meetings, with the PEM responding to decisions and materials produced by a given committee. This is a particularly appropriate role to assume with a specific patient population program committee, especially if the group is functioning effectively.

Coordinator

This role is mandatory, as it is within the overall definition of the PEM's job. One of the main reasons for having someone such as the PEM involved to some degree with all the patient education committees is to ensure that similar information is available to all groups. Having the PEM monitor and coordinate the various patient education committees' activities results in standardized procedures being used, new ideas and resources developed by one group being shared with others, and duplication of efforts being avoided.

☐ Improving Committee Function

In addition to the roles mentioned in the previous section, PEMs have ongoing responsibility for improving committee function. One of the major reasons that committees are sometimes ineffective is that little time is spent at the beginning establishing the processes that will enable future effectiveness. For example, a committee that is not quite sure of what it should be doing will be nonproductive no matter how interested and dedicated its members are. Therefore, it is important that the PEM, working with the chair and the various committee members, plan how each committee will function. (Ideas on how to plan for a committee's first meeting were discussed in the hospitalwide patient education committee section of this chapter.)

The four major management tasks listed in figure 4-1 can help define specific components that will assist the PEM in establishing an effective new patient education committee.[8] These tasks need to be addressed before the first meeting of a newly formed committee.

If the PEM is working with already-established committees that are not functioning effectively, the problems need to be determined and improvements implemented. To assess and make improvements in how a patient education committee is functioning, the following tasks need to be completed:

1. If the PEM is the chair of the committee, he or she should assess its ability to function by answering the following questions:

- How well are people participating in meetings?
- Who is coming to meetings? Are they coming on time?
- Are the committee's objectives being met?
- Have the management tasks described in figure 4-1 been accomplished?
- What should be done to improve the committee's function?

On the basis of this overall evaluation, the PEM should involve the rest of the committee in a self-evaluation process and make recommendations for changes. Depending on the situation, particularly if there are personality conflicts within the group, the PEM may want to talk to each member individually and then report back to the group.

2. If the PEM is not the chair of the committee, he or she should discuss this assessment process with the chair and assist as needed. If this is not possible, the PEM should consider how he or she might intervene during meetings to make the committee more effective, for example, by:
   - Encouraging greater participation by asking specific people for input
   - Asking for clarification if members seem confused
   - Summarizing key points and actions periodically
   - Proposing objectives, deadlines, and the like to help the committee make more concrete action plans and decisions

   It may be necessary to talk with members of the committee individually, outside the meeting, to determine how they feel about the committee. If their concerns are similar, the PEM should work with the chair to find a solution.

☐ Team Interaction Barriers to Interdisciplinary Collaboration and Strategies to Address Them

In *The Interdisciplinary Health Care Team: A Handbook*, Ducanis and Golin[9] describe a number of barriers to interdisciplinary collaboration and team performance that have relevance to patient education committees. The use of the word *team* in this section can apply to any kind of patient education committee or to an interdisciplinary care delivery team.

Effective team functioning is primarily determined by the quantity and quality of interactions among team members. Problems often arise from lack of communication and interprofessional conflicts associated with individual roles within the team, the goals of the group, and issues of professionalism. The following sections describe these barriers and several strategies that PEMs and others can use to address them. The PEM can often reduce or alleviate problems stemming from these factors by providing an environment in which team interactions can be developed and enhanced.

Barriers to Communication

Barriers to communication include communication patterns and communication distance. Others are time, location, record-keeping systems, and language.

Communication Patterns and Distance

Who talks to whom is a major variable in team interaction, and a good deal of research has been done on what determines communication patterns and their consequences in team functioning. A significant factor in communication patterns between team members is who holds the most central physical position in a group when discussion occurs. The person who has the shortest distance when speaking to other members of a group is likely to emerge as the leader. Communication, therefore, is best served by sitting in a pattern that is circular in nature, where all members are seated with equal distance from each other. This pattern leads to a greater feeling of independence, autonomy, and power, resulting in a sense of satisfaction and enhanced team morale.

A decentralized communication network, where all members communicate freely with each other and each has access to all available information, seems to be the most effective for solving complex human problems. This pattern is in contrast to a centralized network where information is channeled to one individual and there is little communication between team members.

Time

There must be sufficient time to share critical information, both formally and informally, if team collaboration is to work effectively. Examining means of communication other than face-to-face meetings and making full use of documented information will help reduce this barrier. For example, if the team makes use of relevant written reports, less time may be required for team meetings. Checklists or work sheets left on the patient's medical record and telephone calls can also enhance communication among team members, thereby reducing the number of face-to-face meetings.

Location

Where team members' work areas are located can stimulate or reduce free and open communication. Work and meeting areas should be located so as to increase the exchange of information among team members as much as possible. Offices adjacent to each other and meeting rooms located in patient care areas where team members work will increase the exchange of information among members.

Record-keeping Systems

Well-developed interdisciplinary records can enhance communication. A record-keeping method should be chosen that focuses on patient problems and integrates all aspects of care. Individual record-keeping methods and forms for the various disciplines should be avoided. (See chapter 9 for more information on documentation systems.)

Language

Language problems revolve around the different disciplines using terms that are not understood by other disciplines or terms that have different meanings depending on the specific professional perspective. The use of professional jargon results in interdisciplinary differences and poor communication. The PEM should recognize that this is a problem and ask that terms be explained. Team members need to check with each other frequently to ensure that they are being understood.

Role Conflict

A common source of conflict for interdisciplinary teams involves ambiguous and overlapping roles resulting from team members responding simultaneously to multiple roles. All team members fulfill three kinds of roles: *personal roles* based on their own attributes and agendas; *professional roles* based on competencies in their discipline; and *team roles* based on behaviors used to maintain the group and fulfill member needs (for example, leader, moderator, evaluator).[10]

Conflicts over professional roles seem to pose the greatest problem in working together for interdisciplinary health care teams where overlapping responsibilities and competencies exist. Figure 4-4 contains an exercise on role conflict, designed by E. Bernheimer, that can be used to help interdisciplinary teams work through professional territoriality.

After working through this exercise, the following steps can be taken to resolve some of these role issues:

1. Clarify role expectations and perceptions where team members share their perceptions of each other's role.
2. Identify professional competencies and explain what their responsibilities entail.

Figure 4-4. Role Conflict Exercise in Patient Education

Health Profession _____

Instructions

Please identify yourself by listing your health profession. Select only *one* of the following multiple choices for each square. Please consider these statements in light of (a) *status quo* (the way it is now) and (b) the way you think it *should be.* There are *no* right or wrong answers. Place the appropriate letter in each square.

1. Determining the amount of information a patient needs about his or her medical status is best done by:

   a. Clinical pharmacist   e. Patient
   b. Dietitian   f. Physical therapist
   c. Health educator   g. Physician
   d. Nurse   h. Social worker
   i. Other   _____
                 ☐ (a)   ☐ (b)

2. Assessing possible obstacles to patient compliance in the home environment is best done by:

   a. Clinical pharmacist   e. Patient
   b. Dietitian   f. Physical therapist
   c. Health educator   g. Physician
   d. Nurse   h. Social worker
   i. Other   _____
                 ☐ (a)   ☐ (b)

3. For patients with a chronic medical condition, assistance in complying with the regimen is best provided by:
   a. Clinical pharmacist   e. Patient
   b. Dietitian   f. Physical therapist
   c. Health educator   g. Physician
   d. Nurse   h. Social worker
   i. Other   _____
                 ☐ (a)   ☐ (b)

4. Assessing the patient's "readiness to learn" is best done by:

   a. Clinical pharmacist   e. Patient
   b. Dietitian   f. Physical therapist
   c. Health educator   g. Physician
   d. Nurse   h. Social worker
   i. Other   _____
                 ☐ (a)   ☐ (b)

5. One-on-one counseling with the patient on his or her prescribed regime is best done by:
   a. Clinical pharmacist   e. Patient
   b. Dietitian   f. Physical therapist
   c. Health educator   g. Physician
   d. Nurse   h. Social worker
   i. Other   _____
                 ☐ (a)   ☐ (b)

6. Counseling a patient on his or her prescribed drug regimen (with attendant possible drug interactions and side effects) is best done by:

   a. Clinical pharmacist   e. Patient
   b. Dietitian   f. Physical therapist
   c. Health educator   g. Physician
   d. Nurse   h. Social worker
   i. Other   _____
                 ☐ (a)   ☐ (b)

(Continued on next page)

Figure 4-4. (Continued)

7. Helping arthritic patients incorporate a prescribed daily exercise plan in the home is best done by:

   a. Clinical pharmacist   e. Patient
   b. Dietitian   f. Physical therapist
   c. Health educator   g. Physician
   d. Nurse   h. Social worker
   i. Other _____

       ☐ (a)   ☐ (b)

8. Helping a patient change his or her eating pattern is best done by:

   a. Clinical pharmacist   e. Patient
   b. Dietitian   f. Physical therapist
   c. Health educator   g. Physician
   d. Nurse   h. Social worker
   i. Other _____

       ☐ (a)   ☐ (b)

From E. Bernheimer. Role conflict exercise, pp. 184–85. In: W. Squyres, ed. *Patient Education: An Inquiry into the State of the Art.* New York City: Springer Publishing Company, copyright ©1980. Used by permission.

3. Examine overlapping roles and misperceptions based on the discussion in the first two steps.
4. Renegotiate role assignments.

Goal Conflicts

Conflicts over goals and their priorities may disrupt collaboration among team members. This is not only true for newly formed teams, but also for those teams that have been in existence for a period of time. The direction in which a group sees itself moving needs to be defined so that members' differing perceptions do not lead to repeated disagreements regarding appropriate actions to take. Goal-setting exercises can provide a structured way for the team to share perceptions about goals and priorities so that areas of consensus can be identified and disagreements discussed. Constructing an affinity chart, which involves group brainstorming and organization of related ideas, is one way to identify differing perceptions about goals.[11]

Professional Barriers

Health care professionals have been educated and socialized to be autonomous and specialized, which supports their impetus to act alone without reference to others. Often the boundaries of professional responsibility are not clear-cut, and individual team members do not adequately understand the skills and competencies of their colleagues.

The question of professional responsibilities and prerogatives concerning who does what and who decides who does what needs to be discussed. In addition to autonomy and specialization, topics for discussion should include division of tasks, delegation of authority, professional stereotypes, specific expertise of the various professions, ethical standards, and legal responsibilities of the various professions. Sessions should be planned regularly for team development purposes to preclude the notion that something is wrong.

Differences in the various professional codes of ethics may be the result of territoriality, where the team approach is ignored and in some cases even precludes some professionals from participating on interdisciplinary teams. Team members need to be able to interpret their professional codes of ethics and discuss the effects on an interdisciplinary approach so that mutual understanding exists among members.

An individual's profession often determines his or her status in a group. Team members with less perceived status tend to defer to others with higher status, even when they have more accurate information about the issues being discussed. Recognizing professional hierarchies and their impact on team function, along with developing clear operational guidelines that reward participation in giving information and making decisions, will help to alleviate this barrier.

□ Organizational Barriers to Interdisciplinary Collaboration

The professionals who constitute an interdisciplinary team and determine how that team operates are markedly influenced by the organizational setting. The hospital's goals, norms and values, structure, sources of authority and decision making, and systems of rules and processes are among those organizational characteristics that affect how a team functions. In most instances, the PEM has no control over these factors. However, analysis and understanding of them and their impact on interdisciplinary team collaboration can help the PEM respond appropriately to situations resulting from these forces. In some cases, the PEM is provided a window of opportunity where he or she can be proactive and recommend ways to improve interdisciplinary team collaboration through organizational changes before conflict arises.

Typically, bureaucratic organizations have hierarchical structures that tend to emphasize and reinforce the divisions between disciplines. Communication, rewards, and sanctions tend to be restricted along these channels. However, organizations that espouse team principles need to be committed to alter themselves so that interdisciplinary team function can be enhanced and nurtured. If the organization cannot change, it will be constantly at odds with its teams.

The PEM needs to examine how interdisciplinary patient education committees and care delivery teams interact with the organization with regard to the following eight functions:[12]

1. *Goals and objectives.* If the organization's goals are not shared by the team, some clarification must be reached. Either the goals are not appropriate or the team does not understand, or has not been integrated into, the organizational structure.
2. *Assignment of tasks and roles.* The relationship between the team's role definition, task assignment, and activity is crucial to the way it functions. Defining what constitutes team membership, assigning appropriate roles, and resolving role ambiguity are important activities within an organization.
3. *Authority structure.* The authority structure must reinforce the team's activities in order to ensure adequate team function. The position of the team leader within the overall organization, the kind of decisions that can be made, and whether the team fits into the formal authority structure or authority evolves from other sources such as member expertise are all important questions that need to be answered.
4. *Communication network.* Communication between the organization and the team cannot be assumed simply because team members come from separate units within the hospital. Integration into the pattern of communication within the hospital improves team performance. Also, record-keeping systems and retrieval of information need to support team efforts by providing interdisciplinary forms in language common to all.
5. *Processes, rules, and procedures.* A hospital's processes, or the way it works to fulfill its goals, can help or hinder team functioning. If these rules, procedures, and processes are organized solely along disciplinary lines of authority, the flexibility needed for the interdisciplinary team to function most effectively is not forthcoming. For example, processes that focus on patient-centered care, interdisciplinary documentation, and case management encourage teamwork.

6. *System of rewards and sanctions.* Important to team success is whether its efforts are rewarded in some way by the organization. The hospital's norms and values influence the way the team functions. These need to be carefully appraised when developing teams.

7. *Spatial relationships.* An organization can significantly influence team operation and efficiency by recognizing that proximity is needed to enhance team interaction and reduce territoriality.

8. *Evaluation procedures.* Evaluation procedures in the organization must take into account the efforts of a professional as a member of an interdisciplinary team and not just as a practitioner within a specific discipline. In an organization, evaluation of activities reflects what is perceived as being valued and rewarded, so the team as a system needs to be evaluated.

□ Conclusion

Effective patient education committees and interdisciplinary team collaboration are essential if hospital-based patient education is to provide the appropriate mechanisms and necessary support to health care providers involved in teaching patients and their families. In order to develop a network of committees and teams at the various levels of patient education programming, the patient education manager must provide the leadership to stimulate interdisciplinary collaboration. This leadership may involve serving as a convener, a committee chair, a facilitator, an advisor, or a coordinator, as well as working to eliminate any barriers or conflicts that may impede the smooth functioning of patient education committees.

Working with interdisciplinary committees can be both frustrating and rewarding. Decision making by committee can be slow, and progress is often hindered by competing responsibilities of individual members. However, any negative aspects are outweighed by the positive effect on patient education program development provided by a well-functioning committee incorporating staff involvement, shared responsibility for making decisions and obtaining legitimacy and support, and input from a variety of perspectives.

References

1. Lee, E. A., Garvey, J., Finnegan, G., and Giloth, B. *Implementing Patient Education in the Hospital.* Chicago: American Hospital Association, 1979, p. 65 (out of print).

2. Lee and others, worksheet 4-1, p. 71.

3. Lee and others, worksheet 4-2, pp. 72-73.

4. Lee and others, worksheet 4-3, p. 74.

5. Lee and others, p. 66.

6. Ducanis, A. J., and Golin, A. K. *The Interdisciplinary Health Care Team: A Handbook.* Germantown, MD: Aspen Systems Corp., 1979, p. 108.

7. Lee and others, pp. 66–67.

8. Lee and others, pp. 67–69.

9. Ducanis and Golin.

10. Mumma, F. S. *What Makes Your Team Tick?* King of Prussia, PA: Organizational Design and Development, 1984.

11. Leebov, W., and Ersoz, C. E. *The Health Care Manager's Guide to Continuous Quality Improvement.* Chicago: American Hospital Publishing, 1991, pp. 154–57.

12. Ducanis and Golin, pp. 75–87, 174–76.

Bibliography

Bernheimer, E. Working through the territorial imperative in a hospital setting. In: Wendy Squyres, editor. *Patient Education: An Inquiry into the State of the Art.* New York City: Springer Publishing Company, 1980, pp. 181–92.

Ducanis, A. J., and Golin, A. K. *The Interdisciplinary Health Care Team: A Handbook.* Germantown, MD: Aspen Systems Corp., 1979.

Goren, S., and Ottaway, R. Why health care teams don't change: chronicity and collusion. *Reward and Recognition* 15(7–8):9–16, July–Aug. 1985.

Hankey, T. L., and Elandt, N. J. Collaborative approaches to patient education in the physicians' office. *Patient Education and Counseling* 12(3):267–75, Dec. 1988.

Hill, R. *Alaskan Adventure: A Team Problem Solving Exercise.* Dexter, MI: Effective Strategies, 1990.

Hopper, S., and Lange, M. Nurses' expectations and the realities of multidisciplinary education. *The Diabetes Educator* 13(2):126–29, Spring 1987.

Huszczo, G. E. Training for team building. *Training and Development Journal* 44(2):37–41, Feb. 1990.

Miller, C. How to construct programs for teams. *Reward and Recognition* 21(8–9):4–6, Aug.–Sept. 1991.

Mumma, F. S. *What Makes Your Team Tick?* King of Prussia, PA: Organizational Design and Development, 1984.

Richardson, A. T. Nurses interfacing with other members of the team. In: *Collaboration in Nursing.* Rockville, MD: Aspen, 1986, pp. 163–85.

Tobis, P. M., and Becker, M. C. Making the most of meeting time. *Training and Development Journal* 44(8):34–38, Aug. 1990.

Zemke, R. Team building: helping people learn to work together. *Training Human Resource Development* 15(2):23–34, Feb. 1978.

Zimberlin, L. Considerations in developing diabetes care teams. *The Diabetes Educator* 14(2):113–16, Mar.–Apr. 1988.

Chapter 5

Gaining and Maintaining Organizational Support

Dorothy A. Ruzicki, Ph.D., R.N.

☐ Objectives

The reader will be able to:

- Explain the importance of gaining hospitalwide support to ensure viability of an organized patient education program
- Identify some factors that influence the level of patient education support
- List specific, practical strategies patient education managers (PEMs) can use to enhance their abilities to influence their organizations
- Describe methods to increase the visibility of patient education both internally and externally

☐ The Importance of Gaining Support for a Coordinated Patient Education Program

Patients, physicians, pharmacists, nurses, and hospital staff and managers all talk about the importance of patient education. In fact, most health care professionals who have direct patient contact have some sort of competency related to patient education in their job descriptions. Regulatory agencies, researchers, third-party payers, and professional organizations all speak to the necessity of patient education. Why, then, if patient education is so critical to care, do those who manage hospitalwide patient education programs need to gain the support of key decision makers and staff?

There are many reasons to promote patient education among patient care staff and at the highest levels of the organization. Without the support of these people, patient education may lose out to many competing priorities. In a time when patients are discharged from hospitals earlier and sicker, when families are expected to care for loved ones during convalescence, when people are encouraged to take charge of their own health and illness, education in how to do so is essential. In addition, if other health care professionals, including managers, do not understand the role of a hospitalwide PEM and how a coordinated approach benefits the delivery of patient education, the position could be targeted for elimination as a cost-cutting measure.

☐ Factors That Affect Support for Patient Education Managers

A number of factors affect the PEM's ability and need to have influence within his or her organization. Several major ones are described in the following sections.

Limited Understanding of the PEM's Role

The role of patient education manager is a relatively new one, having evolved over the past 10 years or so, usually within an education department or a nursing department. Its evolution has been quiet and not well understood by many health care practitioners or other managers. Confusion about the PEM's role can lead and has led to lack of support for its functions. With greater knowledge about the role, key decision makers and staff are more likely to provide necessary support—for both the PEM's role and the patient education programs that are initiated.

Practitioners and line managers may ask why patient education needs to be managed anyway, especially if most health care professionals have some type of responsibility for patient teaching outlined in their job descriptions or their professional codes. In fact, it is often difficult for some professional staff to separate the patient education component from the care they provide, as in physical therapy, for example. A narrow specialty focus coupled with ownership feelings about patient education can undermine the effectiveness of a centrally managed approach, unless administrative support for the function is present. When practitioners understand the PEM's role and it is supported administratively, they will be more likely to participate in a coordinated patient education effort with better outcomes for the patient (for example, better materials, defined educational objectives and a standardized context, limited duplication, and so on).

Furthermore, many people confuse the PEM's job with that of the patient educator. They wonder, "Why isn't the patient education manager teaching the patients? Wasn't he or she hired to do patient education?" They fail to realize that a PEM's responsibilities are broader—to manage and coordinate hospitalwide education efforts—and that a PEM may even lack knowledge or skills to teach specialized patient care or provide other kinds of patient education.

It is somewhat paradoxical that although many health care professionals see themselves as having responsibility for patient teaching, they expect the PEM to do most of it, particularly when their time is limited. If they are busy, they are willing to delegate responsibilities for teaching without realizing that it would be impossible for any one person to singlehandedly teach all types of patients. Thus, many health care professionals do not support the PEM's role because they do not understand how he or she can help them teach patients.

Everyone's Doing It, Yet No One's Responsible for Patient Education

Another factor that influences PEM support is that many people teach patients, but not everyone feels accountable for patient education or for the coordination of patient education efforts. Decision maker support for PEM efforts is critical; without it, the PEM has limited ability to organize and coordinate the efforts of various disciplines and departments. With so many people involved, it is imperative that patient education efforts be well coordinated and managed and that PEMs have the necessary authority to get things done.

Increased Competition for Scarce Resources

An obvious reason why PEMs need the support of key people has to do with the allocation of resources, particularly in today's environment of financial restraint and tight budgets. In order to design and implement necessary programs, PEMs must have the required human and material resources. Without champions at the decision-making level, these resources will not be provided.

High Acuity of Hospitalized Patients

With sicker patients, the need for patient education is less obvious. When patients are so sick, how can they learn? PEMs must persuade both clinical staff and decision makers that their services are necessary even when the need is not blatantly obvious. For example, although patients are obviously sicker while they are hospitalized, they are still not completely well when they are discharged and in a position where they must assume part of their care themselves.

Support for the PEM role enables the PEM to design and implement a hospitalwide approach to help patients learn what they need to know at the most appropriate time during their hospital stay or before or after their inpatient experience. This may include new methods for reaching patients and their families across an entire organization and may require coordinating many different departments, disciplines, and settings.

High-Tech Environment

Hand in hand with heightened patient acuity are the related high-technology equipment and the emphasis on use and support of that technology. When patients require high technology, staff time will be devoted to providing care using complex equipment, making patient education less of a priority. Thus, PEMs need support to keep patient education prominent in this environment.

Organizational Location of PEMs

Another factor in gaining support is the location of most PEM positions within the organization. As mentioned earlier, PEMs are usually part of the nursing or education department. In these departments, they provide staff support to the line organization. Although the PEM staff positions are important, they are limited in power and authority. Furthermore, PEMs are usually buried within their own departments, with many of their colleagues wondering what they actually do. Because of these limitations, PEMs need to be visible so that others in the organization know, value, and support their function.

Use of Authority and Development of Personal Skills

A final factor that can influence support for PEMs relates to their perceptions of their own power and authority within the organization. If they feel powerless in staff positions and uncomfortable with their lack of organizational experience and political savvy, they can unwittingly affect the perceptions of others about their ability to have real organizational clout. This is where key decision maker support is extremely helpful because it will assist in attaining power and influence. However, very often attention and support from decision makers will not be present unless the PEM has already achieved some degree of visibility. It is as necessary for PEMs to develop their own abilities in communication, management, and organizational savvy as it is for decision makers to give them a boost. Both work together to promote patient education throughout the organization.

Obtaining decision maker and staff support assists PEMs in developing, enhancing, and managing successful patient education programs. The following section provides clear guidelines for developing the personal skills necessary for PEMs to obtain support and for planning strategies to obtain support from specific groups.

□ Strategies to Gain Support

A variety of skills and strategies are useful in gaining and maintaining hospitalwide support for patient education efforts. Some of the strategies discussed herein focus on developing personal skills and attributes that will improve communication between PEMs and potential supporters within the hospital. Other strategies explain how to target specific groups, including administration, medical staff, and other patient care staff.

Develop Personal Skills and Attributes

Having strong personal skills (for example, communication skills, organizational savvy) is especially vital to patient education managers, who must use them to gain the support they need to accomplish program goals through others.[1,2] As a first strategy to gaining hospitalwide support, PEMs should assess their personal skills/attributes and establish a plan to address their deficiencies. The personal skills discussed here reflect personal skills that are useful in any position, but are particularly critical for the PEM's efforts to build administrative and staff support.

Learn Communication Skills
PEMs armed with strong communication skills are more likely to gain and maintain administrative and staff support. One reason good communication skills are so important is that PEMs do not usually supervise the staff who carry out patient education programs, and most programs and activities are implemented through other people. PEMs must be able to get along with others, communicate clearly and concisely both orally and in writing, listen well, summarize points, and conduct meetings effectively—all important skills for any manager. These can be learned through courses in management and communication, constructive feedback from supervisors and peers, seeking opportunities to conduct meetings, gaining experience and self-evaluating, and so on.

To get along with others and obtain their support, the PEM must also be fair and objective in dealing with others. It is extremely important that PEMs be able to view situations objectively (or at least to appear to be objective), to remain calm even in emotional situations (territoriality being a hot topic), and to refrain from becoming personally involved in issues. Once support is gained, objectivity helps maintain it.

Expand Knowledge Base
Acquiring a broad knowledge of health care trends and the specifics of patient education is key to working with others in health care and gaining their support and cooperation. This knowledge indicates to others that PEMs are not isolated and are aware of broader institutional and health care issues. The type of knowledge needed by PEMs includes such areas as:

- National and local health care trends
- Patient education trends
- Patient education research with clinical application
- Management functions, especially planning and budgeting
- Specific hospital goals and objectives
- The hospital's management system

Implementing strategic planning for patient education (see chapter 2) is an excellent way of keeping current with many of the preceding topics. Additional methods, some of which will be used for strategic planning as well, include the following:

- Reading newspapers, general health care journals, and nursing and patient education journals

- Participating in patient education specialty organizations, such as the American Society for Healthcare Education and Training (ASHET) or the Society for Public Health Education (SOPHE)
- Attending meetings, conferences, and teleconferences
- Attending institutional management education programs
- Taking management classes at local universities
- Participating in, and providing community service for, voluntary health agencies
- Networking with other hospital managers and community leaders

Develop Organizational Savvy and Political Skills

Before PEMs can even begin a campaign to gain hospital support, they must know their organizations. Health care organizations vary widely, and PEMs must be very familiar with both the formal and informal power structures of their own institutions. This requires determining the organizational culture and learning the traditions of the organization. Some sample strategies are to:

- Make use of the organizational chart. It explains the formal reporting structure.
- Learn and use the formal lines of authority. Though cultivating the informal structure is useful, the PEM should not rely on it exclusively and risk violating any manager or administrator's sense of protocol.
- Observe how things get done and who gets things done. Who makes decisions? Are they centralized or decentralized? How powerful are the physicians in influencing decisions?
- Learn the rules of the organizational game. These vary from institution to institution, because the corporate culture varies. For example, the Veterans Administration (VA) system is very different from that of a private Catholic hospital culture. A state university medical center's rules differ from those of a proprietary, for-profit hospital. Health maintenance organizations (HMOs) have their own sets of rules and traditions. Small community hospitals may have different and less formal relationships with physicians than large teaching hospitals have.
- Listen and observe and network. The PEM should go out of his or her way to meet people from various parts of the hospital. Additionally, he or she should read about the organization.
- If possible, find a mentor. This should be someone who believes in what the PEM is doing—someone who has achieved position and respect and who can provide advice.

Effective PEMs—in fact, all good managers—develop sound political skills (such as those evident in the preceding strategies) in order to cultivate political support so that they can accomplish their goals. And it is important to point out that, contrary to popular belief, political savvy and the use of political skills are *not* synonymous with manipulation.

Develop Negotiating Skills

The ability to negotiate is important, particularly in building support and power. To gain ground, PEMs must be willing to compromise, to attempt to achieve a win–win situation for all involved. Sometimes this is difficult, especially if the PEM is attached to a particular idea, program, or outcome. For this reason, flexibility is another important personal trait to develop.

To learn negotiating skills, PEMs should read some of the books available, such as *Getting to Yes: Negotiating Agreements without Giving In,*[3] or take a course on negotiation. PEMs can practice negotiating in everyday encounters with staff and managers in other departments.

Develop a Winning Attitude

In addition to the skills previously mentioned, a winning attitude can enhance a PEM's personal skills. PEMs with a winning attitude—those who are patient, have a sense of humor, are able to take risks, and are willing to go the extra mile—have a greater chance of establishing successful patient education programs.

As mentioned earlier, the PEM's role is basically that of an internal consultant or facilitator who must work through others to accomplish goals. Thus, PEMs must be patient. They must bear in mind that tasks will eventually get done through other people, *but it will take time.*

Another useful asset for PEMs is a good sense of humor. It is important to laugh a little, share humor with others, and not take one's self too seriously. Otherwise, the PEM role can be very frustrating, and continual frustration can limit the PEM's effectiveness when dealing with others.

Effective PEMs, like other kinds of leaders, are risk takers—in suggesting new and unusual ideas, writing proposals, speaking out as advocates for issues and principles they believe in. Taking risks places the PEM in a noticeable, visible position, politically a good place to be, but also a scary one. Taking chances can help start a new program and increase exposure. Examples could include a proposal for a self-care unit or one where family members are taught, or an outpatient education program for chronic illness. Inherent in proactive behavior is the risk of being perceived as foolish or of not knowing all the answers. The examples just mentioned all require resources and may not enhance revenue. However, without some risk taking, complacency sets in and needed changes will not occur. PEMs should not be afraid to stand up for what they believe in, as long as sufficient homework is done in advance. It is important to learn to be comfortable with some measure of risk taking.

Another attribute that PEMs should develop is a willingness to give some extra effort to accomplish tasks. PEMs who watch the clock, who are unwilling to stay an extra hour or two to finish a report or meet with a vice-president, who refuse to take work home occasionally, or who refuse to volunteer for committee work or take on additional projects may find themselves locked out of truly superb opportunities to build influence and support. Likely, they will be noticed, but not as organizational movers and shakers.

On the other hand, those PEMs who go the extra mile and are willing to sacrifice a bit for the entire organization demonstrate that the goals for which they are working are important. At the same time, PEMs must know how to set priorities and allocate time appropriately to achieve the really important goals.

Develop Strategies for Specific Hospital Groups

Efforts to gain and maintain hospitalwide support are most effective if they are carefully planned and targeted toward specific hospital groups. By tailoring strategies to the unique needs and characteristics of their diverse audiences, PEMs are more likely to achieve greater results and, ultimately, greater support for their efforts.

In all cases, PEMs must be familiar with their target groups—what turns them on, what turns them off, their special languages and professional cultures, what benefits they get from patient education efforts, their hot buttons, their literature, and so on. For example, PEMs will not get much sympathy or assistance from financial personnel if they go to them extolling the virtues of high-quality patient education regardless of cost. Instead, PEMs must talk to financial people in terms of dollars and cents, and indicate an understanding of the organization's financial picture.

The specific groups PEMs must target to gain support are discussed in the following sections, and include administration, medical staff, and other patient care staff.

Administration

Health care administrators are key supporters needed for successful patient education efforts. At first, PEMs may wonder why these busy people would even notice patient education activities. However, PEMs should never be afraid of hospital administrators and should seize opportunities to point out how important patient education is in health care delivery. Administrators will be interested in patient education if its goals are in sync with those of the institution overall.

In order to talk with administrators, PEMs should be very familiar with national and local health care trends that affect patient education. Generally, patient education concerns are the result of other, broader health care issues. For example, implementation of the prospective payment system had a great impact on patient education. By encouraging providers to limit the average length of stay for patients, prospective payment helped enhance and emphasize the role of patient education in preparation for early discharge. PEMs should be aware of the broader health care trends and their impact on patient education.

As mentioned previously, some ways to keep track of health care trends include keeping up-to-date with the literature, reading, talking with administrators about current issues, and attending conferences that discuss implications of national trends on patient education. PEMs who take advantage of these opportunities to point up the value of patient education will find it easier to gain support.

An excellent way to elicit the support of administrators is to point out how patient education supports the hospital's goals. For example, most administrators are concerned about finances. Patient education efforts that cost money but do not show positive results in the quality of care in very tangible or demonstrable ways are doomed to failure. And administrators and financial managers have heard all about the soft or "potential" effects of patient education, especially from clinicians. In a resource-scarce environment, those arguments no longer work and may turn administrators off. To gain administrator support, PEMs must learn about budget and finances, and be able to talk the language of cost containment.

Additionally, PEMs need to research and identify how patient education specifically benefits the hospital. The more specific the information and the better supported it is by real data, the more likely it is that administrators will find reasons to support patient education. Some of the more tangible outcomes of patient education of interest to administrators include the following:

- Preventing untimely readmissions through effective discharge planning
- Meeting JCAHO requirements that relate either directly or indirectly to patient education
- Increasing patient satisfaction
- Increasing productivity and efficiency and using resources more effectively
- Reducing malpractice risk
- Increasing physician satisfaction with care
- Enhancing the community image of the hospital

How the PEM communicates with administrators can influence their responsiveness. The United States Department of Veterans Affairs suggests the following methods for effective communication with administrators:[4]

- Relate patient education issues to existing concerns and the facility's mission statement and priorities.
- Although some additional resources may be needed, focus on better use of money and staff time already being spent.
- Be concise and clear. Lay out issues and options. Don't go with general problems or complaints.
- Do not target specific disciplines or services as problems. Build a case for what needs to be accomplished and what is needed to deliver patient education services.

Before initiating specific strategies, it is useful to identify the one or two administrators who would have the most involvement in patient education activities and then direct most communication to them. At the administrative level of many hospitals, this is the vice-president for patient services and/or the vice-president for nursing.

However, other administrators should not be forgotten when issues arise that might be of interest to them—for example, strategies that could affect finance, those that could result in heightened risk management, those that affect safety issues, and definitely those that affect patients and practitioners in nonnursing departments. Following are examples of specific strategies that the PEM can use to keep administrators aware of patient education efforts:

1. Regularly communicate with them in writing. The PEM should send memos, current articles about the effectiveness of patient education, letters from persons happy with patient education services, and current research/evaluation studies that demonstrate an impact on quality or, even better, on cost. Administration could be provided with an annual report, focusing on results. The PEM might even write a manuscript on patient education and submit it for publication, having first run it by an administrator for input. That will catch the administrator's attention, even if the manuscript is not published.

2. Communicate verbally. The benefits of patient education should be discussed with administrators in meetings and informal conversations. Additionally, administrators should be interviewed when conducting needs assessments.

3. Volunteer to make presentations and reports on patient education at meetings where administrators are present.

4. Urge administrators to serve in key committee positions, such as chair of the hospitalwide Patient Education Committee. Administrators have line authority and most PEMs do not, so this representation is important.

5. Submit proposals or programs to administration that will dovetail with organizational goals.

6. Keep patient education visible throughout the organization, for example, through a patient education recognition program. (Specific strategies for these are mentioned later in this chapter.) Administrators should be involved in those special activities, for example, to hand out certificates, give short speeches at luncheons or receptions, or recognize award winners.

Medical Staff

The medical staff is another important group for PEMs to target. Physicians can be very influential with administration in ensuring the visibility of patient education efforts and obtaining the required resources to implement patient education programs.

Not only can physicians be powerful allies, they can also be even more powerful enemies. Although patient education programs can succeed without physician support, they are doomed if physicians are opposed to them. Therefore, it is a wise PEM who takes the steps necessary to garner their tacit approval, if not their blessing.

Physician support can be gained by offering patient education programs that contribute to high-quality patient care and thus please the patients. Although it is fairly easy to demonstrate whether patients are pleased with the programs, it is not as easy to document how patient education affects patient care. Physicians are schooled in scientific data, and many are skeptical about the real value of patient education programs. To enlist their support, PEMs must be conversant with the research bases of patient education. They must not only feel comfortable talking about how patient education affects quality of care, they must also be comfortable with and knowledgeable about research and evaluation studies that indicate positive patient education outcomes.

It is advisable to keep current with patient education journals that cover original research, such as *Patient Education and Counseling,* as well as to conduct occasional literature searches on patient education topics in general medical journals. Medical staff are more likely to place greater credence in patient education research published in medical journals.

Physicians are also supportive of patient education programs that save them time. For example, informational materials that clearly explain commonly used instructions are often welcomed. However, a word of caution is in order here. Physicians should *not* be asked to write patient education materials. In fact, PEMs should write the materials themselves and then ask physicians to review the content. This is because many physicians write at a level far too advanced for the average patient, and once they have written anything, they often have a sense of ownership that makes it very difficult for the PEM to make revisions.

PEMs will find that physicians who are in some way involved in decision making about patient education programs are far more supportive. They are also more likely to recommend patient education programs to other medical staff. Physician involvement is generally best limited to overall program approval and consultation. For example, it is extremely helpful to have physician advisors to patient education committees, particularly physicians who are widely respected by their colleagues. Their involvement is invaluable in helping to increase the visibility of patient education programs.

In communicating with physicians, both in person and in writing, PEMs should be straightforward and succinct. With heavy demands on their time, most physicians do not take the time to read lengthy information, nor do they respond positively to programs that involve complex protocols.

Some specific strategies to enlist physician support are:

1. Involve physicians in the formal Patient Education Committee structure.
   - Request that the Medical Executive Committee appoint a physician to the hospitalwide Patient Education Committee. This individual would be responsible for occasional reports back to the Medical Executive Committee. It is helpful for the PEM to write summary reports of committee meetings for the physician representative to report back to other staff.
   - Request that medical staff specialty committees, such as the Pediatric Committee, recommend physicians to consult with staff and to review specific programs being developed in those specialty areas. Upon completion, these programs can be reviewed and approved by the appropriate medical staff committee.
2. If involving medical staff directly in the formal committee structure mechanism is not workable, always invite physicians to be consultants and reviewers for patient education programs and materials. Patient education program ideas should be taken to medical staff committees for suggestions. It is important to involve physicians who are respected by their colleagues and who will have influence in maintaining support.
3. Develop an orientation package on patient education that can be used to orient new physicians. If possible, a listing of patient education programs and materials should be included, as well as the names of resource people and how to access them.
4. Provide physicians with a list of patient education materials that they can order for their own office use. (Physicians can also distribute preadmission educational materials to patients prior to admission, as is done with surgical patients prior to surgery.)
5. Ask physicians to help teach patient education classes. Physicians might appreciate the opportunity to formally teach patients in a different setting, and patients will appreciate the added expertise.
6. Survey physicians (with a short, concise tool or a phone call) to gather input on their patient education needs. The medical staff committees should be used to assess the needs for patient education.

7. Send the medical staff newsletters on patient education topics, programs, and materials, or include this information in hospital newsletters that are regularly sent to staff physicians.
8. Communicate any evidence of patient satisfaction with patient education programs to the hospital medical staff and individual physicians with privileges at the hospital. Getting patient support often wins physician support.

Other Clinical Staff

Clinical staff who will implement patient education programs represent another very important target group from which PEMs need support, cooperation, and input. These staff members include all the various disciplines with direct patient contact—nurses, pharmacists, dietitians, and technicians, to name a few.

Clinical staff have many demands on their time, and patient education is just one aspect of their jobs. To gain their support and involvement in patient education programs, PEMs should provide strategies to make teaching easier, develop incentives and rewards for teaching, and encourage supervisor support for staff involved in patient education. Like administrators and physicians, these staff should also be made aware of the tangible benefits of patient education efforts.

Because of the time pressures clinical staff face in carrying out their basic responsibilities, patient education programs must be easy to understand and implement. Complex, lengthy programs are doomed to fail in the current health care environment. Clinical staff appreciate patient education programs that can help them provide better, more consistent care without wasting precious time. Well-coordinated, interdisciplinary programs also eliminate duplication and confusion for both staff and patients.

Some useful methods to make it easier for staff to participate in patient education include preparing practical and appealing patient education literature and videotapes for use at the hospital, in physicians' offices, or even for patients to take home. It is important to mention that patient education programs that incorporate materials such as pamphlets and videotapes need these materials to be easily accessible and available for use as needed and when expected. Staff have little patience for seeking out their own resources. Directories of patient education programs and teaching plans that are practical and easily implemented also serve to ensure staff support of patient education.

Clinical staff who participate in patient education program development are often the greatest program supporters, and their involvement can have many positive outcomes. In addition to their support and participation, these staff generally discuss patient education with other staff, physicians, and patients. They have a vested interest in ensuring the program's success, and they also bring valuable information to the program planning sessions about how the program can best be implemented by staff.

PEMs should always involve hospital staff in program planning and listen carefully to what they have to say. If staff members indicate that a particular program is too difficult to implement, they are often right, and it will be a frustrated PEM who chooses to ignore their counsel. However, this is also an excellent opportunity for the PEM to involve staff in problem solving to develop approaches that will work.

Specific strategies to develop the support of staff members include the following:

1. Identify and invite representative clinical staff to participate on committees planning patient education programs for specific target populations. Be sure to seek permission from the appropriate supervisors/managers.
2. Make sure that all patient education materials and program protocols or guidelines are reviewed by relevant staff.
3. Implement staff development and training programs that focus on patient education. These include:
   - Providing orientation for new employees on patient education programs. New employees should be given orientation to the hospitalwide education program as part of their initial orientation to the hospital and their department or unit.

- In-service training should be provided on how to implement new programs.
- Continuing education programs on how to teach patients should be provided periodically. A continuing education program might be designed to improve basic staff teaching skills, how to develop readable written materials, how to assess learning needs, and so forth. A helpful method is to incorporate patient education as part of a larger, clinically focused conference. Videotapes and opportunities to role-play can be effective tools in teaching patient education. Staff should also be allowed to practice what they have learned during the educational program.[5]

4. Recognize and reward staff for their patient education contributions by:
   - Including their names in publications or videotapes they have helped develop
   - Recognizing them in hospital newsletters, magazines, or patient education displays
   - Honoring them with patient education excellence awards
   - Sending copies of special thank-you letters to their supervisors and their personnel files
   - Asking a vice-president to send a note of thanks to both the employee and his or her direct supervisor
   - Helping them write a manuscript about their patient education activities and submit it to a national journal
   - Asking them to serve as talent in videotapes about patient education—in their own roles
   - Asking them to participate in presentations on patient education, especially those that are highly visible, to administration or the Board of Trustees
   - Sending staff to patient education conferences and programs

5. Evaluate and encourage support structures that offer incentives for staff participation. Ask these questions:
   - Do job descriptions make mention of patient education responsibilities?
   - Is patient education part of the performance appraisal for employees involved in direct patient care?
   - Are employees allowed time to work on patient education committees and to develop and review programs and materials?
   - Are support structures present to help them, such as library staff to conduct computer searches and educational staff to help develop materials and teaching aids?
   - Does the hospital allocate funds to provide the necessary resources to assist staff in implementing patient education and reduce their time spent (for example, video programs and equipment for repetitive content)?
   - Are there funds to send staff to patient education conferences or otherwise provide them with educational opportunities?

It is important to point out that in order to gain support from general hospital staff, PEMs must first cultivate the support of their supervisors or managers. Interest, encouragement, and rewards provided by their direct supervisors go a long way toward ensuring active staff participation in patient education. At the very least, managers need to be approached for permission to involve their staffs in the development of patient education programs. If interested, these supervisors and managers can also participate on patient education committees and may want to conduct program planning meetings in their own departments. They will probably also have suggestions for developing or improving patient education programs and materials.

☐ Methods to Gain Visibility for Patient Education

Which comes first, visibility or support? Being visible in the organization promotes support, but then support also enhances visibility. Needless to say, to remain viable and effective, PEMs and their activities must be prominent and visible throughout the organization and beyond. Many of the strategies mentioned earlier in this chapter are aimed at specific target groups and incorporate methods to increase organizational visibility as well as to elicit support.

What follows in this section is a grouping of strategies that specifically focus on creating greater visibility for patient education. They are organized into two categories: communication methods, including methods of acknowledging staff efforts, and special events.

Communication Methods

Letting others know about patient education activities heightens interest and visibility and demonstrates that patient education is an active department.

Communication methods are limited only by what is possible within each organization. PEMs should identify the normal internal and external routes of communication and use them, but not overlook new ideas that might be attention grabbers. A variety of internal and external communication methods can be used to increase the visibility of patient education, and the following sections discuss some of the more common ones.

Internal Communication Methods

PEMs can increase visibility internally by collecting, monitoring, and publicizing the results of patient education efforts via annual reports, meetings, presentations, and hospital newsletters. If possible, a presentation to the hospital's Board of Directors or administration highlighting particularly noteworthy results of a patient education program can do wonders to strengthen visibility of the overall program.

Most hospitals publish employee newsletters. These newsletters provide excellent forums for reporting patient education events, and are especially effective for giving staff credit and announcing the recipients of patient education awards. Additionally, many hospitals publish a more polished magazine or newsletter for external distribution to such "publics" as supporters in the community, development fund contributors, School of Nursing alumni, volunteers, community leaders, other hospitals, and so on.

Employee newsletters usually come out frequently enough (often once a week) to provide fast, timely information. This means that they can be used for announcements about upcoming patient education programs and events that employees may want to be involved in. However, such information should be succinct and limited to patient education news that employees will find valuable.

Magazines sent to an external mailing list can be used to describe successful programs, relate stories about educational efforts aimed at specific patients, and recognize employee efforts in patient education. These publications can also be very effective in keeping "friends" of the hospital, such as board members and volunteers, up-to-date on patient education. These targeted groups might prove invaluable later in obtaining support for critical programs.

In addition, many hospital departments write short newsletters that are issued several times a year. Departmental newsletters are an excellent way to reach clinical specialists and to promote patient education in specific departments. Whereas many employees may not read the general employee newsletter, they almost always read their own department's publications.

Yet another communication avenue that should not be overlooked is the physician or medical staff newsletter that many hospitals send out regularly to all staff physicians. Although many physicians do not read it thoroughly, they often scan it for pertinent information. Additionally, their office staff may see it. The key here is to keep patient education content concise and related to physician concerns. Content should focus on changes in programs that affect physicians, such as new programs and materials and how they can access them.

Besides the existing channels of communication, PEMs might consider developing a series of standardized patient education newsletters that can be used internally or sent to physicians' offices. These might give advice or provide tips for patient education as well as include information about programs and resources.

External Communication Methods

External communication methods must be explored in order to build public relations for patient education efforts and maintain visibility in the community. An excellent resource for finding out about community communication possibilities is the hospital's public relations director or marketing staff. In fact, before approaching any community news vehicle, savvy PEMs always consult the appropriate in-house public relations manager. Not only will this individual provide invaluable advice, he or she can also provide political guidance (that is, what's appropriate and what's not, what will be viewed positively by administration and physicians and what won't), which is particularly important in these days of heavy competition.

Community newspapers also can be used for communication, particularly in smaller communities. However, because newspapers get so many requests and suggestions for stories from special interest groups, they tend to accept only those that have a vivid human interest theme, such as the story of a very young child who has had major heart surgery and whose parents took advantage of the educational program. Occasionally, small community newspapers will include a story on a special educational event or an employee who has received a major award. However, unless the paper is a very small one, this is often the exception rather than the rule. Sometimes community newspapers list upcoming events, in which announcements of community education classes could be placed. In many communities, radio stations also announce upcoming patient education programs (those open to the public) in their public service announcements.

Visual Display Methods

Some communication methods, such as visual displays, can be used to increase visibility among both internal and external hospital publics. For example, attractive patient education displays placed in areas of high traffic can be very helpful in enhancing both internal and external visibility. They may be either stationary, one-time displays or portable displays that move from area to area or department to department. Display topics can highlight employees who are involved in patient education, spotlight specific programs and personnel, and explain Patient Education Week/Month.

Depending on their topics, stationary displays are most effective if placed in locations where the public cannot miss them, such as the entrance to the hospital or cafeteria or wherever staff members congregate. One excellent location for displays in large institutions is at elevator waiting areas. Displays placed in specific departments can even explain how to implement patient education programs. However, these should be placed in employee classrooms or conference rooms and out of public view.

Displays should be primarily visual with very little printed content. Most people pass by them but do not take time to read them thoroughly. Pictures and colorful displays typically attract more attention than printed material does.

Bulletin boards are similar to stationary displays and may be placed either at employee entrances or in specific hospital departments. As with displays, bulletin boards can be used to convey a variety of patient education information. The design criteria mentioned for displays also pertain to bulletin boards. It is important to use well-designed, colorful flyers and other information to attract attention, so that their message stands out among other material on the bulletin board.

Another idea is to have space specifically reserved for patient education on both general staff and patient bulletin boards. This space can be used to highlight patient education goals and events. If assigned space is used, PEMs need to consistently maintain and update the information or staff will be unlikely to rely on it.

Recognition of Staff Efforts in Patient Education

A discussion on how to gain visibility for patient education would be incomplete without mentioning the importance of involving, and then acknowledging, staff efforts in patient education. In addition, such recognition aids greatly in gaining staff support. One way to do this is to provide Patient Education Excellence Awards, whereby staff members are selected by their peers and/or managers for their expertise and then recognized with special receptions, luncheons, displays with their pictures, badges, buttons, or certificates. This can be done periodically throughout the year and then during Patient Education Week. (See figures 5-1, 5-2, and 5-3 for examples of publicity and nomination forms used in one hospital.)

Figure 5-1. Publicity for Patient Teaching Awards Nominations

November Is Patient Education Month

Who should represent your unit/department by receiving the Patient Education Excellence Award?

Patient teaching—more important than ever these days, but *harder* than ever to fit in. Regardless of the many barriers, do you know someone who does a great job and serves as a super role model? If so, now's your chance to bestow some recognition!

Complete an official ballot that lists criteria for candidates. Separate forms exist for these categories:

1. Registered Nurse
2. Licensed Practical Nurse
3. Other Health Care Professionals

Be sure to mark and turn in your ballot to your nurse/department manager by October 25th. Thanks.

Reprinted from Sacred Heart Medical Center, Spokane, Washington.

Figure 5-2. Patient Teaching Excellence Award: Official Ballot for Health Care Professional

Vote for one of your coworkers to represent your department for the Patient Teaching Excellence Award. Turn this ballot in to your department manager before _____.

Award Criteria:

1. Staff person (not specialty educator) who is dedicated to patient education and who demonstrates this in one-on-one teaching experiences with patients.
2. Staff person teaches patients on a consistent basis by incorporating patient education into day-to-day care, and/or actively participates in development of patient teaching materials and processes.
3. Staff person works well as a team member with all health care professionals to provide effective patient education and discharge planning.

Name of Candidate: _____

Unit/Department: _____

Please provide a comment or two to support your vote:

_____

_____

_____

_____

_____

Reprinted from Sacred Heart Medical Center, Spokane, Washington.

Figure 5-3. Patient Teaching Excellence Award: Official Ballot for RN

Vote for one RN coworker who exemplifies the following characteristics *consistently* and to a *high degree*. Turn this ballot in to your department manager before _____.

RN Criteria:

1. Completes initial discharge planning assessment at time of patient admission.

2. Identifies patient/family learning needs.

3. Develops a plan to meet the assessed needs of each patient; collects subjective and objective data from families and other staff members.

4. Includes patient and family in formulating plan of care.

5. Includes restorative and preventive elements in planning patient care to ensure maximum health potential at discharge.

6. Implements and coordinates a health teaching program appropriate for the patient and/or family's ability and willingness to learn.

7. Evaluates patient's response to teaching provided and documents on appropriate forms.

8. Explains all procedures, treatments, and medications to patient and family as appropriate, and documents these on the proper forms.

9. Encourages the professional development of team members by facilitating their attendance at in-service programs, conferences, and lectures within the medical center.

Name of Candidate: _____

Unit/Department: _____

Please provide a comment or two to support your vote:

_____
_____
_____
_____
_____

Reprinted from Sacred Heart Medical Center, Spokane, Washington.

Products

There are several products—tangible outcomes of patient education efforts—that can be used both internally and externally to create awareness and enhance visibility of patient education efforts. These include such products as patient education literature and videotapes, which can be used in the hospital, physicians' offices, and even patients' homes. Directories of patient education programs and teaching plans also serve to make patient education more visible, particularly if staff can easily see that they are realistic and easy to implement.

Special Events

Numerous special events can spotlight patient education and heighten its visibility throughout the hospital. Some of the most popular include Patient Education Week/Month activities such as patient education health fairs and contests.

Even before national Patient Education Week became official, many hospitals recognized patient education through their own special awareness days, weeks, or months. However, with the first week in November now designated as National Patient Education Week, many more institutions are using this opportunity to recognize patient education efforts, and others have changed the dates of earlier events to coordinate with

111

the national celebration. It is a wonderful opportunity to share accomplishments and promote patient education in general. A packet of information to assist in organizing events can be obtained for a nominal fee from the International Patient Education Council (IPEC), in Rockville, Maryland.

All sorts of activities can be organized, including:

- A specific theme that is woven throughout the week's activities and incorporated in all publications and displays.
- A proclamation from the governor or mayor posted in a display or wherever patients and staff can see it. For example, one hospital placed copies of such a proclamation on meal trays to let patients know about Patient Education Week. (Local patient education interest groups, such as chapters of ASHET often combine efforts to ensure recognition of Patient Education Week.)
- Contests, such as word scrambles, with a patient education focus.
- Awards recognizing hospital staff who have developed unique patient education programs or have supported patient education year-round.
- Buttons highlighting patient education for staff and physicians to wear, such as the "I love patient teaching" button.
- Displays illustrating patient education resources.
- Patient education workshops or special speakers.
- Picture displays or articles in hospital newsletters on patient education committee members.
- Patient education tips printed in departmental newsletters.
- Information on special patient education programs printed in the hospitalwide employee newsletter.
- A patient education fair for visitors, with a table display of resources and services such as simple health screening activities.
- A list of patient education resources for staff published in the employee news sheet.
- A three-minute videotape of staff actively involved in teaching, made to play continuously and used in place of a display.

☐ Conclusion

Gaining and maintaining support is critical to the successful management of patient education programs. As times get tougher and resources scarcer, PEMs will continue to scramble for available resources in health care institutions. For this and other reasons, it is important to develop strategies for gaining support. This often means the PEM must develop or sharpen personal skills, as well as develop specific strategies for gaining support from such key groups as administrators, medical staff, and clinical staff.

Increasing visibility and gaining support go hand in hand. Increasing the visibility of patient education keeps it in everyone's mind, especially when communication efforts highlight its fundamental importance to patient care. Communication methods can include a variety of internal publications, such as newsletters, and external options, such as announcements in community newspapers.

By using a variety of techniques to garner and maintain support and increase visibility, PEMs need not worry about their positions being cut by people who may not understand the breadth and scope of their work. When PEMs have support for patient education, it is easier to develop the programs patients need. And when patients receive high-quality and timely education, they can make an easier transition from hospital to home and are less likely to need to return to the hospital soon after discharge. When the PEM gains support for patient education, both the hospital and its patients are the real beneficiaries.

References and Notes

1. For further information on developing personal skills, see Bartlett, E. E., Advocacy skills and strategies for patient education managers, *Patient Education and Counseling* 8(4):397–405, 1986; and Ruzicki, D., Patient education power, *Patient Education Newsletter* 8(6):1–3, 1985.

2. Fisher, R., and Ury, W. *Getting to Yes: Negotiating Agreement without Giving In.* Boston: Houghton-Mifflin, 1981.

3. Fisher and Ury.

4. A VA Field Task Force. *Patient Health Education: Building Medical Center Commitment (Facilitator's Guide).* Washington, DC: Department of Veterans Affairs, Office of Academic Affairs, Patient Health Education Program, 1988.

5. Devine, E. C., O'Connor, F. W., Cook, T. D., Wenk, V. A., and Curtin, T. R. Clinical and financial effects of psychoeducational care provided by staff nurses to adult surgical patients in the post-DRG environment. *American Journal of Public Health* 78(10):1293–97, 1988.

Bibliography

Giloth, B. Creating greater visibility to strengthen the hospital's patient education program. *Promoting Health* 8(1):6–9, 1987.

Giloth, B. Incentives for planned patient education. *Quality Review Bulletin* 11(10):295–301, 1985.

Kernaghan, S., and Giloth, B. *Working with Physicians in Health Promotion: A Key to Successful Programs.* Chicago: American Hospital Publishing, 1983 (out of print).

Ruzicki, D. Staff involvement in patient teaching: making it happen. *Patient Education and Counseling* 10(1):83–89, 1987.

Chapter 6

Managing Risk through Patient Education

Leah S. Kinnaird, Ed.D., R.N.

☐ Objectives

The reader will be able to:

- Establish the link between patient education and risk management
- Describe ways to manage risk through patient education

☐ Overview of Patient Education and Risk Management

As risk managers search for ways to reduce the number of lawsuits filed against hospitals, they are finding that patient education is one effective measure. Patient education facilitates the sharing of information that contributes to a more cooperative relationship between hospitals and patients, which can influence whether suits are filed. Thus risk managers are often willing to lend strong support to patient education efforts.

Patient educators offer reassurance and psychosocial support to patients. Because patients sometimes base their perceptions of care on how well they are treated by hospital staff, their decision not to litigate may be a direct result of what patient education has done for them.

This chapter begins by examining the malpractice climate that U.S. hospitals face, providing some reasons for patient suits that have implications for patient education, and exploring other factors that influence patient education. It then discusses three types of patient decision-making issues and two kinds of patient education programs related to risk management. Finally, the chapter closes with information on how patient educators can work with risk managers.

This chapter is an expansion of the following article: L. S. Kinnaird. With hospitals' malpractice risk rising, patient education offers positive response. *Promoting Health* 7(4):6–8, July–Aug. 1986. The author wishes to acknowledge the assistance of Kilby Strickland and Yvonne Zawodny, R.N., of the Risk Management Department at Baptist Hospital of Miami; William Bell, general counsel for the Florida Hospital Association; and Robert White of the Physicians Protective Trust Fund.

☐ The Malpractice Climate That Hospitals Face

In understanding the current malpractice climate in the United States, it is helpful to look at the experiences of one state where malpractice has been a major issue. Patient educators and risk managers need to understand that the increased use of technology and the shift toward failure to diagnose as a cause for lawsuits are affecting some hospital practices. Patient education is one of those practices.

The state of Florida is noted for many things—sunshine, time-shares, and centenarians—but one distinction in which it takes little pride is that medical malpractice has been headline news in the state for more than a decade. The situation is so poor that the trauma network in Dade County broke down in July 1987, partly because of the escalating malpractice climate, and has never been rebuilt. Adult trauma is managed only at the county hospital downtown. Physician efforts to limit awards for noneconomic damages have failed. If the number of malpractice cases has declined, it may be because they are being settled through advance arbitration. The gap between health care providers and South Floridians has not improved, and, if anything, 10 years has brought even greater polarization.

What has happened in Florida is now spreading rather quickly throughout the rest of the country. In fact, the public debate about health care reform inevitably includes some discussion of malpractice and defensive medicine. Recently, the "Nightline" town meeting in Chicago, *Emergency: Health Care in America*,[1] provided microphones for consumers, attorneys, physicians, legislators, and others to confront each other. An obstetrician from Texas declared that half the Caesareans done in the United States and one-third of all operative procedures are unnecessary. An attorney from Chicago declared he did not see any defensive medicine. An angry consumer asked why an ambulance can "pass by the fine hospitals, but trauma has to go 25 miles away." And June Osborn, M.D., chair of the National Commission on AIDS, stated that the pressure of the legal system influences her teaching practices as a medical professor. Malpractice is a growing concern influencing the very fabric of the nation's health care system.

Litigation dating back to the 1960s has established that hospitals can be sued as providers of care; that the risk can sometimes be assessed against the "deepest pocket," that is, the party or parties best able to pay; and that employers are responsible for wrongs committed by their employees in carrying out their business. In the past, physicians carried most of the risk as providers of care, but hospitals have become implicated as mutual, if not solely responsible providers.

Consequently, hospitals nationwide have become increasingly vulnerable to litigation. Big buildings, sophisticated equipment, and rigid hospital routines contribute to the kind of atmosphere that separates providers and consumers. People equate big hospital bills with big hospital profits. The complicated dynamics of insurers, medical suppliers, physicians, consumers, and hospitals is poorly understood. But when patients are faced with a big bill, anger toward the sender of the bill rises. Often that sender is the hospital.

Historically, malpractice claims against physicians were for improper treatment cases and the highest awards involved birth-related problems. Currently, failure to diagnose is the leading cause of suits in Florida. "The more technology we have [and] the more diagnostic tools are available to us, the more the public expects people to be able to diagnose illness," said James Haliczer, an attorney.[2] Hospitals are frequently the providers of diagnostic procedures (for example, mammography and magnetic resonance imaging), increasing their vulnerability to litigation, even when the issue is failure to diagnose, seemingly a physician responsibility. In addition, with more technology at their fingertips, physicians, with apparitions of attorneys hovering over their shoulders, order extra procedures to protect themselves from litigious patients. Therefore, costs go up, as do the bill and the anger. A vicious cycle of events continues.

With little relief from these trends in sight, there is cause for concern. These trends quickly get the attention of the hospital's chief executive officers, financial officers, and risk managers, but patient educators should be aware of them as well.

Although patient educators are not usually thought of as risk managers, they play a part in helping hospitals deal with the issue of malpractice. When litigation centers on the patient's understanding or lack of understanding of the care provided, patient education can obviously have an important impact. More and more, malpractice is everyone's concern. Therefore, the better patient educators understand the consumer and the uniqueness of the patient–provider relationship, the more likely they are to provide the information and support that encourages collaboration between the hospital and the patient.

☐ Why Patients Sue

By rights, Americans can sue for practically anything; whether or not they are successful is determined in the courts. In Dade County, Florida, closed-claim experience data show that the number of malpractice cases rose until 1987, but has declined in the past three years.[3] Insiders suggest that, after this brief respite, the number of claims is again on the rise. The cause for the cycle of events is unknown. Some observers have even suggested that excessive payoffs are a cultural phenomenon not unlike huge lottery wins and the enormous salaries of high-profile sports stars. In such an atmosphere there seems no limit to assessing damages for the loss of a limb or a malformation in a child. Assigning a dollar value to health is a cognitive and emotional matter carried out in the courts, reported by the media, and evaluated in the minds of the public with sometimes staggering figures.

Incidence of Litigation

It would seem that studying the incidence and trends of litigation might hold some key to understanding why patients sue and even how patient education efforts could address this issue. However, taking such a simple concept as linking the legitimacy of malpractice claims with the actual incidence of negligence is difficult.

The number of patients who experience adverse events and later sue their physicians is relatively low, relatively stable, and not necessarily related to adverse events that met the criteria for harm established by independent researchers. The legal community would like to think that malpractice litigation is "a means of obtaining civil justice."[4] However, there is room to say that the frequency of claims is excessive and, yet, there are times when a claim might seem legitimate but is not made. Writing in the April 1984 issue of *Law, Medicine and Health Care* on the predisposition of patients to file claims, Irvin Press noted that, although as many as one-third of all patients may experience an iatrogenic incident, fewer than 5 percent who experience harm ever file suit. As he points out, it is not the incident itself, but the patient's perception of what has occurred that determines whether a suit will be filed.[5]

Perceptions and Misconceptions

With so much litigation possible, it would be useful to be able to predict who is likely to sue. In normal, everyday, care-giver transactions, fears of lawsuits, whether conscious or not, influence practice as well as the inclination to participate in giving patients information. In conducting ethnographic research among nurses, one researcher has noted that nurses have certain perceptions of patients that lead them to categorize patients they think are inclined to sue, raising fears of teaching information they expect might be used against them. The categories are as follows:[6]

1. Patients who "take notes and write everything down"
2. Patients who "have a lawyer in the family"

3. Patients who "are lawyers, accountants, or other professionals"
4. Patients who have certain injuries or illnesses (for example, "head injuries, backache")
5. Patients who have serious injuries or illnesses
6. Patients who "are always wanting to know"

A physician malpractice consultant was questioned as to whether all of the above-mentioned patient categories indeed were more inclined to sue. He agreed that some (but not all) were. From his point of view, the characteristics of patients in the first three categories were less likely to have an influence on intent to sue. Patients who write many notes may simply be compulsive rather than suit-prone. Attorneys, professional people, and their relatives may not necessarily be more suit-prone and may receive exceptional care by virtue of their care givers assuming they have higher-than-usual expectations.

What the physician did identify was that certain types of injuries and illnesses might tip off the possibility of a lawsuit. For instance, patients who have severe injuries suffer terrific losses. The more wronged a patient feels, the more likely he or she is to seek restitution from any related, or for that matter even unrelated, source.

A related finding was that the less familiar a patient is with the provider, the less invested the patient is in that relationship. This problem was apparent in the closing of Dade County's emergency departments to trauma. Severely traumatized patients, not having known their physicians in advance, sought restitution for terrific losses from the person who had given them emergency care. According to William Bell, general counsel for the Florida Hospital Association, "People typically find it easy to sue strangers and find it difficult to sue people who are trying their best to care for them."[7] This is corroborated in a *Medical Business* article relating that ophthalmologists are less likely to be sued, probably because they have a long-running history with their patients.[8] Eye conditions may be singled out as more suit-resistant, not because of the condition but because of the long-standing relationship between practitioner and patient.

Patients who "always want to know" pose a special problem, because sometimes there is no explanation for a condition or a failure of treatment. Not everyone is willing to accept "I don't know" as a legitimate response. According to a Miami personal injury attorney, "People run to lawyers when they can't get answers." Some patients make comments as follows: "I could never understand why my loved one died, and I was hoping the lawyers could help me find out."[9] Some patients decide to sue after being encouraged by acquaintances and medical personnel.[10]

Intent to sue is not a highly predictable behavior and certainly more research is needed; but it can be said that when the relationship between provider and patient is poor, when the patient (or family) has unrealistic expectations or does not understand certain issues, and when the patient is angry or grieving over an actual, a severe, or a perceived loss, the chances of litigation increase.

What is important to note in the preceding discussion is that assumptions a practitioner might make about a patient's likelihood to sue may not be based in fact. If there is fear that a lawsuit might occur, the practitioner may be less inclined to talk with, and provide information to, the patient. Such hesitation on the part of the practitioner would only increase the gap in communication and retard the development of a caring attitude—the very factors that are known to reduce the possibility of a lawsuit. Based on the advice of the physician consultant previously quoted, it would behoove practitioners to give compulsive patients pen and paper, welcome their questions as intelligent consumers, and involve them in as much decision making as possible.

As a review of the relevant literature indicates, angry patients are more likely to sue because they received inadequate information than they are because they received too much. Yet, even today, patient educators continue to encounter health care professionals who undervalue the importance of information for patients. As Robert M. Cunningham, Jr., a long-time and well-respected observer of the hospital field, wrote in the December 1,

1978, issue of *Hospitals,* many professionals believe that "teaching patients to take care of themselves is like teaching the passengers to fly the airplane."[11] Although nervous passengers may be comforted by an explanation of why the engines change pitch, they rarely, if ever, request to take over the controls. Research reported in the December 7, 1984, *Journal of the American Medical Association*[12] suggests that the same is true of patients. Comparing the expectations of clinicians to the actual preferences of their patients, the study found that the clinicians underestimated their patients' desire for information, but overestimated their desire to make decisions. Therefore, anger might be triggered if patients receive too little information or feel abandoned when decisions are made.

It has been argued that "the chief method for minimizing the potentiality of patients to make trouble for doctors and nurses by criticizing their work is to withhold information, so the patient cannot argue from adequate knowledge."[13] It would be comforting to think that the decade of the '80s has changed such attitudes, but the gap between providers and patients remains. A review of the kinds of litigation most commonly filed suggests that withholding information is ineffective: People sue because they do not have enough information to understand, not because they have been given too much to understand. Because the public is better educated and better informed than ever before, withholding information is one sure way to encourage the kind of adversarial relationships that result in suits.

☐ Factors Influencing Patient Education and Support

Several factors have made it particularly difficult to meet patients' needs for information as well as for reassurance and other forms of personal support. For example, same-day surgery has exploded as an alternative to inpatient care since the implementation of Medicare's diagnosis-related groups in 1983. Coming into the hospital on the morning of outpatient surgery leaves the patient little opportunity to use various resources that were once available on the days and nights before surgery. Previously, hospitalized patients had the time to learn how to work the simple items that can be problematic (their electric beds, call buttons, and television). They had time to practice incentive spirometry and learn how to cough and deep breathe. Now surgery and actual patient contact have been compressed into sometimes short, wakeful hours for the patient. The patient arrives at the hospital in a rush. Medication is administered with little waiting time, and the teachable moment is gone.

Similarly, patients who are admitted to hospital beds are staying for shorter periods of time. Little time is available to teach good self-management skills. Education has been streamlined to the absolute necessities of care. Thus going home, as it has been said, "quicker and sicker," patients are at greater risk for developing problems.

At the same time, hospital staff members are struggling to care for more acutely ill inpatients. Work loads are greater and less time is available for personal interaction with patients, let alone for the niceties of communication that can help reassure patients. Coupled with the external pressures of tightened insurance dollars and problems with access to care, the situation is not conducive to the establishment of strong positive relationships between health care professionals and patients.

Although the hospital environment is changing, the public's belief that the health care system should be infallible remains constant. Health care professionals do little to encourage a more realistic expectation. For example, during the course of an interview with one physician to determine his interest in a preoperative teaching program, a patient education manager was told that the physician saw no need for such a program. All the physician had to do, he said, was to tell his patients that they "are going to the Baptist Hospital Hotel, where the service is wonderful, and they'll feel fine."

Consider the unrealistic expectations such a statement could raise. The hospital is not a hotel—nurses give patient care, not deliver room service—and patients may feel worse after surgery or some other procedures than they did when they arrived. Well intended though this physician's remarks may be, they open wide the door to a major discrepancy between expectations and reality that can result in patient disappointment and anger, and a desire to find a target for those feelings.

Another factor that may affect patient education and support is the attitude of the hospital staff toward patient involvement. It is no secret that medical care, as traditionally practiced, involves authoritarianism on the part of the provider and dependency on that of the consumer. In the traditional medical model, the professional prescribes and the patient complies. It may take some effort to get staff who are accustomed to this approach to work with patients in a more collaborative manner.

☐ What Patient Education Can Do

Even though some patients sue hospitals for both rational and irrational reasons, the majority of patients do not sue. High-quality care is the rule rather than the exception. Patient educators need to reinforce patient perceptions that the quality of care is high and that the hospital staff provides proper support.

Patient education offers hope for the ongoing litigation crisis largely because of the psychosocial support inherent in the teaching–learning process. Patients evaluate their care according to what they perceive, and although most patients may not be able to evaluate the quality of the medical care they receive, they can make judgments about how they are treated personally.

Patient education offers opportunities to encourage patient independence; sharing information is what patient education is all about. Including patients in an exchange of information also means sharing control and power. Knowledge is power; patients who hold it are more likely to feel in control and less likely to feel disappointment and rage when faced with a situation in which they believe that those in whose hands they have placed themselves have abused their trust.

The process of patient education is ideally a collaborative exchange between the educator and the patient—one that should contribute to the creation of a more cooperative, less adversarial climate. Helping patients through the decision-making processes in health care goes a long way toward developing a therapeutic and nonlitigious relationship.

Involvement in Decision Making

When people are hospitalized, they frequently encounter new types of decisions that they may be poorly equipped to handle. Even a highly intellectual and competent college professor may not really understand the difference between coronary bypass surgery and a valve replacement. For the uninitiated, such simple matters as recognizing medications can be difficult. Some decisions can be so difficult that, without encouragement, patients may withdraw entirely from participating, leaving important, personal matters to others.

Although the idea of involving patients in decision making and encouraging their independence is not new, patient educators are playing a larger role in it than they ever have before. There is increased emphasis on personal decision making through standards for patient rights, awareness of informed consent, and legislation regarding advance directives.

Patient Rights
The American Hospital Association's[14] first statement of patient rights and responsibilities dates back to 1973. Since that time, public interest in obtaining information in a timely and courteous manner has continued to build. Consistent with these demands, provider response for the actualization of patient rights has been on the rise. The Joint Commission

on Accreditation of Healthcare Organizations (JCAHO) has placed renewed emphasis on patient rights by transferring the former introductory statements about patient rights (which have been a long-standing aspect of its *Accreditation Manual for Hospitals*) into a separate chapter.[15] By receiving the same treatment as that of other standards, patient rights are now measured and scored as part of the accreditation process.

The expectations established by the JCAHO serve not only as a guideline for providers in organizing services, but also as a resource for attorneys in planning litigation based on national and local standards. Therefore, the patient education manager has responsibility for understanding the intents and ensuring that hospital policies operationalize those intents. Policies must be in place that protect and exercise "the right of the patient, in collaboration with his/her physician, to make decisions involving his/her health care . . . and the right of the patient to the information necessary to enable him/her to make treatment decisions that reflect his/her wishes."[16]

Too often, there is confusion about the roles of physicians and other staff in the decision-making process. At Baptist Hospital of Miami, the Patient Education Liaison Committee has developed a policy that clarifies the role of the nurse in this process (figure 6-1). The policy gives the nurse responsibility for helping the patient, but with the mutual involvement of the physician, particularly in matters of informed consent.

Informed Consent

The term *informed consent* has received attention in biomedical situations primarily since 1972. It involves the willing and uncoerced acceptance of a medical intervention by a competent patient after there has been disclosure by the physician about diagnosis, prognosis, the nature of the intervention, risks, benefits, and alternatives to treatment.[17] The physician is responsible for providing informed consent.[18,19] However, if there are questions or reasons to believe that the patient has not been adequately informed, other care givers serve as the patient's advocates. "According to many hospitals' policies, making sure that the patient understands what the doctor told him is the nurse's responsibility. So, if you (as the nurse) discover that a patient is confused about the procedure he consented to, you can give him more information; if he remains confused, or if you don't feel qualified to give him the information he needs, document your observations on his chart and make sure the doctor answers his questions."[20]

Informed consent is much more than a ritual of obtaining signatures on forms. It is an opportunity for meaningful instruction and for building rapport between patient and physician through a clear understanding of the diagnosis and course of treatment (including the risks, benefits, and alternatives). Informed consent is the premise on which patients make decisions to participate in treatment.

There can be confusion about informed consent and consent to treat. When patients are admitted to hospitals, they grant permission to be treated, or *consent to treat*—consent to receive the usual services of the hospital (for example, nursing care, intravenous fluids, respiratory treatment). Without the patient's permission, the hospital and its practitioners may be liable for "unconsented touching" or "battery."[21] The patient is giving approval to proceed with the physical and psychological matters unique to routine health care. Without such approval, patients are not admitted.

But such global approval does not apply to the more invasive and risk-prone procedures. Informed consent, then, is used as the way to involve the patient in these specific care decisions. Dialogue about these decisions needs to occur early enough for the patient to have time to absorb the information and consider the alternatives.

Once the physician has informed the patient, the nurse helps by restating the issues. When patients are struggling with treatment decisions, the nurse or other care giver can help by phrasing questions that engage the patient as an individual making a unique and very personal choice: What other information do you need? What do you understand about the risks? The benefits? What other choice(s) do you have? What difference will the treatment make? Must you have the treatment now, or do you have another choice?

Figure 6-1. Baptist Hospital of Miami Policy and Procedure Manual

Policy number: 308.04C
Addendum

☐ Administrative

☒ Divisional Patient Care Services

☐ Departmental

Nursing Generic Manual

Subject:

Patient Education/Discharge Preparation Nursing Functions

Procedure for Implementation:

The professional nurse is independently responsible for "the observation, assessment, nursing diagnosis, planning, intervention, and evaluation of care; health teaching and counseling of the ill, injured, or infirm; and the promotion of wellness, maintenance of health, and prevention of illness of others."*

The professional nurse is responsible for initiating the following Patient Education/Discharge Preparation activities:

A. Support in preparing patient for diagnostic tests and procedures.
   1. Provide information about tests and procedures before they are done.
   2. Explain hospital terminology.
B. Help for the patient/family making decisions about hospitalization and nursing care.
   1. Provide information and support for making decisions related to hospitalization and nursing care within hospital protocols.
   2. Encourage communication with physician regarding treatment issues.
   3. Provide information to promote health and encourage patient, parent, or family attitudes that support the medical plan of care.
   4. Reinforce information provided by the physician regarding diagnosis, prognosis, and topics concerning informed consent. (See Policy 309.02; Consent/Authorization: Nursing Responsibilities.)
C. Continued care/self-management.
   1. Prepare patient/family for continued care at home with regard to hygiene, general nutrition and diet, elimination, skin and wound care, and prevention of the spread of infection/infectious diseases.
   2. Help patient and family develop the skills needed for self-care. This includes medications, activity level, physical care, nutritional support, and other needs identified by the nurse or prescribed by the physician.
D. Documentation of the patient/family response by including:
   1. The patient's attention/participation in care (affective).
   2. What the patient is able or unable to do (skills).
   3. Information that indicates a patient's level of understanding of care (cognitive).
   4. Resources given to the patient and family.

*Florida Department of Professional Regulation, Board of Nursing, Chapter 464, October 1989.

Submitted by: _____   Approved by: _____
              Director, Health Education   (Vice-President Patient Care Services)

              _____
              Patient Education Coordinator

Approval Date: _____

Review Dates: _____

Revision Dates: _____

What else do you need to know? The patient may want to write down questions that remain unanswered. In this role the nurse serves as a reinforcer of the information that has previously been given by the physician and facilitates patient involvement in the choice. Clarity between nurse and physician roles has helped to promote patient participation in choices and care-giver satisfaction and harmony.

Advance Directives

Advance directives is the generic term for statements made by people, when they are competent, to direct health care decisions when they are unable to communicate. The Patient Self-Determination Act of 1990 is federal legislation that was born out of the Omnibus Budget Reconciliation Act to ensure that patients have the right to participate in, and direct health care decisions through, advance directives. The provisions of the law require that hospitals, home health agencies, hospices, and other institutional recipients of Medicare or Medicaid funds follow the laws of each state regarding advance directives and specifically meet the following criteria:[22]

- Provide written information to adult patients about their rights under state law (sometimes established by state legislatures and sometimes by state courts) regarding advance directives
- Document in the patient's medical record whether he or she has an advance directive (in the case of a hospital, at the time of admission; a home health agency, before coming under the care of the agency; a hospice, at the time of initial receipt of care)
- Not discriminate or otherwise respect patient rights differently based on whether he or she has an advance directive

The self-determination law went into effect December 1, 1991. Since that time, hospitals nationwide have written policies, procedures, and literature for patients and provided educational programs about advance directives.

Advance directives are generally of two types:

1. *Living wills.* These are documents that allow people to decide, while they are competent, the degree to which they want to have life-prolonging procedures when they have a terminal illness and death is imminent.
2. *Health care surrogate (also called health care proxy or durable power of attorney for health care).* This is the designation of a person to make decisions for the patient who is so incapacitated that he or she cannot make those decisions.

A health care surrogate has the role of making decisions or refusing or accepting treatments. Essentially, he or she is the individual who makes the informed choices that a patient would otherwise make. Powers of the surrogate are usually limited, do not include all procedures (for example, abortion, sterilization), and sometimes must be renewed after a certain period of time elapses.

The Patient Self-Determination Act has served to increase public awareness of advance directives and, in time, will increase the number of people who are admitted to hospitals with advance directives in hand. To date, the number of people entering hospitals with advance directives in hand has been small. Federal legislation includes the provision for a national educational campaign that will continue to encourage the public to seek information.

Despite this provision, patient education managers (PEMs) would be wise to carefully screen educational literature and media to determine if the terminology and issues apply at the state level. Little can be said generically that the national audience can act on other than the right to have an advance directive or a surrogate. Advance directives are not necessarily transferable to states other than the one of residence. However, some helpful advice is to complete an advance directive now (while there is time to think ahead); give copies to close family members, physicians, attorneys, and others interested in the person's decisions; keep a copy available or maybe a note in a wallet stating where the advance directive can be located; and renew it annually by reviewing and affixing a new date.

Admission to the hospital is hardly the time to talk about end-of-life decisions, because most people are being admitted with the hope of successful outcomes. But providing the documents for advance directives shows the organization's commitment to the law and gives the patient the chance to review them later, at home, with the knowledge that there are people at the hospital who can provide additional information if needed. Hospital boards of trustees, physicians, and the community often have a high degree of interest in this subject, providing the patient educator an opportunity to serve as a resource and to demonstrate the depth and scope of patient education.

Effective Patient Education Programs

Incorporating patient education realistically and sensitively into hospital care can have valuable, but sometimes intangible benefits. After all, the success stories are those that do not end up in court. The failures, of which there are far fewer, are relived in litigation. Therefore, it is not always easy to link the effect of a high-quality educational effort to reduced malpractice. But the people who give care and represent hospitals know of successes. The following ideas, a telephone follow-up system and a bereavement support program, have been successful in providing patients with the information and support they need and in encouraging good relationships between hospitals and patients.

Telephone Follow-up

For more than six years, patients at Baptist Hospital of Miami have been receiving follow-up phone calls at home from their nurses. Whether discharged from the emergency department, a medical–surgical unit, or ambulatory surgery, patients have a chance to ask questions and be reassured that they are progressing. Most often, the conversation is brief and rewarding. A 54-year-old gentleman with diabetes was so impressed that his nurse would check on him at home by phone that it brought tears to his eyes when he talked about it. The phone call was a pleasant and unexpected surprise.

But on occasion, a patient with a problem is encountered. A nurse in cardiac rehabilitation remembers calling a patient routinely, only to find the patient "not quite her former self" and unable to carry on a coherent conversation. Concerned, the nurse had the patient, who was having a stroke, readmitted through the emergency department. Her intervention made an important difference. Telephone follow-up in cardiac rehabilitation is a "good part of my day," according to the nurse who works there—so much so that telephone numbers are readily available and calls are made sometimes in the afternoon, for example, to a patient who was not quite up to par when exercising that very morning.

In establishing a telephone follow-up system, these factors must be considered:

- Determine criteria for which patients routinely are called. Sampling patients is not advisable; rather, it is better to call patients from certain service areas or those with certain conditions.
- Establish a time frame within which calls are made.
- Create policies that communicate the telephone requirements.
- Teach staff questions and information to elicit from the patient, as well as additional information to give to the patient.
- Refer the patient for any identified problems.
- Document date and time of telephone call attempts and patient responses.
- Call another time if a problem is identified.

According to the nurse manager in outpatient surgery, the telephone call program at Baptist Hospital has been highly successful. Every patient who has outpatient surgery and is discharged without being admitted to the hospital is called one to five days after going home. The nurse asks basic questions: "How do you feel? What problems have you had? Have you talked with your doctor?" Patient responses are recorded on either the fact sheet, the nurse's notes, or observation notes, depending on the type of procedure. The dates and times of the calls are noted, as well as specific information and referrals.

Frequently, patients have had problems with pain management, dressings, nausea and vomiting, hematomas—problems that can be relieved by the information the nurse provides over the phone. On occasion, patients are referred directly to the emergency department (for example, if they have changing levels of consciousness or cardiac status), but most often, a problem is referred to the patient's physician. Anesthesiologists are particularly attentive to calling patients when they receive a referral from nurses—such referrals may involve complaints ranging from sore throats and body aches to tightness in the chest and stiff necks. All these contacts and the information provided help to abate more serious complications and relieve the patient's anxiety. This help goes a long way toward maintaining much-needed rapport between hospital and patient.

Bereavement Support

The risk manager at Baptist Hospital of Miami is quick to point out the value of bereavement support in helping patients and families understand loss. The hospital's experience is long-standing—dating back to the early 1980s—with a team of nurses and chaplains giving counseling and support to parents whose children have died at birth. Instead of whisking the baby away in the traditional hush-hush manner, the nurse gives the parents time to hold the newborn who has died and to reflect on their loss. A staff member takes photographs of the baby and footprints for a "memory card," given to the parents before they go home or filed in case they might want the picture in the future.

At first, such intervention was unusual and was questioned by both physicians and nurses, because it was such a diversion from custom. But the team prevailed and gradually taught others that parents' needs are different from those of providers. After a decade of experience, the risk manager is confident that this program has helped parents deal with grief and release their anger. Instead of running into a blank wall of professional silence, parents are surrounded by supportive people who address their questions and provide tangible memories of their lost child. The inpatient program for support has grown into continued group meetings and the organization of SHARE, Pregnancy and Infant Loss, Inc. (a national group).

In addition, bereavement support has become an organized activity for families of oncology patients. A 10-week program meets weekly and is led by a nurse and a social worker. Spouses and other close relatives enroll about three months after the death of their loved ones. The program follows guidelines established by the Grief Education Institute.[23] Those attending have a one-hour interview and assessment prior to enrolling to determine their readiness for participation in the group. Readiness may depend on attention span, emotional health, and willingness to participate. Once the sessions begin, each builds on the previous one with the intent that each person will work on grief and socialization. Members learn how feelings of guilt can get in the way of having a good time and how to deal with extreme anger, sometimes directed inappropriately at physicians or other providers. Essentially, through support and information they learn how to reinvest in life. The program goes a long way toward meeting both hospital and individual goals.

☐ How Patient Educators Can Work with Risk Managers

Patient educators need close working relationships with departments throughout the hospital—from the switchboard to the print shop. Collaborative efforts with risk managers can be especially beneficial in gaining support for patient education. If ever there were an effective argument for patient education, it lies in the risk management office, where the benefits of reduced liability are realized. Risk managers are likely to be strong, internal voices for comprehensive patient education. According to the risk manager at Baptist Hospital, "The informed patient is the best patient."[24] The risk management staff supports patient education for both inpatients and the community, an approach that strengthens the health intelligence quotient of known and potential patients.

Risk managers welcome the hard work of patient educators that builds rapport between care givers and patients. Patient educators are often pioneers within hospitals who write literature, foster new programs, and create advocacy strategies for patients. Dealing with the results of the breakdown of rapport and misunderstandings, risk managers can facilitate change within the hospital system and make it easier for patient educators to find the support they need to implement new programs.

Risk management can provide guidance for the PEM with regard to the following:

- Review of written materials for appropriateness of content to avoid implied guarantees and/or unnecessary statements of standards and to ensure that information is presented objectively
- Identification of key questions that may require legal consultation (for example, Should nursing staff serve as witnesses to signatures on advance directives?)
- Identification of types of litigation that influence hospital practices
- Review of policies and procedures that involve patient education (for example, informed consent policies)
- Special attention for patients who are angry and are seeking restitution

Hospital risk managers can sometimes serve as a "listening ear" for patients who do not know where to direct their concerns. Risk managers have experience in dealing with basic human needs and emotions when people are overstressed.

Risk managers also have an "eye" for effective documentation, rarely a favorite subject of busy practitioners who are more interested in being face to face with a patient than having their heads buried in a written record. Giving patients written information to take home goes a long way toward helping them understand and toward creating the idea that someone cared enough to put it in writing. In the past, it was not uncommon for patients to take home notes scribbled on the bottom of tissue boxes, paper towels, and any plain piece of paper conveniently found. Now, discharge instructions need to be written and readily available for many kinds of patients, but especially for the high-volume, high-risk patients.

Although documentation is important throughout the hospital stay, the need for adequate discharge instructions and documentation of those instructions cannot be overstated. Because short-stay, emergency care, and ambulatory treatment represent such brief encounters in the hospital, patients need written information to remind them of care directions. The nurse must note the patient's ability to comprehend the information and ensure that medication effects do not confuse the patient. Often it is best to provide the information before the procedure is done. When the patient is being discharged, information must be provided to the person who will be staying with the patient, including a review of the signs and symptoms that should be reported to the physician. The information and the patient's or care giver's response must be written in the medical record carefully. The risk management staff is a useful resource in helping drive home the point about the importance of documentation in short-stay areas.

When care givers have taken the initiative to listen carefully and discuss the sensitive and complex subject matter of health care, the possibility for litigation diminishes. In a telephone conversation, Robert White, director of claims and loss prevention for the Physicians Protective Trust Fund, clearly stated: "Patient rapport and good documentation are the only two things that matter in loss prevention. Many people like to think it's much more sophisticated than that. But it all comes down to those two basic things in the end."[25] In two words, that is patient education.

☐ Conclusion

With the increased incidence of litigation against hospitals and the greater need for information on patient rights, informed consent, and advance directives, it has become more important for patient educators to foster good relationships with patients and to work closely with risk managers. Patient educators can foster good patient relations through formal patient education programs as well as through daily interactions that provide information and psychosocial support.

References

1. Koppel, T. Emergency: Health Care in America [Television program]. Washington, DC: Nightline, 1992.

2. Class, P. Suit pursuits: failure to diagnose is leading cause of lawsuits. *Medical Business* 3(2):10, Jan. 16, 1990.

3. White, R. E. *Loss Prevention for the 90's.* Coral Gables, FL: Physicians Protective Trust Fund, 1991.

4. Localio, A. R., Lawthers, A. G., Brennan, T. A., Laird, N. M., Hebert, L. E., Peterson, L. M., Newhouse, J. P., Weiler, P. C., and Hyatt, H. H. Relation between malpractice claims and adverse events due to negligence. *The New England Journal of Medicine* 325(4):245–51, July 25, 1991.

5. Press, I. The predisposition to file claims: the patient's perspective. *Law, Medicine and Health Care* 12(2):53–62, Apr. 1984.

6. Kinnaird, L. S. Nurse participation in patient education in a community hospital. Doctoral dissertation, *Dissertation Abstracts International* 48(12):3532-B, part I, Florida State University, Tallahassee, FL, June 19, 1988.

7. Bell, W. Telephone communication, Mar. 5, 1992.

8. Class, P. Patient profile: the patient who sues. *Medical Business* 3(2):10, Jan. 16, 1990.

9. Class, P. Patient profile: the patient who sues.

10. Hickson, G. B., Clayton, E. W., Githens, P. B., and Sloan, F. A. Factors that prompted families to file medical malpractice claims following parental injuries. *Journal of the American Medical Association* 267(10):1359–63, Mar. 1992.

11. Cunningham, R. M., Jr. Forty years of trial and error. *Hospitals* 52(23):91–93, 127, Dec. 1, 1978.

12. Strull, W. M., Bernard, L., and Charles, G. Do patients want to participate in decision-making? *Journal of the American Medical Association* 252(21):2990–94, Dec. 7, 1984.

13. Jaco, E. G. *Patient, Physicians, and Illness: A Sourcebook in Behavioral Science and Health.* 3rd ed. New York City: The Free Press, 1979, pp. 202–3.

14. American Hospital Association. A Patient's Bill of Rights. Chicago: AHA, 1992 (Catalog no. 157759).

15. Joint Commission on Accreditation of Healthcare Organizations. *Accreditation Manual for Hospitals.* Oakbrook Terrace, IL: JCAHO, 1992.

16. JCAHO, pp. 103–4.

17. Beauchamp, T. L., and Childress, I. F. *Principles of Biomedical Ethics.* 3rd ed. New York City: Oxford University Press, 1989.

18. Informed consent: opening the doors to physician–patient communication. *Minnesota Medicine* 73:35–39, Oct. 1990.

19. White.

20. Rabinow, J. Avoiding legal risks in the short procedure unit. *Nursing Life,* 1986, pp. 24–25.

21. Informed consent: opening the doors to physician–patient communication, p. 35.

22. McIntyre, R. L. Congress passes "patient self determination act." *Info Trends: Medicine, Law & Ethics* (Newsletter published by the University of Medicine and Dentistry of New Jersey, Robert Wood Johnson Medical School, Piscataway, New Jersey) 6(2):1, 3, Winter 1991.

23. Grief Education Institute. *Bereavement Support Groups: Leadership Manual.* 3rd ed. Denver, CO: GEI, 1988.

24. Personal communication with Baptist Hospital, Feb. 18, 1992.

25. Phone conversation with Robert White, director of claims and loss prevention for the Physicians Protective Trust Fund, Mar. 26, 1992.

Chapter 7
Financing Patient Education

Barbara E. Giloth, M.P.H., C.H.E.S.

☐ Objectives

The reader will be able to:

- Review the current status of third-party reimbursement for patient education
- Identify strategies to maximize third-party reimbursement
- Identify strategies to increase resources overall for patient education

☐ The Challenges in Obtaining Financial and Other Resources for Patient Education Programs

Locating resources to support patient education programming continues to pose major challenges. The fact that most patient education activities are not separately reimbursable by third-party payers has made it difficult for patient education managers (PEMs) to clearly identify a revenue stream that could justify budget increases. The extent to which everyone in the hospital can contribute to a patient education program makes it impossible to focus all resources in one or two cost centers. The degree to which effective patient education must be integrated with clinical service delivery makes it more difficult to answer the question: What does it cost to provide patient education?

The guidance in asking the right questions about financing that is provided in the following section is a good starting point for meeting these challenges. This information, coupled with the useful strategies for increasing third-party reimbursement and other resources described later, can help PEMs to form an overall approach for maximizing resource support for patient education.

☐ Questions to Ask about Financing Patient Education Programs

Depending on the hospital and the role of the PEM within that hospital, the financing questions to be answered will vary. If the PEM's role is primarily coordinative and consultative, the financial questions to be addressed are likely to be the following:

- What is the most efficient and effective way to deliver patient education services to different target populations?
- What amount of resources is needed to deliver such services?
- Which program delivery option is most cost-effective; that is, which option will result in the largest impact for dollars spent?[1]
- Where are the additional resources that will be needed to support a new or expanded service?

If, on the other hand, the PEM heads a department that delivers a series of services such as cardiac rehabilitation, prenatal education, diabetes education, and so forth, a whole different series of questions comes to the fore:[2]

- Is the patient education department's budget on target with the chief financial officer's (CFO's) expectations?
- How can expenses be managed more effectively (for example, through contract staff, staff incentives to accumulate billable hours, clarification of overhead allocations, and so on)?
- Will revenue streams be adequate to meet revenue projections?
- Is the pricing for services appropriate for the local market?

This broad range of questions cannot be answered in only one chapter. For questions related to financial management, including budgeting, the reader should turn to health care financial texts.[3] For questions related to research on the effectiveness and efficiency of various patient education strategies, the reader is referred to chapters 13, 14, and 15 of this book.

☐ Current Status of Reimbursement for Patient Education Services

Although the financing of health care has changed substantially since the landmark document *Financing for Health Education in the United States* was written in 1980, there has basically been little change in the overall status of reimbursement for patient education. Patient education that is integral to care, part of the treatment plan, and delivered under the supervision of a physician has been and continues to be allowable as an administrative expense under nearly all third-party payer policies; yet it is still rare to find specific patient education programs, other than diabetes patient education, reimbursed as a separate service.

Although *Current Procedural Terminology* (CPT) codes currently exist for group counseling sessions, most public and private insurance plans do not provide separate coverage for these services. Codes only establish a mechanism for billing; they cannot guarantee third-party reimbursement. The recent change in physician payment via the resource-based relative value scale does not increase separate reimbursement for patient education, but does increase the relative value of payment to physician groups such as family practitioners who are likely to provide such cognitive services.

Diabetes patient education stands out as the major patient education reimbursement success story for a variety of reasons:

1. Diabetes is a condition that requires daily self-management if it is to be treated successfully. Serious problems are likely to occur if the self-management regimen is not followed regularly. The patient education required for this self-management is substantial. The benefits of diabetes education programs can be measured quickly, and there are likely to be significant changes in emergency department use and hospital admissions that can be translated easily into cost savings.

2. The American Association of Diabetes Educators (AADE), along with the American Diabetes Association and the Centers for Disease Control's diabetes initiative, has provided a large and visible lobbying force at the national and state levels. Physicians have played active roles in these organizations.

3. Under the guidance of the National Diabetes Advisory Board, this diabetes community was able to develop a set of standards for diabetes patient education programs. Although these became the focal point for a formal recognition program under the auspices of the American Diabetes Association, they have also been used by state diabetes control programs and insurers as a basis for quality assurance and as a condition for reimbursement.[4] Third-party reimbursement for diabetes patient education was received by 40 percent of the respondents to a 1988 AADE membership survey.[5]

4. State Diabetes Control Programs took the lead in approaching Medicare and other third-party payers with a plan to reimburse diabetes outpatient education. Maine was the first state to get all four major insurers (Blue Cross/Blue Shield, Medicare, Medicaid, and commercial insurance companies) to approve diabetes patient education as a separate, reimbursable charge. They did this through a three-year pilot program at 24 health centers that tracked reductions in length of hospital stay and overall cost savings.[6] Current data suggest that there is at least some reimbursement for diabetes outpatient education programs by all major third-party payers in a majority of states.[7]

Although much can be learned from the diabetes example in terms of standards development, coalition building, approaches to third-party payers, and estimating costs of patient education programs, the health care delivery and financing issues have changed sufficiently so that it is less likely that other diseases and conditions can follow the same path. It is clear, for example, that managed care of one sort or another is likely to become the rule rather than the exception.[8] Although it might seem that the visibility of patient education should increase under such a system, the incentives are toward bundled payment, continuity of care, efficient use of services, and measurable outcomes of care rather than toward separate reimbursement for services.

As part of documenting the status of third-party reimbursement for patient education, the following section reviews more specifically the extent and type of reimbursement provided by each of the major third-party payer groups.

Medicaid

Medicaid is the federal–state government program that finances health care for specified low-income individuals. By federal mandate, certain basic services must be offered by states to all categorically needy Medicaid enrollees.

Although patient education is allowable as part of covered inpatient and outpatient services, few patient education services are covered separately. Emphasis is on prenatal programs, which usually include prenatal education. Under the Early Periodic Screening, Diagnostic, and Treatment (EPSDT) Program enacted by Congress in 1967, states are required to provide health assessments and examinations and immunizations to all Medicaid-eligible children under the age of 21. Many states have done a limited job of informing eligible parents of the availability of this program, and restrictions on access to services and provider qualifications have limited the number of children receiving services.

In 1989, under Omnibus Budget Reconciliation Act (OBRA) legislation, Congress mandated outreach to bring potential beneficiaries into the program and specifically included health education and anticipatory guidance as a covered service, mandated treatment of conditions identified through screening, and expanded access to children not currently covered by the program.[9] Implementation of these expansions appears spotty because of the cost implications for strained state budgets.

Several key reimbursement problems are specific to Medicaid. First, many states have set reimbursement rates so low that hospitals lose money for every Medicaid patient they service.[10] It is currently estimated that on the average Medicaid pays $.80 for every dollar of care provided.[11] Second, the Medicaid program currently covers a smaller and smaller percentage of those below the federal poverty level; in 1976, 35 percent of such persons were not covered. By 1991, this figure had soared to 60 percent.[12] Therefore, no matter what policies the actual state Medicaid program chooses to implement, a growing percentage of the poverty population has no coverage for basic medical care, let alone patient education services. With an estimated 36 million people without health insurance,[13] the question of whether patient education services are reimbursed is not relevant to this population.

Medicare

Medicare is the federal government program that provides health care to elderly and disabled individuals. Since its inception in 1965, Medicare reimbursement has been limited to care that is "reasonable and necessary for the treatment of an illness or injury."[14] In general, Medicare does not cover primary preventive services for people who are well.

Although more than 450 bills have been introduced since 1965 that have sought to add various preventive benefits under the Medicare program,[15] the only ones that have been enacted reflect a bias toward immunization and screening rather than education and counseling. Currently the only preventive services covered broadly include immunizations for beneficiaries at high risk of contracting hepatitis B, pneumococcal pneumonia immunizations, pap smears, and mammograms.

Medicare, however, will expand access to preventive services for eligible patients using Federally Qualified Health Centers receiving a grant under Sections 329, 330, and 340 of the Public Health Service Act. According to regulations published in the June 12, 1992, *Federal Register*,[16] preventive primary services—including nutritional assessment, preventive health education, and immunizations—will be covered when provided in these settings. Specifically *excluded* are group or mass information programs, health education classes, or group education activities including media productions and publications. Related Medicaid rules are being developed separately.

The introduction in 1983 of the prospective pricing system and diagnosis-related groups (DRGs) essentially put an end to hopes that inpatient education might be reimbursable as a separate line item. Concern about patients being discharged "quicker and sicker," however, has resulted in more attention being paid to discharge preparation. Diabetes continues to be the major outpatient education service that is reimbursed separately given that the program meets preset guidelines such as the national standards mentioned earlier. Although never enacted, legislation introduced in 1991—the Medicare Prevention Benefits Act—would provide reimbursement for risk assessment, preventive interventions, and counseling for persons first becoming eligible for Medicare.

As with the Medicaid program, hospitals can expect to lose a significant amount of money caring for Medicare patients. Newly released data by the American Hospital Association suggest that hospitals will pay out $9 billion more than they receive in fiscal year 1993 for taking care of hospitalized Medicare patients.[17]

Private Health Insurance Plans

Traditionally, private health insurance plans have covered patient education and related services in one of four ways. Most commonly, such services have been covered through incorporation into administrative costs.[18] Less frequently, insurers have offered a benefit package that includes specified patient education benefits, for example, cardiac rehabilitation. They may also offer incentives to maintain healthy behavior or provide health education programs.

In 1991, Blue Cross and Blue Shield Association issued guidelines designed to serve as the basis for a model preventive services benefit. Based on screening guidelines developed by the U.S. Public Health Service and the American College of Physicians, coverage includes well-baby care, childhood immunizations, and routine adult medical screening tests for cancer, heart disease, and other preventable illnesses.[19] The Health Insurance Association of America (HIAA) followed suit in 1992, announcing "a campaign to encourage employers to promote benefit packages that cover preventive services of demonstrated effectiveness."[20] Although it is too soon to tell how widely this benefit will be adopted, particularly given employer concern with rising health care costs, this does represent an opportunity for plans to expand their emphasis on prevention, although not necessarily on patient education.

Another way that private insurers have supported patient and health education programs is through the use of financial incentives to encourage the adoption of healthy behaviors, such as premium discounts to nonsmokers or health club discounts for policyholders. Still others are providing health education programs directly to policyholders. For example, *Healthtrac* is a series of consumer education/health management programs that provide health risk appraisals and other health education interventions via the mail to subscribers of participating Blue Cross and Blue Shield plans as well as other employer groups. Some of the programs, such as *Babytrac*, are targeted to specific consumer groups—in this case, pregnant women and those interested in becoming pregnant—and behaviors particularly relevant to that group, such as ongoing prenatal care, smoking cessation, and adequate nutrition.[21,22]

Finally, insurance companies have supported a variety of research and demonstration projects designed to test the feasibility of implementing new benefits for patient education and preventive services and/or the effectiveness of these services. For example, in 1979, the Blue Cross and Blue Shield Association of Greater New York began reimbursing for care provided in New York University's Cooperative Care Unit; it also cooperated in the evaluation of this program by providing utilization and financial data to the university. The INSURE project began in 1980, funded by insurance companies, private foundations, and the federal government to study preventive services as a health insurance benefit. The preventive services provided were appropriate for different age, sex, and risk factors and included physical examinations, laboratory tests, immunizations, and patient education.[23] After five years and at least one preventive care visit to a participating physician, the at-risk study patients had significantly reduced four risk factors compared with the control patients. A greater proportion quit smoking, began to exercise regularly, and always used seat belts, and the female patients began to perform monthly breast examinations.[24]

State governments have increasingly enacted legislation establishing requirements for coverage of selected benefits under private health insurance plans. These "mandated benefits" apply to group health insurance plans purchased by employers from private health insurance companies. They do not apply to companies that self-insure, nor do they apply to employers who provide no health coverage to their employees. A 1988 survey of state health care coverage laws showed that the most commonly mandated services are mammography, well-baby care, diabetes education, cytologic screening, preventive care for children, and cardiac rehabilitation.[25] Because of the extent of self-insurance, it is not clear how much impact this legislation has had on actual access to health education and preventive services.

Health Maintenance Organizations and Preferred Provider Organizations

Health maintenance organizations (HMOs) are responsible for providing a comprehensive range of services for a defined population for a preset fee. The capitation payment gives HMOs a financial incentive to keep patients healthy; they conserve resources if their members' use of lower-cost primary care services, including health education, prevents utilization of more expensive secondary or tertiary services. There is considerable variation, however, in the health education and preventive services offered by different types of HMOs, with group or staff models such as Kaiser Permanente and Group Health of Puget Sound often investing substantial resources in patient education and health promotion. Independent practice organizations (IPOs) appear less likely to offer such services. A 1988 survey of HMOs by Group Health Association of America found that over 73 percent of the respondents reported that they cover health education classes.[26]

A 1986 survey of preferred provider organizations, or PPOs (organizations in which patients obtain discounted health care by visiting only the group's designated providers), documented a substantial interest in health education and preventive care. More than half of PPOs cover periodic preventive checkups, and almost half reimburse physicians and other health providers who teach patients how to minimize risks to their health.[27] In other surveys of insurance coverage for preventive services, HMOs are the most likely to cover preventive services, followed by PPOs, and followed further by traditional indemnity plans.[28]

Despite broader coverage of preventive services, many consumers avoid HMOs and PPOs because of the restrictions they impose on the selection of providers. However, managed care and capitation appear to be two strategies that are playing increasingly important roles in the health care reform debate.

☐ Strategies to Increase Third-Party Reimbursement

Although the overall third-party reimbursement climate is not favorable for the separate reimbursement of patient education, there are some opportunities to increase payments for services that are largely educational in nature. The challenge for PEMs is to work with their CFOs and administrative staff to assess the potential for additional reimbursement given the local financial context and the range of hospital services. There is a real risk that enormous amounts of time can be spent for a minimal return. Some patient education services, for example, are of such short duration and relatively small expense that the administrative costs of a separate billing would render this impractical.

The following five steps offer an opportunity for PEMs to assess and tap local opportunities for reimbursement before moving on to the wider range of financing strategies. Although somewhat dated because of changes in health care financing in the past five years, *Third-party Reimbursement for Diabetes Outpatient Education*, published in 1986 by the American Diabetes Association, offers helpful step-by-step guidance regarding approaches to third-party payers:[29]

1. *Assess extent of current patient education reimbursement.* This first step involves data collection to determine the current status of reimbursement for patient education services offered by the hospital. Some of this information may already be available through routinely generated financial reports. Some may be available through patient education department records if the department provides direct patient services. Some of the questions may never have been asked before and may require meetings with the business office and the CFO. It is also important at this time to assess the interest by the hospital in actively pursuing reimbursement opportunities for patient education. If there is no such interest, the PEM's time would best be spent looking at other strategies to increase resources for patient education. The following data should be gathered:
   • What charges are currently generated from patient education services?
   • What proportion of these charges are currently paid for by patients themselves?
   • Are any of the charges for patient education services submitted for third-party reimbursement?

- Of the charges submitted for third-party reimbursement, what proportion are reimbursed?
- Do any of the managed care contracts negotiated by the hospital include patient education services? If so, was any consideration given to the amount of resources required to implement these services?
- Does the CFO think it would be useful to pursue additional reimbursement for patient education services?

2. *Assess the overall payer environment.* This information is critical to identifying opportunities for potential expansion of reimbursement. The most likely sources of information are again routine financial reports and the CFO. The strategic planning department may have data regarding local employers and their health care benefit plans. The Chamber of Commerce and/or local business coalition also may be sources of employer information. State, local, and county health departments can provide data on poverty indices, extent of Medicaid coverage, and existence of state-mandated benefits. Because much of this information will have relevance for a broad range of hospital services, it is recommended that the PEM work with key financial and administrative staff to coordinate its collection and analysis. The following data should be gathered:
   - What is the hospital's payer mix? Are patients primarily covered by public programs, or is there substantial private coverage?
   - Who are the largest insurers for the hospital's major services? Be as specific as possible.
   - Do any employer groups comprise a significant component of the hospital's inpatient or outpatient caseload?
   - To what extent are HMOs and managed care plans a significant part of the hospital's market share?
   - How are EPSDT (see p. 131) services provided in the community?
   - Are there any state-mandated patient education or preventive service benefits?
   - To what extent are the major employers, including the hospital, self-insured?
   - To what extent do the physicians on the hospital medical staff offer patient education services, and to what extent are they reimbursed for them?

3. *Assess payer interest.* Although the third-party payer policies described in the previous section represent overall directions for reimbursement, individual commercial insurers and individual Blue Cross/Blue Shield plans set local priorities. State Medicaid plans differ, and the fiscal intermediaries for Medicare often interpret regulations differently. An initial strategy in reaching these payers is to meet with their appropriate staff members to gather the following information:
   - How does each payer view the scope and importance of patient education?
   - Does the payer ever reimburse separately for a patient education service? If so, under what conditions?
   - Does the payer reimburse for an education service, such as a smoking cessation program, if it is part of cardiac rehabilitation?
   - Would the payer consider reimbursing for a patient education service in the future?
   - Would the payer consider a pilot project to look at such reimbursement?
   - Do local payers offer patient education or health promotion services directly to subscribers? If so, is there an opportunity to contract with hospital staff as providers?
   - Are local payers willing to support hospital-sponsored patient education or community health education programs through financial or in-kind contributions?

4. *Focus on patient education services with a high likelihood for reimbursement.* There is little reason for a PEM to try to increase reimbursement for inpatient services. There was never much opportunity for separate reimbursement of inpatient education, but the advent of DRGs ended what little there was. Reimbursement is

most likely for outpatient chronic disease services that seek to ensure that the patient and family have the skills they need to manage the condition in question.

Diabetes education has received the most reimbursement, accelerated in the 1980s by the development of national standards and a recognition program, as described earlier in the chapter. Diabetes educators have been particularly successful at demonstrating to insurers the positive cost impact of outpatient diabetes education services. Other similar types of services include cardiac rehabilitation, pulmonary rehabilitation, ostomy management, IV therapy, physical therapy, and occupational therapy. Like diabetes patient education, these services are all very treatment-oriented, and although they have substantial education components, they appear to have had some success with reimbursement because they are "rehabilitation" or "management" services.

Prenatal education continues to receive substantial emphasis because of the nationwide interest in lowering infant mortality. This interest does not usually translate into direct reimbursement for such services, but rather into increased availability of grant funds such as through the national Healthy Start initiative, into special programs at the state level that increase the working poor's accessibility to prenatal care, and into an expansion of prenatal education programs sponsored at the worksite.

Health promotion programs such as smoking cessation and weight reduction are more likely to be reimbursed if they are seen as treatment for an already-existing condition; however, some commercial insurers and Blue Cross and Blue Shield plans offer limited reimbursement for these types of services. Again, health promotion programs are more likely to be directly sponsored by the employer or insurer than reimbursed as part of a third-party agreement.

5. *Integrate patient education into outpatient care.* A large percentage of outpatient education services are activities that should be integrated into the routine delivery of outpatient care, especially primary care. Patient education for hypertensives, for example, requires assessment, problem solving, and reinforcement over time at every visit. PEMs can work with physicians and outpatient staff to look for ways to ensure that these services are integrated efficiently. For example, Kaiser Permanente in Northern California has been studying ways to develop a "learning environment" in which the practitioners are able to easily access educational tools and resources.[30] Other ambulatory care managers are identifying ways that they can develop systems and incentives that will support implementation of patient education and, more broadly, preventive services.[31-33]

Some innovative ambulatory care managers are developing new types of outpatient services that address the patient education, counseling, and limited medical management that specific groups of chronic disease patients need. For example, the Department of Neurology at Good Samaritan Hospital and Medical Center, in Portland, Oregon, began their Continuing Care Clinics to provide comprehensive outpatient care that focuses on the impact of Alzheimer's disease, multiple sclerosis, and amyotrophic lateral sclerosis (ALS), also called Lou Gehrig's disease, on the family unit as well as the patient. Care plans may include individualized education regarding the course of the illness, its effects and options to consider in future planning, guidance in managing specific symptoms, supportive counseling, referral to community resources, triage to appropriate medical specialists, and introduction to essential legal/financial decisions. These clinics are run as physician offices using common procedural terminology (CPT) codes for billing purposes. Visits with the RN are billed as a minimal visit because only physician supervision is required.[34] (For more on these clinics, see chapter 18.)

☐ Strategies to Increase Resources

Although maximizing existing third-party reimbursement for patient education is important, a total focus on this activity will not only lead to frustration, but it may also jeopardize overall resource support within the institution. Instead of this approach, an overarching resource identification and implementation strategy should be identified. The following eight steps lay out the scope of such a strategy.

Clarify the Organization's Financial Goals

It is important to identify the organization's financial expectations for the patient education program. In general, because of the integration of patient education into a wide variety of roles and departments, it is next to impossible for the hospital coordinating function to generate enough revenue to cover even direct expenses. Individual program areas such as cardiac rehabilitation or diabetes education may, in and of themselves, generate enough revenue to cover direct costs or perhaps break even.

Pressuring administration to specify financial goals (rather than waiting for them to cut programs when they lose money) provides PEMs with a context in which to negotiate. For example, if the goal is unrealistic, a PEM then has an opportunity to negotiate, trading unrealistic financial expectations for the expected impact of patient education on factors such as length of stay, quality indicators, use of other hospital services, or community image. Look for the answers to the following questions:

- Are prenatal education services viewed as a community benefit, or are they viewed as a revenue-producing service?
- What is the expectation of the Board and/or administration regarding the overall direct financial contribution of patient education to the organization?
- To what extent are other benefits of patient education seen as critical enough to outweigh scant revenues?

These questions must be answered if PEMs wish to avoid spending enormous amounts of time trying to cover all financing options.

Specify Needed Resources

An early step in any financing strategy is to know what resources are needed to accomplish the desired objectives. Yet this step is often left out in the early stages of resource development for patient education. This happens partly because PEMs do not usually come to their positions with a financial background and may be intimidated by such analysis. It may also occur because PEMs are afraid to identify the multitude of resources that are contributing to patient education programs for fear that this may be ammunition for staff and program cuts. The extent to which the details of the financial analysis can be shared has to do with the relationship established with the CFO and how patient education is viewed by senior management in the hospital. In any case, such an analysis must be done in order to be able to move ahead with a successful financing strategy.

It seems intuitively obvious that resources cannot be generated to finance an activity until their amount has been specified. Yet patient educators are often unable to say how much time it takes to accomplish specific patient education objectives. Determining this is an important first step in calculating the costs of a patient education program, because staff time is usually a significant component of total costs. An example of time analysis for cancer education is presented by Patricia Agre and colleagues at Memorial Sloan-Kettering Cancer Center in New York.[35] This step feeds directly into a broad cost analysis that seeks to estimate the cost of a program so that decisions can be made about implementation feasibility.[36]

The way costs are presented, especially to others, depends on the financial systems in the particular hospital. The way in which the patient education program overall is organized also has an impact on the way needed resources are identified. For example, if the hospital has a patient education department, part of the costs of any individual program may be a percentage of the department's expenses. Although accumulating information on the resources to plan, run, and evaluate all patient education programs takes time, beginning such analysis with the next program to be developed will provide a jumping-off point for future analysis.

Generally, program costs can be separated into two parts: development costs and ongoing program expenses. Development costs include planning time, purchase of package programs, purchase of materials, staff training, and initial promotion. These costs vary depending on whether the organization develops its own program or purchases an already-existing program. Ongoing program expenses include staff teaching time, documentation time, registration time, secretarial time, equipment use, materials, and space/janitorial services and other indirect costs.

Increase Administrative Support for Patient Education

Lack of adequate resources for patient education can be related to general resource constraints faced by all hospital services as well as to the difficulty in identifying visible revenue streams. However, an overriding challenge for PEMs is the chronic lack of administrative support for implementation of a coordinated and hospitalwide patient education program. Although it is important to take advantage of opportunities for increasing resources through third-party reimbursement and other funding sources, demonstrating the impact of patient education on organizational goals such as patient outcomes, patient satisfaction, efficient use of resources, and risk management is critical to the success of the program.[37] Not only is this likely to result in increased budget, but it is likely to result in the hospitalwide support that is necessary for multidisciplinary collaboration and multidepartmental cooperation.

Several studies on the utilization of preventive services suggest the importance of institutional strategies broader than increased reimbursement in order to ensure that such services are utilized. The Rand Health Insurance Study, for example, showed that even when care was 100 percent reimbursed, enrollees did not receive adequate preventive care, which suggests that reimbursement in and of itself is not sufficient to ensure that services are delivered.[38] More recently, data from a survey of primary care physicians suggest that the new Medicare reimbursement for mammograms will not increase utilization until physicians are convinced that such screening is effective for this population.[39]

Identify Other Management Opportunities to Influence Budget

On the downside, revenue is difficult to identify for patient education because of its ubiquity: It is everywhere in the hospital. The continuous presence of patient education, however, can make it impossible to ignore when resource allocation is being considered. For example, patient classification systems can be used to document the amount of time that patient education of different types of patients requires. Once the amount of time is known, it can be multiplied by the salaries of various involved staff members to find out the cost of providing patient education. Estimates for managed care contracts should include patient education because of the potential impact of this service on the efficient use of resources by patients. The Centers for Excellence concept also offers another opportunity to increase visibility and therefore resources for patient education; such centers may contract with a patient education department to provide target population-related services. For example, a cardiology center may contract with patient education for smoking cessation and stress management programs.

Increase Efficiency

PEMs have three major opportunities to demonstrate an impact on organizational efficiency. First, they can show that implementation of many specific patient education interventions have positive impacts on resource utilization. For example, appropriate test or surgical preparation can reduce the number of canceled procedures due to misunderstood instructions.

Early and well-planned patient education interventions with patients who have complex behaviors to implement at home can decrease length of stay, reduce follow-up calls, and reduce emergency department visits.[40] Second, they can work through hospitalwide management of patient education to reduce duplication of activity, materials, and equipment; streamline procedures; and consolidate donated services. For example, the Department of Patient and Community Services at Kent General Hospital in Dover, Delaware, prepares an annual cost savings report that documents the value of donated materials and services (see figure 7-1). Use of targeted print and visual materials can save clinician teaching time that may be more effectively utilized for individualized teaching. Third, they can recommend elimination of services that are not well utilized, that consistently fail to meet objectives, or that are being done more effectively by other organizations in the community.

Collaborate Internally and Externally

There should be little question that internal and external collaboration is the most powerful source of resources for patient education. This is partly because of the nature of patient education—a part of everyone's job description. The effectiveness of educational interventions is likely to increase with the synergy of health care providers working together. These interventions are a function that is strengthened by a variety of techniques, most of which taken by themselves are not high-cost items.

Chapter 2 has already addressed the process of identifying internal and external resources. This information can be used as a basis for a more targeted look at the time, space, and material resources that are available to accomplish a specific patient education program. On the other hand, chapter 4, which deals with interdisciplinary collaboration, provides a guide to team development as a strategy to increase resource availability for, as well as effectiveness of, patient education programs. More specific examples of external partnerships are described in the following section.

Diversify Funding Sources

In order for patient education to flourish, especially in the outpatient setting, a diversified set of funding sources have to be tapped. These include the following:

Partnerships

Partnerships offer the widest number of options because the range of organizations that are potential sponsors is almost limitless. The objective here is to find other organizations that have similar objectives and will therefore be willing to contribute money, staff, or other in-kind resources to the project. Such organizations may include other health care providers, voluntary health organizations, schools, government agencies, churches, civic groups, community development corporations, self-help organizations, social service agencies, and others.

For example, the National High Blood Pressure Education Program has been very successful in engaging churches in high blood pressure prevention and control programs.[41] Voluntary health organizations offer a particularly rich source of resources. Although they do not usually have large grant resources, they do often provide financial support for the development of print and audiovisual materials, as well as targeted program support, and supplies of educational materials. In addition, organizations such as the American Cancer Society work cooperatively with hospitals and other health care providers to deliver nationally developed patient education programs such as "I Can Cope" and "Look Good, Feel Better," as well as patient support programs such as "Reach to Recovery."

Other important community organizations may also offer unique kinds of partnerships. The Stanford Arthritis Center, for example, has worked out a win–win relationship with the California community college system. The center manages 30 to 40 arthritis

Figure 7-1. Cost Containment Report, Kent General Hospital Patient Education Department (January 1 through June 30, 1988)

I. Volunteer Hours

	Hours	Cost	Savings
Volunteer Personnel—PCE	391	$4.25	$1,661.75
Volunteer Personnel—CL	133	$4.25	$ 565.25
		Subtotal:	$2,227.00
		Section I Total:	$2,227.00

II. Donated Employee Mileage

	Miles	Rate	Savings
Trips to Smyrna–Clayton Round Trip: 26 miles × 26 trips	676	$0.27	$182.52
Trips to Felton Round Trip: 16 miles × 26 trips	416	$0.27	$112.32
		Subtotal:	$294.84
		Section II Total:	$294.84

III. Pharmaceutical Paid Presentation

OB Classes Ross Laboratories	$400.00	$400.00
Endometriosis Forum Tap Pharmaceutical	$150.00	$150.00
Asthma Update Schering Pharmaceutical	$200.00	$200.00
	Subtotal:	$750.00
	Section III Total:	$750.00

IV. Teaching Equipment/Materials

A. Diabetes

	Quantity	Cost	Savings
Chemstrip bG	1	$ 35.00	$ 35.00
One Touch Strips	2	39.00	78.00
Smart Start Kits	11	25.95	285.45
Heart Decisions for Life VCR tape	1	295.00	295.00
Cholesterol & Your Heart	50	0.65	32.50
Cholesterol Watch—Pads/Tear Sheets	50	5.00	250.00
Test Strips	3	36.00	108.00
ID Cards	45	0.50	22.50
DE Identification Tags	10	1.00	10.00
Gestational Diabetes Booklet	11	5.00	55.00
Self-Test Diary	17	1.50	25.50
Cards—Hypo/Hyperglycemia	25	1.50	37.50
Take Home Kits	40	25.00	1,000.00
Gift Pax	100	1.00	100.00
Glucofilm Test Strips	3	60.00	180.00
Managing Your Diabetes Booklet	15	10.00	150.00
Rulers	40	0.50	20.00
ID Cards (ICN)	40	0.50	20.00
VCR Tapes (Spanish)	2	249.00	498.00
VCR Tape (Lifescan)	1	39.99	39.99
Flip Chart	1	100.00	100.00
Life Style Lesson Books	15	9.95	149.25
Here's to Health (Eng—Spanish)	5	7.45	37.25
Humulin Starter Kit	10	20.00	200.00

Figure 7-1. (Continued)

	Quantity	Cost	Savings
Ultra Blood Glucose Meter	1	120.00	120.00
Ultra Test Strips	1	32.00	32.00
Ultra Control Solution	1	15.00	15.00
Blue Starter Kits (Bags)	5	8.00	40.00
A Path to Healthy Living	25	9.95	248.75
Autolet Lite	1	28.00	28.00

Subtotal: $4,212.69

B. Ostomy	Quantity	Cost	Savings
Multiple dressings	10	$ 6.00	$ 60.00
Kaltostaf (Calcium Alegenate)	4	25.00	100.00
Optipore	10	2.50	25.00
Skin Clens	10	5.00	50.00
Epilok	15	5.00	75.00
2½″ pouches & flanges	20	15.00	300.00
Perineal foam cleanser	1	15.00	15.00
Modern Management of Pressure Ulcers	2	75.00	150.00
(Video & Manuals)			0.00
Skin cleansers, various types	7		200.00
Dressing, various sizes	10		100.00

Subtotal: $1,075.00

C. Pt/Comm Education	Quantity	Cost	Savings
The Brain at Risk Video	1	$250.00	$250.00
How to Care for Your Parents Book	1	5.95	5.95
Medication Tear Sheets	25	0.50	12.50
Special Diet Cookbook: MS	1	7.95	7.95
Assess Peak Flow Meter	2	20.00	40.00
Helping Patients Breathe a Sigh of Relief	1	500.00	500.00
(Asthma Wellness Teaching Packet)			0.00
The Beat Goes On Video	1	39.95	39.95
The Numbers Don't Lie Video	1	39.95	39.95
Chicken Pox Cards	275	0.25	68.75
Strep Throat Cards	275	0.25	68.75
Hand Foot and Mouth Disease Cards	275	0.25	68.75
Anatomical Guide Flip Chart	1	100.00	100.00
Infant Formula Cards	25	2.20	55.00
Infant Feeding Video with books	24	25.00	600.00
When Your Loved One Has Alzheimer's	1	8.95	8.95
Disease—A Caregivers Guide			0.00
A Parents Guide to Asthma	1	17.95	17.95
Business Leadership in Aging	1	15.00	15.00
Aging America: Trends & Projections '91	1	20.00	20.00
You & Your New Baby Video	60	25.00	1,500.00
Getting the Most Out of Your Theophylline Therapy Video	1	20.00	20.00
Your Lungs: The Tree of Life	1	20.00	20.00
Aspects of Respiratory Medicine Manual	1	10.00	10.00
Azmacort Demonstrator	1	20.00	20.00
Opti Haler: Drug Delivery System	3	20.00	60.00
Introduction to Opti Halers Video	1	20.00	20.00
Asthma Wellness Center	1	200.00	200.00
Inspiraease	4	25.00	100.00

Subtotal: $3,869.45

D. Child Life	Quantity	Cost	Savings
Little Tikes Toy Box	1	$ 60.00	$ 60.00
My Shape and Stir Pot	1	10.00	10.00
Kiddie Craft	1	7.95	7.95

(Continued on next page)

Figure 7-1. (Continued)

Big Bird in the Box	1	12.95	12.95
Teddy Bear Pop Up	1	12.95	12.95
Disney Typewriter	1	9.00	9.00
45 Records	8	1.00	8.00
Albums	8	9.95	79.60
Videos	2	14.95	29.90
Space Rockets Card Game	1	3.00	3.00
Lion Head Puppet	1	4.75	4.75
Small Teddy Bear	1	6.00	6.00
Robo Cop Game	1	8.95	8.95
Scrabble Sentence Game	1	8.75	8.75
Book of 1,000 Jokes	1	2.95	2.95
Walter Payton Book	1	2.95	2.95
William Perry Book	1	2.95	2.95
Multiplication Flash Cards	1	2.99	2.99
Christian Family Bedtime Book	1	11.95	11.95
Bears Book	1	1.95	1.95
Grover Sleeps Over Book	1	4.95	4.95
Coloring Books	3	1.49	4.47
Small Cars	10	6.00	60.00
Big Bird Rocker	1	29.75	29.75

Subtotal: $ 386.71

Section IV Total: $9,543.85

V. Literature

A. Diabetes

	Quantity	Cost	Savings
Publications: January	160	$1.25	$ 200.00
Publications: February	759	1.25	948.75
Publications: March	263	1.25	328.75
Publications: April	145	1.25	181.25
Publications: May	250	1.25	312.50
Publications: June	95	1.25	118.75

Subtotal: $2,090.00

B. Enterostomal

	Quantity	Cost	Savings

Subtotal: $ 0.00

C. Pt/Comm Education

	Quantity	Cost	Savings
Publications: January	210	$1.25	$ 262.50
Publications: February	1,700	1.25	2,125.00
Publications: March	301	1.25	376.25
Publications: April	125	1.25	156.25
Publications: May	645	1.25	806.25
Publications: June	325	1.25	406.25

Subtotal: $4,132.50

Section V Total: $6,222.50

Grand Total: $19,038.19

Reprinted, with permission, from Kent General Hospital, Dover, Delaware, 1992.

self-management courses that are coordinated through this system. The center receives a set amount per student per hour of state reimbursement, whereas the consumer pays only a nominal fee to participate.[42]

Consumer Payment

Although consumer payment is associated with decreased likelihood of utilization of patient education and preventive services among low-income populations,[43] it is also a source of revenue that should be tapped where possible. For example, several PEMs have noticed that their weight reduction classes are full, even given a registration fee and a generally low-income population. These kinds of revenues can begin to support other programs for which the intrinsic demand is low. PEMs should be careful to identify the size of the population that can begin to pay for services, while at the same time building resources for those who cannot pay, such as through scholarship funds.

Business Sponsorship

The business community in general is very concerned about skyrocketing health care costs. Local business leaders are likely to be interested in opportunities to positively affect these costs through more effective involvement of consumers and their families in health care decision making and prevention programs.

Although business and industry have become somewhat disillusioned about the ability of general health promotion programs to have a measurable impact on productivity and health care costs, there is considerably more interest in the positive effects of targeted programs such as prenatal education, high blood pressure education, and back injury prevention programs. For example, the Johnson and Johnson "Live for Life" health promotion program documented that absenteeism for participating employees declined significantly over the three-year study period.[44] Approaches for support of specific business leaders, health committees of the Chamber of Commerce, or Wellness Councils should be accompanied by documentation of expected impact, reasonable and measurable program objectives, and a plan to track program results.

Physician Donations

Physicians are becoming more aware of the importance of patient education to accomplish informed consent objectives and to increase the likelihood of effective patient self-management. They can and should be tapped to contribute to the ongoing implementation of education programs for their patients. Most often, patient education staff have asked for resources to purchase print or audiovisual resources or equipment. Offering a broader basis of support, the medical groups representing most of Stanford University Hospital's medical staff cosponsored the development of the Health Library.[45]

Another way to approach the resource question is to ask physicians to purchase educational materials, consistent with the hospital-based program, to use in their offices. Several PEMs have developed prototype print materials that the physician's office can print, adding the physician's name to the cover.

There is the potential for a hospital-based patient education program to negotiate contracts with physician practices to provide specific types of patient education services such as diabetes education, prenatal education, chemotherapy classes, arthritis self-management, and so forth at their offices. However, the prevalence of the use of this strategy is not known. Although this strategy might not bring in unencumbered revenue, the resources it generates can be used to cover existing personnel costs. It also has the advantage of strengthening ties with area physicians.

Finally, special outreach efforts directed toward physician office staff may have an indirect resource-generating effect, in that these staff are often the most effective way to reach physicians themselves. Strengthening these relationships is also likely to result in more consistent and effective patient education programming if the hospital-based and office-based staff are coordinating efforts.[46]

Grants

Effective grant seeking can substantially extend the resources available to PEMs; unfortunately, the majority of them have not used it successfully. Grants are most effectively used to try out new innovative ideas or to develop a specific program component that requires a one-time cost. Most granting agencies, with the exception of special local, state, or federal service delivery grants, are not interested in providing long-term funding for a project. Many are also unwilling to provide grant funds to cover routine costs that look as if they should be covered by the grant seeker.

Grant seekers also often make the mistake of heading immediately for the big funders—The Robert Wood Johnson Foundation or the W. K. Kellogg Foundation. Although these foundations do fund local projects, they also reject hundreds of applications each year. PEMs are much more likely to be successful by utilizing local contacts, a recent copy of *The Foundation Directory,*[47] and *Locating Resources for Healthy People 2000 Projects*[48] to identify those organizations to approach within their county or state. Additional homework about promising donors can be used to determine if their interests are at all congruent with the PEM's needs.

The following organizations should be considered in searching for grants: city, county, and state agencies; Chamber of Commerce; civic groups; churches or interfaith councils; voluntary organizations; local foundations; The Junior League; and chapters of professional associations such as the American Association of University Women. The *Encyclopedia of Associations*[49] might also be used to identify those organizations that may have a special interest in the program area for which the PEM is seeking funding. If there is a development office at the hospital, meet with the director before proceeding with grant writing. This office often functions as the hospital traffic cop, trying to ensure that multiple departments are not tapping the same source at the same time. There are likely to be hospital policies and procedures that support this department's role. In addition to avoiding potential interdepartmental conflict, an early discussion with development staff is also likely to yield useful advice regarding promising grant options.

Taking a locally offered grant-writing seminar can sharpen the PEM's writing skills and provide familiarity with strategies to cultivate funders and design proposals that address their priorities. Figure 7-2 provides some additional ground rules for effective grant seeking culled from the experience of a health education manager in a small Ohio hospital who has been very successful in attracting a wide range of grant resources.

Volunteers

Effective use of volunteers is an extremely important strategy for expanding resources available for patient education programming as well as for increasing the impact of the program. The use of peer volunteers as instructors, assistants, and outreach workers for a variety of programs provides a measure of credibility with a target population that no amount of training and preparation can provide.[50] Although such positions require recruitment, job descriptions, training, and supervision, they offer a substantial opportunity to extend the reach of program personnel.

Program managers of all types have tended to underutilize volunteers, often relegating the volunteers' time to filing and other uninteresting tasks. Successful PEMs are looking for ways to tap volunteers by utilizing their individual skills to design jobs that will be personally rewarding.

For example, one manager of a community health education center has focused on recruiting retirees with specific skills such as public relations, library, and nursing to accomplish specific roles in the center. Managers interested in pursuing such an option should discuss this strategy with the hospital's legal counsel to be sure that no applicable labor agreements, laws, or regulations proscribe the development of such volunteer roles.[51] Our Lady of Lourdes Hospital in Camden, New Jersey, which serves a very poor community, has recruited and trained community members to serve as companions, offer helping hands (especially transportation and shopping to newly discharged or homebound patients),

Figure 7-2. Ground Rules for Effective Grant Seeking

1. Get into the grant information network. Although the *Foundation Directory* may be one source of information about agencies that fund patient education programming, many other sources are often more accessible and closer to home. The National Health Information Center describes a long list of such sources in *Locating Funds for Healthy People 2000 Projects* cited earlier. Patient education managers (PEMs) should scour their professional literature and the notices distributed by state and local agencies for any relevant news about forthcoming grants. They should also make themselves known to the government agencies that frequently administer grants, discussing with agency staff the kinds of special activities that their hospitals are interested in developing or continuing.

2. Like the old puzzle about the chicken and the egg, there is no one answer to the question about which comes first, identifying a need for a program or seeking grants to support a need that is only suspected. It is not wise to wait for the right grant to be announced before investigating suspected program needs. Resourceful PEMs know their communities well enough that appropriate gaps can often be matched with requests for new grant proposals (RFPs). It may be that more current statistics must be gathered quickly in order to complete a grant application, but a program manager should periodically assess community needs to ensure that all programs are on target, no matter what their current or potential sources of financing.

3. Although the general intention of a grant can sometimes bear annual interpretation, a grant proposal should always follow the strict administrative rules outlined by the granting agency. If, for example, an RFP indicates that money will be made available for new programs only, there is little point in applying for operating funds for programming that is already established. If purchase of equipment or covering travel expenses are strictly prohibited, the grant application budget should not reflect expenditures for such activities. Almost all RFPs have some specifications of this kind, and the applicant should read them carefully before beginning to develop the proposal and its budget.

4. If the proposed program cannot reasonably operate without the elements that are prohibited in funding, it is very useful to let the granting agency know that these elements will be financed. In doing so, the applicant can demonstrate that other funding sources are committed to the project. Sometimes major support can be identified, possibly from other grants already in hand. Often, however, a manager must refer only to such basic but essential support as office space and telephone expenses donated to the project by the hospital, or services donated to the project by the hospital, or services donated by physicians, hospital staff members, or others. If the value of these can be quantified, the granting agency can clearly see that others beside itself view the project as important and are investing resources to help the proposed project achieve its goals.

5. Arranging for any kind of financial support from the hospital demands that the PEM fully inform administration and sometimes the Governing Board about the intent of the grant proposal and convince these decision makers of its value. Unless they make this limited early commitment of funds to a program, it is unlikely that hospital executives will consider assuming more of its financial support if and when grant monies are depleted. Granting agencies invariably ask how a program plans to continue operations after the grant period is over and are often favorably impressed if the institution expresses its intent to support the program in whole or in part, once the early expenses of establishing a program have been covered by a grant. The more these considerations are discussed with decision makers before the proposal is written, the firmer the foundation will be for their actually assuming a major portion of program support at a later time.

6. When in doubt about a grant's requirements, a program manager should always feel free to call the grant administrator and ask. Information gained through such personal inquiry can make the proposal-writing process easier and more rewarding and can often help the manager avoid mistakes in operating the program, once the grant is received. Establishing a personal relationship with the granting agency can also give a program manager a better sense of the kinds of proposals that would be more attractive to that agency. At the same time, it will give the grant administrator a better idea of the kinds of grant activities that the program manager would be interested in and capable of undertaking.

7. Granting agency and hospital executive support will be further strengthened by periodic reports about grant project activities. A final report is almost always required by a granting agency, which tends to make decisions about future proposals on the project manager's past track record. In addition to a careful accounting of expenditures, a program manager should include as much information as possible about the numbers of people served, any improvement that could be demonstrated in their status as a result of the program, and any evaluations that were gathered among participants or from other agencies cooperating in the grant project. Finally, it is helpful if the program manager can demonstrate that the funded project has afforded both the funding agency and the hospital some positive publicity in the media; copies of articles and a list of the coverage the project received on radio and television should be attached to the report that is sent to both the funding agency and hospital administration.

This material is adapted from *Health Promotion for Low-Income Groups: Programming Strategies.* Chicago: American Hospital Association, 1989, pp. 20–22. The original text was based on an interview with Karolyn Wilson, Health Education Department, Madison County Hospital, London, Ohio.

enrich after-school programs in the city, work with children with learning and other disabilities, and hug premature babies in the neonatal intensive care nursery.[52] The Patient Education Section at M. D. Anderson Cancer Center in Houston, Texas, has extensive experience in developing volunteer positions with job descriptions and then recruiting individuals to fill these roles. (See figure 13-12 in chapter 13 for an example of such a job description.)

Fund-raisers

The number of options for fund-raisers is only limited by the creativity and energy of program planners. PEMs have reported walk-a-thons, swim-a-thons, senior olympics, dances, bake sales, and auctions as a few of the opportunities for program fund-raisers. All these have as a side benefit an increase in knowledge and support for the hospital and its patient education programs among community members.

The Lakewood Commission on Aging in Lakewood, Ohio, for example, raised money for its Alzheimer's respite program through its "Steppin' Out" celebrity tap dance. A volunteer choreographer worked with 24 politicians, television personalities, and business owners to produce the "wackiest evening of community spirit to hit the North Shore of Lake Erie."[53]

The Senior Care Network of Huntington Memorial Hospital in Pasadena, California, developed a thrift shop in the hospital funded by hospital auxiliary volunteers. The community is asked to donate secondhand clothes and artifacts that are then sold in the shop. The net revenue from this venture is used to support the operating budget of Senior Care Network.[54]

Product Sales

Hospitals are more likely now to consider product sales as a way to at least cover the costs of product development. Entrepreneurial managers are able to extend this strategy to bring in revenue to support other program activities. Most commonly, PEMs offer hospital-produced audiovisuals, program packages, and print materials for sale to help recoup production costs. Some institutions have developed health promotion calendars or packaged patient-designed greeting cards as a way to generate new revenue. Obviously, this latter type of product requires a more substantial market analysis and plan because it offers little benefit other than revenue to the hospital's patient education program.

Contribute to Health Care Reform

Trying to figure out how to identify revenue streams for patient education under the current health care financing policies is a daunting challenge. Because of multiple, inefficient, non-patient-focused payment mechanisms, patient education is devalued as part of the current health care system.

Although the DRG system put in place a positive incentive to reduce length of stay—a goal to which patient education can make a major contribution—other incentives within the system still encourage hospitalization, discourage collaboration with other health care providers, discourage home care services, and discourage patient involvement in decision making. However, supporting policy changes that contribute to health care reform is one strategy PEMs can use to offset some of these problems.

In the long run, substantial changes will be needed in both financing and health care delivery systems if incentives are to be created that support patient education. As the health care reform debate widens, it will be important for all health care providers to take an active role in helping to make institution-based changes as well as in advocating for policy changes to support patient-centered and community-focused care.

The reform strategy currently under development by the American Hospital Association offers a vision of the future of health care that combines universal access, economic discipline, and a restructured delivery system that is both community- and patient-focused. A cornerstone of this vision is community care networks that would provide patients with integrated care organized at the community level. Several important characteristics of networks can offer incentives for patient education programming:[55]

- Their focus on community health status
- Their focus on patients
- Their focus on prevention and primary care
- Their focus on community-level solutions to community problems

☐ Conclusion

This chapter has attempted to lay out a broad strategy that patient education managers can use to tap resources to support their programming. Although the question "When will patient education be reimbursed by third-party payers?" has been one of the most common queries raised in the field, an intensive focus on the pursuit of such reimbursement within the current delivery system is likely to result in much frustration and inadequate dollars. A more productive approach is to access the limited opportunities for reimbursement that are available, while tapping a wide variety of other internal and external opportunities to increase resource support for patient education.

References and Notes

1. In cost-effectiveness analysis, two or more ways of doing something are compared in order to identify the one that produces the greatest impact per unit cost. This term is often used erroneously to refer to a program's ability to reduce health care costs. See, for example, Warner, K., and Hutton, R. Cost-benefit and cost-effectiveness analysis in health care. *Medical Care* 18(11):1069–84, Nov. 1980.

2. See, for example, Burke, B. Financial management not easy in hospital-based health promotion programs. *Outreach* 11(6):4–5, Nov.–Dec. 1990.

3. See, for example, Cleverly, W. O. *Essentials of Health Care Finance.* 2nd ed. Rockville, MD: Aspen Press, 1986.

4. Wheeler, M. L., and Warren–Boulton, E. Diabetes patient education programs: quality and reimbursement. *Diabetes Care* 15 Suppl. 1:36–40, Mar. 1992.

5. 1988 member needs assessment profiles AADE members, identifies needs, concerns. *AADE News* 15(5):1,7, May 1989.

6. Diabetes Control Project for Maine. Reimbursement Pilot Study for the Ambulatory Diabetic Education and Follow-up Program, Final Report. Augusta, ME: State of Maine, 1983.

7. Tobin, C. T. Third-party reimbursement coverage for diabetes outpatient education programs. *Diabetes Care* 15 Suppl. 1:41–43, Mar. 1992.

8. See, for example, Iglehart, J. K. Health policy report: the American health care system—managed care. *The New England Journal of Medicine* 327(10):742–47, Sept. 3, 1992.

9. New opportunities for preventive health care for poor children: Medicaid's EPSDT program after 1989 federal legislation questions and answers. Unpublished briefing. Washington, DC: Children's Defense Fund, Feb. 1990.

10. Fraser, I., Narcross, J., and Kralovec, P. Hospital care for the poor, 1980–1989: participation, unreimbursed costs, and implications for access. Paper presented at the Association for Health Services Research annual meeting. Meeting of the Association for Health Services Research, San Diego, July 1, 1991.

11. American Hospital Association, data collected from the Annual Survey of Hospitals for various years.

12. Current population survey, annual March income supplement. Table prepared by the Congressional Research Service and published in the *1991 Green Book* (background material and data on programs within the jurisdictions of the Committee on Ways and Means), U.S. Government Printing Office, May 7, 1991.

13. Issues and trends: number of uninsured hits 35.7 million. *Business and Health* 10(3):22, Mar. 1992.

14. U.S. Department of Health and Human Services, Health Care Financing Administration. Services incident to a physician's service. *Medicare Carrier Claims Manual*. Part III, Chapter II, sections 2030.1–2050.5. Revision 922, June 1982.

15. Schauffler, H. Health promotion and disease prevention policy under Medicare: an historical and political analysis. Paper presented at the 119th annual meeting of the American Public Health Association, Nov. 11, 1991.

16. *Federal Register* 57(114):24980, June 12, 1992.

17. American Hospital Association. Seven of ten hospitals will lose on Medicare inpatients in 1993. Press release, Sept. 15, 1992, unpublished, Chicago.

18. LeBrun, P., Gendel, T., Woodward-Rice, K., Gerber, D., and Raichel, T. *Blue Cross and Blue Shield Plan Support for Health Education Services: A Discussion of Issues.* Chicago: Blue Cross and Blue Shield Associations, 1982.

19. Blue Cross and Blue Shield backs paying for health screening. *Federal and State Insurance Week,* July 21, 1991.

20. Somerville, J. Insurers group issues preventive health guides. *American Medical News,* May 25, 1992, p. 6.

21. For more information on *Healthtrac, Babytrac,* and others, write to Healthtrac, 2 North Point, San Francisco, CA 94133, or phone 415/445-5217.

22. See also Fries, J. F., Fries, S. T., Parcell, C. L., and Harrington, H. Health risk changes with a low-cost individualized health promotion program: effects at up to 30 months. *American Journal of Health Promotion* 6:364–71, May–June 1992.

23. Logsdon, D. N, and Rosen, M. A. The cost of preventive health services in primary medical care and implications for health insurance coverage. *Journal of Ambulatory Care Management* 7(4):46–55, Nov. 1984.

24. INSURE. Final report of the INSURE project. Washington, DC: Health Insurance Association of America, Sept. 1988.

25. Intergovernmental Health Policy Project. *Clinical Preventive Services: A Survey of State Mandated Benefits.* Washington, DC: George Washington University, 1988.

26. Group Health Association of America, Inc. *HMO Industry Profile: Volume I—Benefits, Premiums, and Market Structure, 1988.* Research and Analysis Department, Group Health Association of America, Inc., June 1989.

27. Logsdon, D. N., Rosen, M. A., Thaddeus, S., and Lazaro, C. M. Coverage of preventive services by preferred provider organizations. *Ambulatory Care Management* 10(2):25–35, May 1987.

28. Gabel, J., DiCarlo, S., Sullivan, D., and Rice, T. Employer-sponsored health insurance, 1989. *Health Affairs* 9(3):161–75, 1990.

29. Task Force on Financing Quality Health Care for Persons with Diabetes. *Third-party Reimbursement for Diabetes Outpatient Education.* New York City: American Diabetes Association, 1986.

30. Larson, P. The educational environment: learning through design. *Outreach* 10(4):3–4, July–Aug. 1989.

31. Boumbulian, P., Smith, D., and Anderson, R. COPC model creates environment for prevention. *Outreach* 12(2):7–9, Mar.–Apr. 1991.

32. Giloth, B. Prevention spells opportunity for hospitals. *Outreach* 12(2):1,3–4, Mar.–Apr. 1991.

33. Kernaghan, S. G., and Jones, L. D. *Prevention Strategies in Ambulatory Care: A Manager's Guide.* Chicago: American Hospital Association, 1992.

34. McKinney, E., and Beedle, J. Continuing care clinics meet needs of patients with chronic diseases. *Outreach* 11(1):5–7, Jan.–Feb. 1990.

35. Agre, P., Bookbinder, M., Cirrincione, C., and Keating, E. How much time do nurses spend teaching cancer patients? *Patient Education and Counseling* 16(1):29–38, Aug. 1990.

36. Lairson, D. R., Mains, D. A., Mullen, P. O., and Velez, R. Estimating the cost of education and counseling programs. *Patient Education and Counseling* 18(2):179–88, Oct. 1991.

37. Kernaghan, S., and Giloth, B. *Tracking the Impact of Health Promotion on Organizations: A Key to Program Survival.* Chicago: American Hospital Publishing, 1988.

38. Lurie, N., Manning, W. G., Peterson, C., Goldberg, G. A., Phelps, C. A., and Lillard, L. Preventive care: do we practice what we preach? *American Journal of Public Health* 77(7):801–4, July 1987.

39. Burg, M. A., and Lane, D. S. Mammography referrals for elderly women: is Medicare reimbursement likely to make a difference? *Health Services Research* 27(4):505–16, Oct. 1992.

40. Giloth, B. Incentives for planned patient education. *QRB* 11(10):295–301, Oct. 1985.

41. National Heart, Lung, and Blood Institute. *Churches as an Avenue for High Blood Pressure Control: Guidelines for Developing Church-Sponsored High Blood Pressure Programs.* Bethesda, MD: National Heart, Lung, and Blood Institute, 1989.

42. Personal communication with Kate Lorig, Ph.D., Stanford University.

43. Woolhandler, S., and Himmelstein, D. U. Reverse targeting of preventive care due to lack of health insurance. *JAMA* 259(19):2872–74, May 20, 1988.

44. Jones, C., Bly, J., and Richardson, J. A study of worksite health promotion program and absenteeism. *Journal of Occupational Medicine* 32(2):95–99, Feb. 1990.

45. Kernaghan, S. G., and Giloth, B. E. *Consumer Health Information: Managing Hospital-Based Centers.* Chicago: American Hospital Association, 1991, pp. 14, 27–29.

46. Griffith, N. Joining hands with physicians' offices to meet changing patient education needs. *Promoting Health* 6(4):6–8, July–Aug. 1985.

47. The Foundation Center. *The Foundation Directory.* 1992 Edition. New York City: The Foundation Center, 1992.

48. Office of Disease Prevention and Health Promotion. *Locating Resources for Healthy People 2000 Projects.* Washington, DC: Department of Health and Human Services, 1991.

49. Burek, D. M., editor. *Encyclopedia of Associations.* 1993 Edition. Detroit: Gale Research Inc., 1992.

50. *Health Promotion for Low-Income Groups: Programming Strategies.* Chicago: American Hospital Association, Division of Ambulatory Care and Health Promotion, 1989, pp. 48–51.

51. See, for example, Brown, N., and Rhodes, R. Understanding the law and volunteer services. *Volunteer Service Administration* 16(6):1,6–8, Nov.–Dec. 1989.

52. Site visit to Our Lady of Lourdes Hospital for the Hospital Community Benefits Standards Program, Feb. 27–28, 1992.

53. Five award-winning fundraisers. *Community Health Funding Report* 7:1–3, Apr. 9, 1992.

54. Kimble, C. S., and Longe, M. E. *Health Promotion Programs for Older Adults: A Planning and Management Guide.* Chicago: American Hospital Publishing, 1989, p. 247.

55. National health care reform: refining and advancing the vision. Document by the Board of Trustees of the American Hospital Association for public circulation and discussion, May 1992.

Bibliography

Abourezk, N., Reardon, G., and Schnatz, J. D. Establishing and operating a third-party reimbursed outpatient diabetes care center. *The Diabetes Educator* 14(1):25–29, Jan.–Feb. 1988.

American Diabetes Association. *Third-party Reimbursement for Diabetes Outpatient Education: A Manual for Health Care Professionals.* Alexandria, VA: ADA, 1986.

American Hospital Association. Strategy emphasizes therapeutic benefits to obtain coverage. *Outreach* 5(2):2, Mar.–Apr. 1984.

American Hospital Association, Division of Ambulatory Care. *Financing Reimbursement and Access to Preventive Services: A Member Briefing.* Chicago: AHA, 1992.

Bartlett, E. Accomplishing more with less under PPS using patient education. *Healthcare Financial Management* 39(7):86–94, July 1985.

Bartlett, E. Which patient education strategies will pay off under prospective pricing? *Patient Education and Counseling* 12(1):51–91, Aug. 1988.

Brackenridge, B. P. Third-party reimbursement: what can we do? *Diabetes Educator* 15(3):208, May–June 1989.

Bransome, E. D., Jr. Improving the financing of diabetes care in the 1990s. Recommendations of the 1989 Conference on Financing Diabetes Care. *Diabetes Care,* Suppl. 1, Mar. 15, 1992, pp. 66–72.

Burke, B. Financial management not easy in hospital-based health promotion programs. *Outreach* 11(6):4–5, Nov.–Dec. 1990.

Cherkin, D. C., Grothaus, L., and Wagner, E. G. The effect of office visit copayments on preventive care services in an HMO. *Inquiry* 27:24–38, Spring 1990.

Cioffi, J. Prospective payment: a view from the trenches. *Patient Education and Counseling* 11(10):295–301, Oct. 1984.

Davis, K., Bralek, R., Parkenson, M., Smith, J., and Vellozzi, C. Paying for preventive care: moving the debate forward. *American Journal of Preventive Medicine* [Supplement to 6(4)], 1990.

Financing for Health Education Services in the United States. Atlanta: Center for Health Promotion and Education, Centers for Disease Control, 1980.

Fox, E. E., Daughtry, D., and Sugg, Z. Reimbursement and diabetes self-care programs in North Carolina. *North Carolina Medical Journal* 49(7):370–71, July 1988.

Giloth, B. Prospective pricing and the implications for patient education. *Promoting Health* (4(6):4–5,11, Nov.–Dec. 1983.

Goeppinger, J., and Walter, J. Financing patient education in arthritis and musculoskeletal and skin diseases. *Arthritis Care and Research* 2(2)80–82, June 1989.

Goldsmith, J. A radical prescription for hospitals. *Harvard Business Review* 67(3):104–11, May–June 1989.

Havlicek, P. L., and Olson, L. Health education in medical group practices: promoting health or business? *Health Education Quarterly* 17(2):129–39, Summer 1990.

Hosakawa, M. Insurance incentives for health promotion. *Health Education* 15(6):9–12, Oct.–Nov. 1984.

Hospital smoke-free policies and nicotine dependency treatment—a good match. *Outreach* (11)1:3–4, Jan.–Feb. 1990.

Hunt, C. Introduction to health insurance and reimbursement issues: options and resources. *Diabetes Educator* 16(4):282–83, July–Aug. 1990.

Intergovernmental Health Policy Project. *Clinical Preventive Services: A Survey of State Mandated Benefits.* Washington, DC: George Washington University, 1988.

Jonas, S. Viewpoint: how to incorporate health promotion into national health insurance. *American Journal of Health Promotion* 3(4):73–74, Spring 1989.

Kernaghan, S. G. Responding to the prospective pricing challenge: 1984 patient education leaders point the way. *Promoting Health* Suppl. 5(6):1–12, Nov.–Dec. 1984.

Kinnaird, L. S. Learning to live with prospective pricing: a patient education challenge. *Promoting Health* 6:6–8, Jan.–Feb. 1985.

Kinnaird, L. S. Small fees, collected regularly, add up. *Patient Education Newsletter,* (Birmingham, AL) June 1985, pp.4–5 (no longer available).

Lairson, D. R., and others. Estimating the cost of education and counseling programs. *Patient Education and Counseling* 18:129–88, 1991.

Lebrun, P., and others. *Blue Cross and Blue Shield Plan Support for Health Education Services: A Discussion of Issues.* Chicago: Blue Cross and Blue Shield Association, 1982.

Logsdon, D., and others. Coverage of preventive services by preferred provider organizations. *Journal of Ambulatory Care Management* 10(2):25–35, May 1987.

Logsdon, D., and Rosen, M. The cost of preventive health services in primary medical care and implications for health insurance coverage. *Journal of Ambulatory Care Management* 7(4):45–55, Nov. 1984.

Lurie, N., Manning, W. G., Peterson, C., Goldberg, G. A., Phelps, C. A., and Lillard, L. Preventive care: do we practice what we preach? *AJPH* 77(7):801–4, July 1987.

Martinez, N., and Deane, D. Impact of prospective payment on the role of the diabetes educator. *The Diabetes Educator* 15(6):503–9, Nov.–Dec. 1989.

McKinney, E., and Beedle, J. Continuing care clinics meet the needs of patients with chronic disease. *Outreach* 11(1):5–7, Jan.–Feb. 1990.

McPhee, S., and Schroder, S. Promoting preventive care: changing reimbursement is not enough. *AJPH* 77(7):780–81, July 1987.

Mullane, M., and others. Patient education reimbursement: an experiment in Maine. *International Quarterly of Community Health Education* 1(1):87–102, 1980–81.

O'Donnell, M. P. Viewpoint: health promotion must be incorporated into national health insurance proposals. *American Journal of Health Promotion* 3(4):71–72, Spring 1989.

Office of Disease Prevention and Health Promotion. *Locating Funds for Healthy People 2000 Projects.* Washington, DC: Department of Health and Human Services, 1991.

Office of Technology Assessment. *Preventive Health Services for Medicare Beneficiaries.* Washington, DC: U.S. Government Printing Office, 1990.

Points of view: reimbursement for patient education services—a move forward? backward? or nowhere? *Patient Education and Counseling* 5(1):2–12, 1983.

Russell, L. B. *Is Prevention Better Than Cure?* Washington, DC: The Brookings Institution, 1986.

Schauffer, H. H., and Parkinson, M. D. Health insurance coverage for smoking cessation services. *Health Education Quarterly* (Forthcoming, 1993).

Sinnock, P., and Bauer, D. Reimbursement issues in diabetes. *Diabetes Care* 7(3):291–96, May–June 1984.

Smith, S. A. Patient education financing under Medicare. *Patient Education and Counseling* 8(3):299–309, Sept. 1986.

Somers, A. Sounding board: why not try preventing illness as a way of controlling medical costs? *The New England Journal of Medicine* 311(13):853–56, Sept. 27, 1984.

Third-party reimbursement for outpatient diabetes education and counseling. *Diabetes Care* Suppl. 13 1:36, Jan. 1990.

Tobin, C. T. Third-party reimbursement coverage for diabetes outpatient education programs. *Diabetes Care* 15 Suppl. 1:41–43, Mar. 1992.

Weinberger, M., Ault, K. A., and Vinicor, F. Prospective reimbursement and diabetes mellitus: impact upon glycemic control and utilization of health services. *Medical Care* 26(1):77–83, Jan. 1988.

Wheeler, M. L., and Warren-Boulton, E. Diabetes patient education programs—quality and reimbursement. *Diabetes Care* 15 Suppl. 1:36–40, Mar. 1992.

Woolhandler, S., and Himmelstein, D. U. Reverse targeting of preventive care due to lack of health insurance. *JAMA* 259(19):2872–74, May 20, 1988.

Chapter 8

Linking Patient Education with Discharge Planning

Kathy L. Menke, M.A., B.S.N.

☐ Objectives

The reader will be able to:

- Identify the importance of linking patient education and discharge planning in different hospitals
- Identify some of the management approaches and vehicles used to integrate the two functions
- Identify means of overcoming obstacles to integrating the two functions
- Describe program strategies to enhance the effectiveness of patient education as part of discharge planning
- Describe ways to extend patient education beyond the hospital inpatient setting

☐ The Importance of Linking Patient Education and Discharge Planning

It is important to establish strong linkages between patient education and discharge planning in any hospital setting. Strong links between these two functions help ensure that the two areas complement rather than overlap each other. More important, these linkages establish a framework to consistently provide the right level of discharge planning and patient education for every hospital patient. Integrating and linking patient education with discharge planning provides a number of benefits to both hospitals and patients, including the following:

- Patient education linked with discharge planning *empowers* patients and ensures that upon discharge, they have the necessary information to care for themselves and make sound decisions regarding their future care.
- Patients who receive adequate patient education linked with discharge planning may mean fewer unnecessary return visits to the hospital and fewer phone calls to health care professionals.[1] This is because educated patients are better able to

differentiate between normal recovery symptoms and more urgent issues requiring medical attention.

- Patients are reassured if they know what to expect during recovery and what goals they need to achieve to fully recover from their illness or injury.
- Practitioners such as physicians and nurses can be reassured that the care provided during a patient's hospital stay is continued following discharge and that patients have the education they need to recover at home.
- Hospitals benefit by avoiding situations where personnel duplicate each other's efforts. Once the functions of patient education and discharge planning are linked, communication among practitioners in each of the areas increases, resulting in a better understanding of what is being accomplished with the patient.

In many hospitals patient education and discharge planning are frequently viewed as separate and distinct functions, unrelated to each other. However, they in fact share many functions and responsibilities. One way they are linked is that an important component of preparing the patient and family for discharge is ensuring that the patient understands his or her condition, medications, anticipated level of activity, and general posthospital health care needs. The patient also may need specialized education on specific equipment, treatment, and follow-up procedures. However, patient education and discharge planning are not synonymous. In addition to preparing patients for discharge, patient education is concerned with such things as preparing patients for surgery and diagnostic procedures, whereas discharge planning includes such responsibilities as obtaining equipment and discharge placement.

Patient education and discharge planning already have a strong *theoretical link*. Patient and family education is identified as one of *six essential elements* of discharge planning according to American Hospital Association (AHA) guidelines. AHA guidelines state that patient and family education is critical to successful discharge planning and that patient education must be integrated into discharge planning in order to facilitate self-care after discharge.[2]

Despite this theoretical link and the reasons given here for linking discharge planning and patient education, in many hospital settings they are not linked at all and continue to be organized as distinct and separate functions. One reason for this is that for many health care organizations, the term *discharge planning* is equated with only extreme interventions, such as discharge *placement*, say, into a nursing home or other facility. However, this narrow view of discharge planning excludes the majority of patients— those who are discharged directly home from the hospital and who do not need the following services:

- Discharge placement
- Referral to a home health agency
- Special arrangements for medical equipment to be brought into the home

Evidence of the numbers of patients who are discharged home rather than to other facilities can be found in statistics published by the Health Care Financing Administration (HCFA): More than 80 percent of Medicare patients were discharged to their homes during the first year of the prospective pricing system.[3] Other recent research suggests that, in general, patients who were transferred to institutional settings, rather than home after discharge, had more adequate discharge plans than did those who returned home following hospitalization.[4]

These findings suggest that large numbers of patients going directly home from the hospital may not receive the benefits of complete discharge planning, including patient education. Obviously, discharge planning efforts concentrating mainly on discharge placement, and without firm links to patient education, cannot fully meet the needs of significant numbers of patients. An obvious solution is to link the two functions more formally within the hospital, and the logical person to establish this linkage is the patient education manager (PEM).

The importance of patient education during the discharge planning process has also increased dramatically in recent years because patients are discharged at an earlier stage of recovery, and they or their families must assume responsibility for their own care once they are home. Formally linking patient education with discharge planning helps ensure that patients have all the information they need to make a smooth transition from the hospital to the home.

The following section provides some general strategies that the PEM may use to integrate and link discharge planning and patient education. Specific references are made to the efforts of integrating the two functions at the University of Nebraska Medical Center (UNMC), in Omaha.

□ Strategies for Linking Patient Education and Discharge Planning

It is important to mention that, regardless of the methods for linking discharge planning and patient education, the pace of this process depends on the organizational culture and structure of the hospital. The process of integrating patient education and discharge functions and linking the roles may be either gradual or accelerated. In more established hospitals a gradual linkage of patient education and discharge planning by the PEM may be more successful than implementation of a new, fully integrated program. This is because gradual integration of the two functions is generally less threatening to those involved.

Various methods can be used to integrate patient education and discharge planning. These methods may be used independently or in combination with others that seem appropriate.

Patient education managers at some hospitals regularly attend weekly, multidisciplinary *rounds*. When this is the case, the PEM is able to ensure that the patient education aspect of discharge planning is addressed. As patients near discharge, in addition to their discharge plans, these rounds may include discussion of plans for providing patients with education to help ensure their recovery. The PEM's participation in these interdisciplinary rounds helps establish the vital link between the two functions (discharge planning and patient education) for key staff from various departments.

Staff development workshops may be a good place to begin the integration process. When patient education workshops for nursing staff are held, including a discussion of discharge planning and presentations by discharge planning staff is key to integrating the functions.

The patient education manager (PEM) and discharge planning coordinator (DPC) at UNMC alternate teaching the new nurse orientation class on patient education and discharge planning. Topics include UNMC resources, policies, documentation, and community resources.

A hospital's *quality assurance/improvement program* is another vehicle for integrating patient education and discharge planning. The development of monitoring activities and indicators that evaluate patient education as a piece of discharge planning is one way to link the two functions.

Patient education and discharge planning are two of the five indicators monitored in the unit-based quality assurance/improvement program at UNMC. In addition, in-house monitoring of patient education and discharge planning is accomplished at the department level. In-house monitoring includes readmission studies, telephone interviews with recently discharged patients, and reviews of medical records. Findings from these monitoring and evaluation activities from the unit and department levels have highlighted the need for the PEM and the DPC to collaborate closely on continually improving existing programs and/or implementing new ones.

One example of this monitoring activity was to review medical records of patients readmitted within 30 days of a previous hospitalization. One patient who was readmitted had received a tracheostomy during his initial hospitalization. The documented patient education on his tracheostomy was less than adequate, and he was readmitted because of complications that a well-informed patient could have handled.

Consequently, the teaching protocol for tracheostomy was revised, and a preprinted documentation form and printed discharge information were developed. The results of the monitoring activity and the changes were subsequently communicated to nurses at their staff meetings and through the nursing newsletter.

Integrating patient education activities in *discharge planning policies* is yet another useful way for the PEM to integrate the two functions. As discharge planning policies are developed or revised, they should include patient education as an important component.

The specific *documentation forms and manuals* for patient education and discharge planning also can be integrated. For example, nursing data bases can include questions related to both areas, and discharge summaries frequently include discharge instructions for patients. Combined patient education and discharge planning forms are already used by some hospitals, and these ensure strong links between the two functions. Referral forms to home health agencies and other health care facilities should state the education that has been provided and list patient education goals.

Strengthening the relationship between the PEM and the staff member(s) responsible for discharge planning is yet another way to help integrate the two functions. An integrated approach requires frequent, regular communication between the PEM and the CDP. One strategy is for each to serve on the other's committees. Another strategy is for each to be available to the other for informal consultation as needs arise. These strategies can help ensure both effective discharge planning and patient education, and avoid duplication.

At UNMC, the PEM reports to the discharge planning coordinator, who in turn reports to the associate hospital director of nursing. This close formal relationship also enhances communication and integration of the functions.

Nurses are the frontline care givers in most hospitals. It is important that patient education and discharge planning be linked in the eyes of *nursing staff* so that they become routine parts of the nursing role. Integrating these functions helps ensure that nursing staff provide patients with the right level of patient education and appropriate discharge planning.

If primary care nurses are to be responsible for discharge planning, they must have information or access to discharge planning tools and resources. At UNMC, every nursing unit has a discharge planning manual that includes listings of home health agencies, resources, guidelines for discharge planning forms, and policies and procedures. The discharge planning coordinator (DPC) has access to a computerized resource listing for the state of Nebraska that is managed by the Nebraska Department of Social Services.

Before effective links between the two functions can be established, it is important to recognize that obstacles to their integration exist in most hospitals. The following section describes some of these obstacles and, more important, addresses how to overcome them.

☐ Obstacles to Integrating the Two Functions

There are a number of organizational and cultural obstacles to integrating patient education and discharge planning, and determined patient education managers must recognize them and devise strategies to overcome them.

One important obstacle to integration is the narrow definition people within the hospital may have of each role. If the hospital has a discharge planner, and his or her role is primarily to arrange for discharge placements for certain patients, it will be difficult to coordinate efforts. Integration will be possible only if there is a broader perspective of discharge planning and patient education.

Another obstacle to the integration of patient education and discharge planning is the threat of encroaching on another's territory. By addressing their concerns directly and trying to develop a realistic description of their roles, the involved staff members can collaborate more successfully. At UNMC, this was accomplished through a meeting of representatives from various disciplines to develop a list of each discipline's responsibilities within the hospitalwide discharge planning policy. In addition, the division of discharge planning into four levels based on AHA's position statement further clarified each discipline's accountability for patient education and discharge planning needs, such as discharge placement (see table 8-1).

The hospital's organizational structure can pose yet another obstacle to integration of the functions. If the managers of these two functions are in different departments, and if the lines on the hospital's organizational chart are very formal or inflexible, linking patient education and discharge planning will be difficult. In these cases, taking small steps toward integration, partial integration, or simply improving collaborative efforts may be more successful.

Still another obstacle to integrating the two functions is the level and quality of communication between interdisciplinary personnel in other health care facilities or home care agencies who see patients before and after hospitalization. Poor communication between discharge planners and personnel in other facilities can result in incomplete discharge planning and inadequate patient education. Communication among the disciplines can be enhanced through the use of specific referral forms and, more informally, through phone calls. Referral forms also help ensure that complete information is sent from one level of care to another. Additionally, it is helpful for the various care givers to be aware of the different agencies that discharge planners work with. This helps ensure that patients receive consistent referrals.

Table 8-1. Levels of Discharge Planning

Level	Scope	Accountable Department	Involved Professions/Departments
1	In conjunction with the medical plan of care, facilitate patient and family understanding of illness/condition, discharge medications, anticipated medical follow-up, anticipated level of functioning, and posthospital care needs.	Nursing	1. Physicians 2. All other allied health care providers as needed
2	Specialized education so that patient and/or family members can provide posthospital care.	Nursing	1. Physicians 2. All other allied health care providers as needed
3	Arrangement and coordination of community support systems that enable patient to return home. (Refer to *The Role of the Social Worker* for specific functions.)	Social Work/ Nursing	1. Physicians 2. All other allied health care providers as needed
4	Relocation of patient and coordination of support systems or transfer to an appropriate health care facility.	Social Work	1. Physicians 2. Nurses 3. All other allied health care providers as needed

Source: Adapted from the position statement, The Role of the Social Worker in Discharge Planning, published by the American Hospital Association, 1985.

There are also obstacles to working with nursing staff to integrate the two functions. Because nurses tend to be task-oriented due to the amount of daily work they must accomplish for each patient, they may feel overwhelmed when reminded of their responsibilities for patient education and discharge planning. However, the tasks for both processes can be so integrated that they become part of routine patient care, rather than perceived as one more isolated task the nurse has to do. In addition, when the processes are integrated, the *patient* is the focus and not the tasks related to patient education or discharge planning.

Another serious obstacle to integration is the time constraints many nurses feel. Higher patient acuities and highly demanding tasks mean that the physical needs of patients take priority over patient education and discharge planning. As already stated, standardized teaching tools can help in overcoming that obstacle. Additionally, they can help nursing staff overcome the relatively common obstacle of not knowing what to teach. If standardized plans highlight or include only the information that must be taught, the nurse is much more likely to be successful in accomplishing the necessary education with the patient.

Finally, managers of hospital departments or units can make many obstacles to integrating discharge planning and patient education simply disappear. How patient education and discharge planning issues are supported is frequently related to the quality of patient education and discharge planning being performed in individual departments or units. Department managers who set expectations for patient education and discharge planning functions and who hold staff accountable for their roles in these areas are key to the success of both functions.

☐ Strategies for Enhancing Patient Education and Discharge Planning

Merely linking patient education and discharge planning is not in itself going to address the changing needs of patients. Methods are needed to enhance both functions in order to meet the needs of all patients who are discharged from the hospital, including outpatients.

Changes in the health care system such as reduced length of stay have been the impetus for a shift away from what was once considered an ideal patient education approach—one that included educational topics as broad as anatomy and disease pathology—toward a more specific focus on teaching the most basic and practical knowledge and skills. It is no longer realistic to routinely teach general prevention (for example, breast self-examination) in the inpatient setting, when that information is unrelated to the inpatient stay. The focus of the education that occurs in the hospital is related directly to the reason for the patient's hospitalization and to the patient having the necessary knowledge to care for himself or herself after discharge. However, preventive patient education is expected in matters directly related to the patient's diagnosis. For example, a surgical patient is taught wound care in order to prevent infection.

As already mentioned, delaying patient education until the perfect educable moment is no longer realistic. If the perfect moment does not come during the inpatient stay, the teaching—and the learning—must occur anyway. This calls for a variety of educational strategies geared to patients who have shorter lengths of stay, but who require patient education in order to ensure their full recovery.

Streamlining and standardizing the educational content is one time-saving strategy. The likelihood of patients receiving consistent, accurate information increases with standardization, and content can still be individualized to meet the specific educational needs of each patient. In many cases, the "nice-to-know" information, including some anatomy, has typically been dropped or shortened in patient education programs. Programs focus more on the "need-to-know" information—that information the patient requires for recovery.

A variety of formats for standardized patient education increases effectiveness and the likelihood of success. Examples include teaching protocols, inclusion of patient education goals in critical paths, standardized care plans, reference books, prepackaged packets developed for specific diagnoses, and preprinted documentation forms. For example, on the preprinted patient/family education record used at UNMC, an asterisk is placed by those items that are essential topics to be discussed prior to discharge (see figure 8-1). This provides staff with a useful checklist.

The need for standardized formats has also increased the need for printed material to reinforce one-on-one patient education. Instructions that patients must follow after discharge are often complex. Both patients and their families are frequently anxious and upset when receiving explanations, so having printed materials that review instructions is critical. Instruction sheets developed for those subjects taught repeatedly on a particular unit (for example, the use of digitalis on a cardiac unit) are also a reassurance for staff.

However, it is important that staff resist the temptation to rely totally on printed material when providing patient education. Printed material serves primarily as backup and reference; *it does not replace face-to-face education.*

Audiotapes, flip charts, and videotapes are also useful supplementary materials for providing patient education. Some hospitals lend or provide educational audiotapes and videotapes to patients for use at home. This is an ideal way to supplement the patient education received in the hospital because the patients and/or families have control over the learning process. They can stop the tape when they need a break, and they can replay it as needed.

A useful form to ensure that patients receive all the necessary instructions prior to discharge is the *discharge summary,* a copy of which is given to patients. The discharge summary usually includes the patient's final instructions under the following categories: medications, activity, and diet. It may also include a list of supplies or equipment needed for home care, any referrals that have been made, and dates and times of subsequent appointments. Finally, it usually has a telephone number the patient can call if questions arise. There is often space for the patient or family member to sign the form indicating that the information has been reviewed and is understood.

Some effort has been made to increase patient independence and individual self-management while patients are hospitalized. For example, leaving medications at the bedside was unheard of 20 years ago, but that has changed with organized self-medication programs. Of course, self-management is only possible with certain diagnoses and at certain times during recovery, and many patients are too weak early in their hospital stay to participate. Self-management techniques include enlisting family members, as well. For example, parents of pediatric patients are often encouraged to provide care and some education for their child throughout his or her hospitalization. Health care professionals are then able to provide gentle, daily guidance and reinforcement rather than a more formal educational session.

Cooperative care units such as the one at New York University Medical Center have gone even further toward self-management during hospitalization as a way to better prepare patients for discharge.[5] Patients must be admitted with a care partner (for example, a family member, a friend, or someone they have hired to stay with them throughout their hospitalization). The care partner assists with the patient's care, observes the patient on an ongoing basis, and participates in patient education activities. To be admitted to a cooperative care unit, the patient must be well enough not to require continuous direct nursing care and must be mobile with limited assistance. In some of the cooperative care units, patient education classes are scheduled into the patient's day along with appointments for other activities such as blood pressure checks and lab work.

Another successful approach to enhancing discharge planning and patient education has been used at the University of Minnesota Hospital and Clinic's Learning Center.[6,7] Here, the definition of a learning center has expanded from merely a room with reference materials to a lablike environment where patients receive instruction from

Figure 8-1. Patient/Family Education Record

		Reg. no.
DATE PRIMARY NURSE ASSESSMENT(S) OF TEACHING NEEDS		
_____		Location
_____		
_____		Date
_____		
_____		
_____		Page 1 of 1

Postoperative Mastectomy

SPECIFIC TEACHING SUBJECT	1. *Phantom pain	2. *Pain meds.	3. *Incision care, for example, drains, dressings, shower, bath	4. *Returning to normal activity, for example, work, driving	5. *Signs and symptoms of infection arm/incision

GENERAL TEACHING SUBJECT	Date Name Unit or Clinic
	Date Name Unit or Clinic
Patient or significant other verbalizes understanding or returns demonstration	Date Name Unit or Clinic

SPECIFIC TEACHING SUBJECT	6. Lymph edema precautions for affected arm	7. Prosthesis and shopping	8. Exercise, for example, range of motion	9. Reach to Recovery	10. Reconstruct surgery

GENERAL TEACHING SUBJECT	Date Name Unit or Clinic
	Date Name Unit or Clinic
Patient or significant other verbalizes understanding or returns demonstration	Date Name Unit or Clinic

Figure 8-1. (Continued)

SPECIFIC TEACHING SUBJECT	11. Patient psychosocial needs	12.*Family and spouse psychosocial needs	13. Breast care BSE and mammography	14. When to notify doctor	15.

GENERAL TEACHING SUBJECT	Date Name Unit or Clinic				
	Date Name Unit or Clinic				
Patient or significant other verbalizes understanding or returns demonstration	Date Name Unit or Clinic				

TEACHING TOOLS (Pamphlets, Films, Flip Chart) USED: Mastectomy Packet
Document: Date, Title, Name, Unit or Clinic.

*Important items

TEACHING PROTOCOL USED: Mastectomy (Springhouse)

MAKE ENTRIES IN BLACK INK

DATE   COMMENTS (Knowledge base, attitude, educational level, response to teaching, etc.):

Postmastectomy Educational Packet

Breast cancer: understanding treatment options—NIH

After breast cancer: a guide to follow-up care—NIH

Breast reconstruction: a matter of choice—NIH

Adjuvant therapy facts for women with breast cancer—NIH

Reach to Recovery packet—American Cancer Society

Mastectomy: a treatment for breast cancer—NIH

Home care of your wound/incision—University of Nebraska Medical Center a registered nurse about a particular skill. The staff nurse on the unit can make the initial assessment and referral. Often this skills training can take 30 minutes or more of teaching time—time that inpatient nurses can no longer afford. The learning center ensures that the patient and family receive consistent, hands-on training. Later, the nurse can follow up to reinforce the teaching, individualize the information, and problem-solve with the patient.

Rehabilitation services at some hospitals include EASY STREET ENVIRONMENTS™, replicas of real-life environments where the activities of daily living can be relearned. This environment provides practical experience during the educational process. Practicing activities such as getting in and out of a car or grocery shopping while the rehabilitation patient is still in the hospital can make the transition to the home smoother.

As already stated, an important consideration in any program strategy for discharge planning is the need to shift some of the care-giving responsibilities for patients from hospital staff to family and friends. For example, many patients receiving intravenous antibiotic therapy are now cared for at home and, in many cases, this care is provided by family members. Consequently, family members are often the primary recipients of patient education.

Including family members in the educational process enables them to support the patient in a variety of ways, such as providing positive feedback, removing obstacles, and in some instances providing the total care. This is a change from traditional practice. For example, nurses used to ask family members to leave the hospital room when patients' dressings were changed, nasogastric tubes were placed, and so forth. Today, however, family members are often encouraged to stay because they are likely to need to continue the care in the home. (See chapter 18 for further discussion on involving family members in patient education.)

Even if family members do not provide the majority of the patient's home care, their influence on his or her cooperation with the prescribed regimen is substantial and may be positive or negative. Health care professionals need to be alert to the effect of the family's influence.

As staff focus on continuity of care for patients, communication between hospital staff and physician's offices or outpatient clinics can often be a problem. However, it is a problem that can be overcome. At UNMC, patient education contact nurses, one from each unit and one from the outpatient clinic, meet monthly. Although the focus of their meetings is not on individual patients, this communication process enhances patient education, discharge planning, and the continuity of care. This is because outpatient nurses help determine the content being covered in the hospital, and vice versa. Clinics use the same teaching protocols and documentation forms that the hospital does. The very first tab in the patient's medical record contains his or her cumulative education records so that a quick assessment can be made of the content that has been covered.

However, many patient education managers are not in hospitals with connecting outpatient clinics. For example, Saint Joseph Hospital in Denver took the initiative to develop and supply patient education teaching packets for distribution in the outpatient setting.[8] Meetings with office staff members focused on orienting them to the appropriate use of the packets and on developing a partnership to ensure success of this activity.

Patient readiness is another area of concern. It is unrealistic for the patient educator to wait for the educable moment or to expect that he or she will be able to keep the patient in the hospital until the patient is deemed "educationally" ready for discharge. Shorter lengths of stay and the greater use of outpatient services mean that more patients are discharged to continue their recovery at home. Patient educators can meet the educational needs of these types of patients by using some of the following tactics:

- Streamlining patient education content to focus on survival skills
- Developing supplemental materials to support face-to-face education
- Extending the boundaries of the education process beyond the hospital walls
- Working with family members to ensure that the patient is ready for discharge

☐ Ways of Extending Patient Education beyond the Hospital

Patient education should no longer begin and end at the hospital door. Traditionally, the hospital was the only place where patient education was appropriate. For example, 15 years ago, when a patient with diabetes was admitted to the hospital, health care professionals had the luxury of delaying his or her discharge until the necessary patient education was complete. As already stated in this chapter, in many cases it is no longer possible to complete all aspects of education during the inpatient stay, and educational referrals may be needed. This is especially true for patients with chronic conditions such as diabetes, who may have to undergo life-style changes. In these cases, other ways must be found to extend education beyond the critical days of hospitalization. Patients may be referred to a support group or service agency, classes held in the outpatient setting, and/or a home health agency.

Hospitals, outpatient offices and clinics, and community groups and agencies offer classes and support that can extend the education that began in the inpatient setting. That is when the education to equip patients with more than just basic survival skills can really begin. That is where patients can learn practical, day-to-day skills and expand their knowledge of their illness beyond what they learned in the inpatient setting. Self-help groups, individuals, and families who are experiencing the same condition can provide patients with additional information and support.

Referrals to home health agencies to provide further care and continue the educational process also may be appropriate. Home health visits are advantageous because they allow for more thorough family assessment, and patients usually feel more comfortable in familiar surroundings.

When referrals to home health agencies are made, the nurses' communication and documentation must be thorough. It is ideal if the hospital consistently uses one agency or has its own home health department. Then the patient education standards or teaching protocols can be the same or at least can be available to each group.

One paradoxical way of extending patient education is to do it before the need arises, even before hospitalization. For example, *preadmission education* has been found to be very effective with orthopedic patients who are taught how to walk with a crutch prior to surgery.[9] For patients who are admitted to the inpatient setting directly following surgery, preadmission education has become a necessity and has required a dramatic increase in communication between PEMs and outpatient staff. This communication helps facilitate discharge planning.

Telephone follow-up programs with patient education objectives are another way to extend patient education beyond the hospital. In settings such as outpatient surgical centers, telephone communication may be the most reasonable way to provide education, both before and after surgery. Telephone programs are an ideal way to follow up with patients and have been implemented in some hospitals. However, because they can be very time-consuming, they may not be practical. In addition, there are concerns regarding the need for documentation and for the telephone communication to be as consistent and comprehensive as the communication that takes place in the inpatient setting.

Given today's constraints, the challenge in preparing patients for their discharge from the hospital is to determine the most effective patient education method and the most logical, efficient, and effective setting. In many cases, this means extending patient education beyond the hospital.

☐ Conclusion

The strength of the link between patient education and discharge planning varies from institution to institution. The degree of integration considered appropriate in one setting may be totally unrealistic in another. Yet, some integration is important to ensure that all patients receive the appropriate level of patient education and discharge planning. Integrating and enhancing these two functions helps ensure that patients can continue to recover at home. In addition, better-educated patients are less likely to return to the hospital or require further care.

Further, integrating discharge planning and patient education ensures that staff in these areas are not working at cross-purposes or duplicating effort. Fragmented patient follow-up is usually the result of a failure to integrate the two functions. The patient education manager is in an ideal position to decrease the fragmentation of patient care by initiating communication about the integration of patient education and discharge planning.

References

1. Falvo, D. *Effective Patient Education*. Rockville, MD: Aspen, 1985.

2. American Hospital Association. *Guidelines: Discharge Planning*. Chicago: AHA, 1985.

3. Health Care Financing Administration. HCFA background paper, Department of Health and Human Services. Washington, DC: Government Printing Office, 1985.

4. Morrow-Howell, N., Proctor, E. K., and Mui, A. C. Adequacy of discharge plans for elderly patients. *Social Work Research and Abstracts* 27(1):6–13, 1991.

5. Bills, S. S. Cooperative care: an educational ideal whose time has come. *Promoting Health* 7(3):8–11, 1986.

6. Sumpmann, M. An education center for patients' high-tech learning needs. *Patient Education and Counseling* 13(3):309–23, 1989.

7. Goldstein, N. L. Patient learning center reduces patient readmissions. *Patient Education and Counseling* 17(3):177–90, 1991.

8. Griffith, N. Joining hands with physicians' offices to meet changing patient education needs. *Promoting Health* 6(4):6–8, 1985.

9. American Hospital Association. Revising procedures for hip surgery cuts costs, LOS. *Hospitals* 59(12):75-77, 1985.

Chapter 9

Designing and Implementing an Effective Patient Education Documentation System

Sandra J. Cornett, Ph.D., R.N.

☐ Objectives

The reader will be able to:

- Identify the legal basis for patient education documentation
- Describe documentation requirements in the Joint Commission on Accreditation of Healthcare Organizations (JCAHO) standards
- Describe the elements of an effective patient education documentation system
- Identify strategies to implement and manage an effective patient education documentation system

☐ Preparation for Effective Documentation

"In God We Trust—everyone else must document." In many ways, this tongue-in-cheek statement sets the tone for the way documentation of patient education is currently approached. Patient education managers (PEMs) are constantly trying to find just the right form or system that will take all their documentation woes away.

Unfortunately, simply initiating a documentation form is rarely the answer. Certainly, making the process as easy as possible and streamlining procedures is important if staff are going to effectively document, but what needs to change is a mind-set. Staff need to become aware of, and value the importance of, documenting the education they give when caring for patients and families, just as they value documenting other aspects of the care they give. The mind-set should become: Take credit for what you do! To effect a change in staff behavior, educational opportunities need to be provided on the legal aspects of patient education documentation and how to properly educate patients and their families. Becoming familiar and comfortable with the language and process of patient education will help professionals document their patient teaching. Patient/family education needs to be viewed as an integral component of care and thus documented along with other care given.

☐ Purpose of Effective Patient Education Documentation

There are two main reasons why documentation needs to be done. The first is to meet complex legal requirements, and the second is to meet the standards of the JCAHO. In addition, effective documentation provides a meaningful way for the team members to communicate with each other, thereby enhancing the team's patient education efforts and collaboration.

The basis for patient education documentation encompasses professional practice acts, standards of practice from professional associations, institutional policies, informed consent, quality and continuity of care issues, and program evaluation considerations. The following sections briefly review these issues.

Professional Practice Acts

Virtually all health care providers have language in their professional practice acts that set a legal precedent for them to render adequate and relevant patient education. Health care providers can be held liable for negligence if a patient does not understand what is necessary for effective management of his or her health condition. This liability challenges health care professionals to develop accurate and reliable methods to evaluate a patient's understanding and to document their educational efforts.

Standards of Practice from Professional Associations

Standards of practice delineated by the various professional associations often outline the responsibilities of a particular professional group to teach the patient and family information about their specific health care needs and how to appropriately modify behavior. Again, implicit in providing information to help patients make decisions and choices about promoting, maintaining, and restoring health is documentation of these educational efforts and their results. If patient teaching is not documented, it is considered not done. These statements and standards for practice from professional organizations provide a basis upon which the professional will be held accountable should there be a question of practice in a court of law. Figure 9-1 contains an example of excerpts of standards from one professional organization that speak to patient education and documentation.

Institutional Policies

Most hospitals have policies and procedures or standards within the various departments that guide health care providers in delivering care. Often these standards and policies include the professionals' role and responsibilities in providing patient education and documenting this process. These documents are important to discuss with staff to help change the mind-set, so that patient education documentation is seen as an expectation of performance and, therefore, is more likely to be valued.

Informed Consent

Informed consent is the legal duty of disclosure and is primarily a liability issue for physicians. It is based on the principle of self-determination, that is, a person's right to decide what should be done to his or her body.[1] It occurs when an individual voluntarily agrees to allow someone else to do something to him or her after information is received. For the individual to exercise this right to decide, appropriate information must be provided about the kind and purpose of the treatment or procedure and its expected outcomes; the benefits and risks or complications of the procedure; any alternatives and their risks and benefits; and the prognosis if treatment is refused.[2] As part of this educational process, the physician must determine the patient's ability to understand the explanation.

Involvement of staff, other than the physician, in the informed-consent process includes the following three elements:

1. Observing the interaction between the physician and the patient, thereby witnessing the signatures
2. Validating that the patient had the capacity to understand and was not coerced to consent
3. Assessing the patient's understanding and clarifying any misunderstandings

To validate understanding of the information, staff need to ask the patient to explain in his or her own words what the physician said. If there seems to be a basic misunderstanding about diagnosis or treatment and prognosis, the physician should be asked to explain all the information once more. Staff should document the results of this process and any actions taken.

Figure 9-1. 1991 American Nurses Association Standards of Clinical Nursing Practice That Apply to Patient Education

---

Standard I: Assessment

The nurse collects client health data.

Measurement Criteria

5. Relevant data are documented in retrievable form.

Standard II: Diagnosis

The nurse analyzes the assessment data in determining diagnoses.

Measurement Criteria

3. Diagnoses are documented in a manner that facilitates the determination of expected outcomes and plan of care.

Standard III: Outcome Identification

The nurse identifies expected outcomes individualized to the client.

Measurement Criteria

2. Outcomes are documented as measurable.

Standard IV: Planning

The nurse develops a plan of care that prescribes interventions to attain expected outcomes.

Measurement Criteria

4. The plan is documented.

Standard V: Implementation

The nurse implements the interventions identified in the plan of care.

Measurement Criteria

3. Interventions are documented.

Standard VI: Evaluation

The nurse evaluates the client's progress toward attainment of outcomes.

Measurement Criteria

2. The client's responses to interventions are documented.
5. Revisions in diagnoses, outcomes, and the plan of care are documented.

Note: Numbers refer to each item's place in the complete standards of practice.

Reprinted, with permission, from *Standards of Clinical Nursing Practice*, copyright ©1991, American Nurses Association, Washington, D.C.

Quality of Care Issues

A foremost method used to monitor the quality of care provided is to audit patient medical records. Audits of records to identify patient education documentation have shown major deficiencies in the medical records of many hospitals.[3,4] Accrediting agencies list lack of documentation about education for self-care and preparation for discharge as the most common charting deficiencies.[5,6] Record audits help define strengths and weaknesses in all patient education efforts, not only the problems of documentation.

Continuity of Care Issues

Effective documentation provides direction for all interdisciplinary team members so that there is continuity and consistency in their patient education efforts. This is particularly important when interdisciplinary team members may not have frequent contact with each other every day. To accomplish this goal, documentation records need to be interdisciplinary in scope. Separate care plans and documentation sheets for each discipline can no longer be afforded if continuity of care is to be achieved. A patient education documentation system must also be developed to communicate the relevant information in an understandable way to those persons responsible for the patient's care after discharge.

Program Evaluation Considerations

Aspects of the patient education process can be studied by using the documentation to help define actual practice against standard criteria. For example, a patient education manager (PEM) may want to know what assessment data are being collected by nurses to identify a knowledge deficit or what methods are being used by staff to evaluate patient response to teaching. The answers to questions such as these can often be determined by auditing the medical record. Results from this process can be used to help formulate changes in a patient education program and the way it is implemented.

JCAHO Standards Addressing Patient/Family Education Documentation

The 1993 JCAHO standards for patient and family education are presented in a separate chapter of the JCAHO's *Accreditation Manual for Hospitals,* for the first time (see figure 10-1). The overall focus is on the instructions given for self-care and the patient's understanding of these instructions at discharge. The standards state that specific knowledge and/or skills must be provided to meet the patient's ongoing health care needs, including teaching safe and effective use of medication and medical equipment, potential drug–food interactions, diet counseling, and when and how to obtain further treatment, if needed. Emphasis is also on providing any discharge instructions given to the patient to the individual or organization responsible for continuing care. There are four major areas (explained in the following sections) for documenting patient education as reflected in JCAHO standards.[7]

Relevant and Adequate Information for Self-Care
Evidence in the medical record needs to indicate that the patient's educational needs pertaining to self-care are assessed, identified, and addressed. Relevant and adequate information for self-care includes the following elements:

- Explanation of the condition
- What to do to manage the condition and how to do it
- When the physician should be consulted
- When the treatment regimen should be discontinued

- Special precautions to take
- What to do when the regimen is not followed
- What to do if new symptoms occur
- How to get clarification of instructions

Information provided on self-care needs to be documented in such a way that other staff know specifically what was taught so that follow-up can occur. For example, the statement "diabetic teaching done" is not acceptable; however, "insulin injection demonstrated as per teaching plan, but not practiced by patient" is appropriately documented so that follow-up can occur.

How the Teaching Was Done

Standard PF.1.1 states that the education received is given "in ways understandable to the patient and/or his or her significant other." This suggests that how the teaching is done is an important factor. It is not sufficient to simply hand out instructional material or have patients watch audiovisual aids as the sole method of teaching. Evidence needs to be documented that learning differences among patients were considered when giving patient education information. Again, use of the word *taught* does not enable staff who read the patient's medical record to adequately follow up using an appropriate teaching method. Words such as *explained, discussed, read, demonstrated, reviewed, practiced,* and *problem-solved* more accurately describe how the teaching was done. Health care professionals must be available to answer questions the patient may have and to give needed explanations.

Evaluation of Learning

Even if the information is relevant and communicated well, the patient's understanding and ability to apply the information for effective self-care needs to be documented. Specific measurable evidence of learning outcomes or the attempted evaluation of learning must be documented. Examples of terms used to indicate measurable, behavioral outcomes include *states, identifies, applies, independently performs, chooses, verbalizes,* and *returns demonstration.* If the patient is unable to answer questions or perform a skill, a statement that there was no evidence of learning and a proposed reason as to why needs to be written.

Characteristics of Educational Process

Throughout the standards, the identification of specific learning needs is stressed. Measurable goals or expected outcomes, stated in behavioral terms, are formulated from this assessment. The educational plan needs to be individualized, and reflect patient and family involvement in the development and implementation of the plan. If the PEMs keep in mind these four areas of emphasis in the standards when helping their organizations to revise patient education documentation, there will be less of an opportunity for problems to occur in meeting these standards.

☐ Plan for an Effective Patient Education Documentation System

To establish an effective patient education documentation system, a process of planned change can be used. Ideally, going through this process will identify only minor weaknesses in the current system, and vastly improved patient education documentation can be achieved with only minor revisions. In some instances, however, analysis of the current system reveals that documenting patient education seems to be an afterthought. Often a teaching–learning form for documentation is haphazardly developed and added to the overall system with little attention given to how to integrate it into the whole documentation system. The most effective system is one where patient education is valued as an integral part of patient care and documentation is thus integrated into the total record-keeping system.

Six major steps need to be considered when developing an effective patient education documentation system. They are:

1. Assess the current system.
2. Formulate goals and objectives for the planned change.
3. Develop strategies for the planned change.
4. Educate the staff to document patient education.
5. Obtain organizational supports for patient education documentation.
6. Evaluate the new or revised documentation system.

Assess the Current System

The first step in the planned change process is to evaluate the degree to which patient/family education is being done and the effectiveness of this education as reflected in the medical record. Most hospital departments are already collecting quality improvement data that monitor institutional and external standards, such as those from the JCAHO. It is important to ensure that the standards used for the record audits are criteria based and measurable. To get a picture of the current status of patient education documentation, both process and outcome indicators need to be assessed. Figure 9-2 gives an example of a generic audit tool that includes both components. The outcome statements are those knowledges and skills expected at the conclusion of the patient teaching. These statements are listed in the form across the top of the boxes in the categories of therapeutic procedures and diagnostic studies and down the right-hand column for the rest of the categories. Process indicators include learning needs assessed, teaching plan identified, education provided, and response noted.

A medical record audit can provide information on how patient education is documented, but it does not necessarily define the causes of any deficiencies in the documentation. Chapter 11 notes a number of causes of inadequate documentation that revolve around four categories of problems: (1) system problems, (2) training problems, (3) performance problems, and (4) material problems. Once the actual causes of documentation deficiency are determined, strategies can be developed to resolve the problems.

Formulate Goals and Objectives for the Planned Change

Results from the assessment phase will determine whether a change in the current documentation process is needed or whether inadequacies in the process are related to performance or training problems. If a system change is needed, the choice becomes whether to make changes in what is currently being done to better integrate patient education activities or to totally build a new documentation system. Regardless of which choice is made, the goal is to implement a documentation system that reflects patient education activities as an integral part of assessing, planning, implementing, and evaluating patient care.

Specific objectives of this planned change may include:

- To standardize the method for documenting patient education
- To provide a written format that reflects use of the educational process
- To implement a documentation system that uses a systematic and comprehensive approach regardless of construct

Develop Strategies for the Planned Change

Specific strategies for implementing the planned change will depend on its goals, the methods and written materials used in documentation, and whether the system is computerized. Before implementation of the new or revised system of documentation occurs,

Figure 9-2. Sample Generic Audit Form for Patient Education Process and Outcome

This form is an evaluation tool used by the Patient Education Evaluation Subcommittee.

Hospital Number: _____

Age: _____ Sex: _____

Date of Admission _____

Nursing Unit: _____

Date of Evaluation: _____

Service: _____

Date of Discharge: _____

Evaluator: _____

Diagnosis/es: _____

	Procedure	Able to state reason for procedure	Able to state patient responsibilities	Provides return demonstration
Therapeutic Procedures	1. _____			
	2. _____			
	3. _____			
	4. _____			
	5. _____			
	6. _____			

	Study	Able to state reason for study	Able to state patient responsibilities	Instructions for Use
Diagnostic Studies	1. _____			1. Indicate + in corresponding blocks if documentation is present in permanent record.
	2. _____			2. Indicate − in corresponding blocks if no documentation is present.
	3. _____			3. Circle numeral (1, 2, 3, and so on) in the last column if documentation is present.
	4. _____			
	5. _____			
	6. _____			
	7. _____			

(Continued on next page)

171

Figure 9-2. (Continued)

	Learning needs assessed	Teaching plan identified	Education provided	Response noted	Patient/family able to:
Health Alterations					1. State reason for hospitalization 2. Describe understanding of health alteration 3. Identify signs/symptoms of potential complications
Medications					1. State name, dosage, and schedule 2. State purpose or actions 3. State major side effects
Nutrition					1. Describe type of diet, restriction, or modification 2. State reason for diet, restriction, or modification

Activities of Daily Living					1. Describe limitations/modifications in
					  a. Ambulation/mobility
					  b. Hygienic measures
					  c. Life-style
					2. Demonstrate use of equipment and/or assistive devices as applicable

Coping Behaviors					1. Demonstrate effective coping behaviors 2. Recognize inappropriate coping behaviors
Discharge Plans					1. Describe follow-up care 2. Identify available resources

Reprinted, with permission, from The Ohio State University Hospitals, Columbus, 1992.

policies, procedures, and forms need to be examined and integrated into the patient care process. If new forms need to be developed or if a computerized system needs to be set up, the guidelines in the following sections should be followed.

Policies, Procedures, and Forms for Documentation

The hospital's documentation policy and procedures should include information to guide staff on the mechanics of documentation and the content of documentation for documentation forms. The *mechanics of documentation* delineate how to record entries in terms of:

- Recording the time
- Indicating activities or interventions rendered by each individual providing care
- Signing the entry
- Writing legibly with appropriate color ink
- Writing chronological events with no blank lines between or within entries
- Using approved hospital abbreviations
- Identifying patients appropriately
- Correcting errors
- Keeping forms in proper sequence

The *content of documentation* reflects a well-defined, standardized process of assessment, planning, intervention, and evaluation used by all health care professionals in the care of patients. This approach includes gathering information, making a diagnosis or defining the problem, establishing the goals or desired outcomes, delivering an individualized intervention, and evaluating the effectiveness of the intervention.

Documentation procedures and forms need to be developed for each phase of the patient care process. The procedure for documenting each phase specifies when documentation is to be completed; what forms to use to document information for each phase; the frequencies of entries; what elements to document; where information is recorded; who can make what entries; and resources to use to help with documentation.

It is imperative that patient education documentation be integrated into each phase of the process rather than be separated. In this way, patient education is more likely to be assessed, planned, implemented, and evaluated within the context of the patient's total care. The following sections describe how documentation is affected during each phase.

Assessment Phase

Patient/family education and discharge planning needs should be evaluated upon admission as part of the patient's overall assessment. Preferably, the assessment form is interdisciplinary so that it truly reflects all the patient care needs and not just those recognized by one member of the team. Usually the initial assessment data are recorded within eight hours of admission. Throughout the patient's hospital stay, an ongoing assessment is done and documented at least every eight hours.

Data collected during this phase fall into two categories: subjective data, or those that are gotten from interviewing the patient and/or family; and objective data, which come from making observations about the patient's behavior. A list of sample questions and observations for collecting subjective and objective data regarding learning is found in figure 9-3. Of course, not all these questions are asked of each patient.

This data base is used as the basis for making a judgment or diagnosis about the patient's responses to actual and potential health problems and life processes. The patient's needs, including those that are educational in nature, are then prioritized. They provide the basis for selecting interventions that achieve patient outcomes for which the health care provider is accountable.

The educational needs documented as a diagnosis are those specific understandings, skills, and attitudes that are lacking and are required in order to attain a more

Figure 9-3.   Assessment of Learning Needs and Readiness to Learn

S = Subjective data (from interviews of patients or family); O = Objective data (from observations about the patient's behavior)

Ability to read/write and educational level

S: Can you read and write English? Another language?

What is your educational background (grade school, high school, technical, or college)?

Do you have a reading problem?

O: Observe evidence of the patient's ability to read or write, for example, read signs, read admission brochure, complete written questionnaire.

Attention span

S: What kinds of things do you find difficult to remember?

What helps you to understand and remember what you have heard or read?

To what degree do your surroundings (noise, presence of others) influence your ability to concentrate?

O: Observe for behaviors that indicate memory loss or lack of concentration.

Comprehension/application

S: What, if anything, don't you understand as well as you would like to?

Once you understand something, to what extent do you try to apply it to everyday situations?

Is your usual tendency to follow directions as given or to change them to suit yourself?

What helps you to understand and remember what you have read?

What do you think would happen if _____ (give a situation such as failure to take medications or adhere to dietary restrictions)?

What do you think accounts for changes in _____?

Why do you think your physician _____?

O: Give an instruction and ask the patient to restate it; observe for his or her ability to explain what to do.

Learning needs and readiness

S: What would you like to know more about?

What have you heard about the likely outcome of this condition?

What have you been told about the treatment/tests planned for you?

What do you think may be the major effect of this illness or condition on you and your family?

Do you know what classes/educational programs are available here? In your community?

Past health instruction/experiences

S: Tell me a little about your way of life.

What do you know about your illness/disease/problem?

How did you find out about it?

Have you ever attended any classes on _____?

Do you have any reading material on _____?

How do you usually react to being ill?

How do you like others to treat you when you are ill?

What things do you do or try to do to keep healthy?

What things in your life seem to make it difficult to stay healthy?

Skill performance

S: How do you _____ (give your own insulin, change your dressing, give your tube feeding)?

Figure 9-3. (Continued)

How would you describe your ability to learn this skill?

How would you describe your feelings about learning this skill?

How would you describe your reaction to using _____ equipment?

How would you describe your manual dexterity at present?

How much practice do you usually need to learn a new skill?

O: Observe the patient or family member as he or she demonstrates a particular skill. Observe for correct use of equipment and supplies, sequencing of procedural steps, recording.

Level of self-care

S: What kind of care have you or someone else needed (for example, dressing, IVs, ADL, Hickman care, medications, and so on)? Are you able to perform any of the care? Describe what you are able to do (start with wounds or something specific that will need to be done after discharge).

How do you feel about the care? What kinds of problems do you experience when doing your own care? What additional help or teaching do you feel would help you to either start, improve, or maintain your ability to care for yourself?

O: Observe the patient performing any of the care he or she is expected to perform.

Reprinted, with permission, from The Ohio State University Hospitals, Columbus, 1992.

desirable condition. These needs must be capable of being satisfied by means of learning experiences. Usually the patient has a knowledge deficit about health conditions, testing, treatments, prognosis, and/or a lack of skill to perform prescribed therapeutic or rehabilitative interventions for long-term health maintenance.

Planning Phase

During the planning phase, a patient care plan based on the assessment is developed and the expected patient outcomes and interventions that are required, given the specific problem, are identified. This care plan is sometimes separate from the assessment form.

An expected outcome is an anticipated result, derived from the problem or diagnosis, that describes a patient's behavior or clinical changes indicating that either the problem has been resolved or progress has been made toward resolution. Patient outcomes need to describe a specific, measurable, observable behavior that will be accepted as evidence that the patient has achieved the desired results. The expected outcome is written using an action verb with few interpretations and a statement describing what the patient is expected to achieve. When applicable, any special conditions under which the behavior is to occur or an acceptable level of performance is included in the statement. Examples of behavioral terms used to document learning outcomes for knowledge, skills, and attitudes are provided in figure 9-4.

The interventions written in the patient care plan are statements of what actions to take to achieve the expected outcomes. Interventions for patient education should include the following components:

- Identity of the learner (it may not be the patient)
- Content to be taught (topical outline or reference to standardized teaching plans that are individualized)
- When teaching is to be done (if appropriate)
- How teaching is to be done
- Teaching material to use
- How learning is to be evaluated

Figure 9-4. Behavioral Terms Used to Document Learning Outcomes

Expected learning outcomes state the knowledge, skills, or attitudes the patient must have or do to demonstrate learning. Each learning outcome statement must include who will do what, when, and how. The use of action verbs identifies when the desired outcome has been accomplished.

Action verbs that identify what learners can do to demonstrate *knowledge:*

- defines
- identifies
- indicates
- labels
- lists
- names
- reviews
- selects
- states

Action verbs that demonstrate *comprehension:*

- applies
- calculates
- chooses
- classifies
- compares
- contrasts
- describes
- discusses
- distinguishes
- explains
- formulates
- gives examples
- interprets
- locates
- reports
- restates

Action verbs that demonstrate a *skill:*

- administers
- applies
- assembles
- changes
- completes
- demonstrates
- injects
- irrigates
- manipulates
- measures
- operates
- performs
- practices
- prepares
- solves
- uses
- walks

Action verbs that identify *attitude* changes:

- accepts
- appreciates
- asks
- attends to
- is aware of
- completes
- contributes to
- cooperates
- engages in
- enjoys
- has interest in
- listens
- looks for
- participates
- prefers
- responds
- is sensitive to
- values
- shows willingness to

Figures 9-5 to 9-8 (pp. 177–186) provide several examples of patient care plans that reflect patient education activities. In figure 9-5, a preprinted generic care plan on post-discharge care that is not disease-specific is presented. Note in figure 9-6 that a learning need can be written as a separate educational diagnosis that is self-contained as one part of a series of care-planning documents. This technique is often used when there is a structured interdisciplinary disease-specific patient education program that prepares the patient and family for complex self-care management at home. On the other hand, patient teaching may be documented as only one of many interventions such as implementation of a medical treatment, actions taken not requiring a physician's order, and ongoing collection of data. When this occurs, the education component of patient care is part of a number of expected outcomes and interventions related to a diagnosis that does not specify an educational need per se (see figure 9-7). Other times, the educational diagnosis is listed as a separate diagnosis, but one of many within the care plan (see figure 9-8).

Input from the patient and family should occur to ensure that the patient outcomes are relevant, realistic, and mutually negotiated. Likewise, educational interventions need to be planned with the patient and family. Involvement of the patient and family in the planning process needs to be documented in the medical record. Planning and/or revision of the expected outcomes and interventions will be ongoing as more data are collected, new problems or diagnoses are identified, and priorities change.

Figure 9-5. Generic Preprinted Patient Education Care Plan That Is Not Disease Specific

R/T = Related to
DHS = Duration of hospital stay
DC = Discharge
Tr = Transfer

No.	Educational Diagnoses (include date/initials)	Expected Outcomes (include date/initials)	Time Frame	Educational Interventions (include date/initials)	Time/s
	Knowledge/skill deficit in postdischarge care of R/T ☐ Lack of experience or instruction ☐ Lack of interest in learning ☐ Cognitive/psychomotor limitation ☐ Request for no information	Patient/ _____ will be able to perform these procedures: _____ _____ _____ • State frequency for performing procedures. • Identify signs and symptoms of possible complications. • State when and how to contact a health professional. • State how to obtain and care for equipment needed at home. • Name medications, dosage, reason for taking, schedule, and side effects. • Describe home diet (preparation and restrictions). • Describe activity level and restrictions at home. • Identify time and place for follow-up care.	by DC by DC by DC by DC by DC by DC by DC by DC	1. Determine who will give care at home and schedule appointments for instruction. 2. Create environment conducive to learning by reducing noise, providing privacy, providing comfort measures. 3. Demonstrate *how* and *when* to perform these procedures: _____ _____ _____ 4. Give handouts: _____ _____ _____ 5. Show audiovisual programs: 6. Explain how to obtain equipment: Item From Phone no. 7. Explain signs and symptoms of these possible complications: _____ _____ 8. Instruct which signs and symptoms require attention from a health professional. 9. Instruct how to contact physician or nurse. 10. Observe return demonstration of procedures	 on on on on on on

Initials	Signature	Initials	Signature	Initials	Signature

(Continued on next page)

Figure 9-5.   (Continued)

No.	Educational Diagnoses (include date/initials)	Expected Outcomes (include date/initials)	Time Frame	Educational Interventions (include date/initials)	Time/s
				11. Patient/_____ to assume routine care of	on on on on on on
				12. Explain purpose, dosage, side effects, and schedule of each medication prescribed postdischarge.	
				13. Instruct on following diet:	
				14. Instruct on following activity level at home:	
				15. Send continuity of care referral to _____ for _____	
				16. Instruct in follow-up care.	

Reprinted, with permission, from The Ohio State University Hospitals, Columbus, 1992.

Implementation Phase

Once care plans have been developed, implementation and documentation of educational interventions can begin. Documentation of educational interventions consists of identifying the learner, topically outlining the content taught, and specifying the teaching method(s) and instructional materials used. It is not necessary to be detailed when documenting what was taught to the patient, particularly if there are standardized teaching plans and guidelines for staff to follow. Teaching methods and instructional materials often fall into the following choices:

- Audiovisual
- Handout
- Explanation
- Demonstration
- Practice
- Role-play
- Group class
- Individual instruction

The reasons for failing to implement certain interventions or for deviations in implementing the care plan need to be noted in the patient's medical record.

Documentation of the patient teaching done and the patient's responses can be included in the progress notes where other patient care interventions are recorded. Often, however, a separate teaching–learning form is used to document what teaching occurred and the evaluation of patient/family learning.

Figure 9-6. Preprinted Disease-Specific Care Plan with a Patient Education Focus

R/T = Related to
DHS = Duration of hospital stay
DC = Discharge
Tr = Transfer

No.	Educational Diagnoses (include date/initials)	Expected Outcomes (include date/initials)	Time Frame	Educational Interventions (include date/initials)	Time/s
	Knowledge/skill deficit in cardiac rehabilitation postdischarge care R/T ☐ Lack of experience or instruction ☐ Lack of interest in learning ☐ Cognitive/psychomotor limitation ☐ Request for no information	Patient/_____ will be able to: • Describe effect of myocardial infarction on home care and life-style. • Identify signs and symptoms of complications (angina, congestive heart failure). • Name discharge medications, dosage, reason for taking, schedule, and side effects. • Describe activity-level progression and restrictions at home. • Take pulse before and during activity and monitor effort symptoms. • Describe appropriate action to take if pulse increases greater than _____ beats per minute during activity. • Describe home diet (preparation and restrictions). • Identify personal risk factors and plan for actions to reduce risk. • Identify coping mechanisms to take during recovery period. • Identify time and place for follow-up care.		1. Determine who will assist with care at home and schedule appointments for instruction. 2. Obtain physician order for cardiac rehabilitation program (CRP) and activity progression as tolerated. 3. Send consults to: ☐ Physical therapy ☐ Occupational therapy ☐ Dietetics (as needed) ☐ Clinical nurse specialist (as needed) 4. Give CRP learning packet and introduce patient to CRP. 5. Discuss effects of myocardial infarction on home care and life-style. 6. Explain signs and symptoms of complications. Emphasize patient actions to take. 7. Monitor activity tolerance to progressive self-care activities. 8. Reinforce pulse taking and monitoring of effort symptoms with activities. 9. Explain name, purpose, dosage, side effects, and schedule of each medication prescribed postdischarge. 10. Instruct on prudent use of cholesterol/saturated fat and sodium. Discuss how to restrict certain foods in diet. 11. Assist patient with identifying personal risk factors. Provide information on reduction techniques. 12. Assist patient with identifying those psychosocial factors that can help or hinder rehabilitation. Explore ways to help patients cope.	
Initials	Signature	Initials	Signature	Initials	Signature

(Continued on next page)

Figure 9-6. **(Continued)**

No.	Educational Diagnoses (include date/initials)	Expected Outcomes (include date/initials)	Time Frame	Educational Interventions (include date/initials)	Time/s
				13. Instruct on how to call physician/nurse and acquire needed resources for follow-up care. 14. Give handouts: 15. Show audiovisual programs: 16. Send continuity of care referral to _____ for _____	

Reprinted, with permission, from The Ohio State University Hospitals, Columbus, 1992.

Evaluation/Revision Phase

The patient's and family's response to the teaching must be documented in terms of the evidence of learning. In most instances, the evidence of learning can be evaluated by using one or more of the following responses:

- States or identifies key points or facts
- Verbalizes understanding
- Applies the information to own situation and correctly responds to complex questions
- Correctly performs a skill, with some prompting, after seeing it demonstrated
- Correctly selects equipment and consistently performs a skill independently
- Inadequately or incorrectly answers questions or performs a skill

These categories are often coded so that a check mark, letter, or number can be used on the teaching form. A column for evaluation comments may be necessary to explain some of the information that was coded.

A review of the patient's and family's response often dictates that a revision is needed in the care plan. Follow-up that is often needed when the patient and family have not met the expected outcomes usually requires one or more of the following revisions to the teaching plan:

- Reteach the information or skill in a new manner
- Reinforce the content in the same way it was taught
- Repeat a demonstration of the skill
- Assist the patient with practicing the skill
- Other: Collect additional data; determine that expected outcomes are not realistic or relevant; determine that learning needs or readiness to learn has changed

Several examples of teaching–learning forms or flow sheets that describe the intervention and evaluation of the learning are found in figures 9-9 through 9-11 (pp. 187–191). Figure 9-9 is generic and not disease-specific and figures 9-10 and 9-11 are preprinted for a specific patient population.

Figures 9-12 to 9-15 (pp. 192–195) show examples of documentation of the entire educational process for a patient needing home care instruction for a G-tube, from assessment of the learning need through revision, including a progress note (see figure 9-15).

Figure 9-7. Preprinted Care Plan That Includes Patient Education as Part of a Noneducational Diagnosis

Start D/C

Etiological factors (related to)

Nursing diagnosis: _____

1. Cardiac factors
   a. bradycardia
   b. tachycardia
   c. heart block
   d. reduced stroke volume
   e. myocardial infarction
   f. congestive heart failure
   g. cardiogenic shock
   h. valvular stenosis
   i. cor insufficiency
   j. hypertension

2. Pulmonary disorders
   a. COPD
   b. cor pulmonale

3. Endocrine disorders
   a. adrenocortical insufficiency
   b. diabetes mellitus
   c. hypothyroidism

4. Hematological disorders
   a. polycythemia
   b. anemia
   c. clotting alterations

5. Fluid and electrolyte imbalances
   a. hypovolemia
   b. hypervolemia
   c. hypocalcemia
   d. hypercalcemia
   e. hypokalemia
   f. hyperkalemia

6. Situational
   a. sepsis
   b. hypothermia
   c. hyperthermia
   d. dialysis
   e. surgery, anesthesia
   f. medications
   g. allergic response

7. Maturational
   a. tetralogy of fallot
   b. septal defects
   c. patent ductus arteriosus
   d. coarctation of the aorta

8.
9.
10.
11.
12.

Start	D/C	**Goals/Outcome**

1. Patient will achieve/maintain optimal hemodynamic function while hospitalized as evidenced by:

   a. Pulse: Rate: _____   Rhythm: _____
   b. Respirations: Rate: _____   Depth: _____
   c. Blood pressure: _____
   d. Skin color   _____
   e.
   f.

2. Fluid balance will be maintained during hospital stay as evidenced by:
   a. Clear breath sounds/adventitious sounds minimized.
   b. Stable dry weight maintained. Weight: _____
   c. Urine output is greater than _____ cc/hour or _____ cc/shift.
   d.
   e.
   f.

3. Patient and/or significant other will identify factors that increase cardiac output by discharge as evidenced by patient stating the following factors that increase cardiac output:
   a.
   b.
   c.
   d.

(Continued on next page)

Figure 9-7. (Continued)

4. Patient and/or significant other will identify and appropriately utilize adaptive techniques needed to perform ADL by discharge as evidenced by patient verbally identifying and demonstrating use of adaptive devices:
   a.
   b.
   c.
   d.

5. Patient and/or significant other will understand prescribed diet by discharge as evidenced by:
   a. Stating the prescribed diet (appropriate foods/rationale).
   b. Stating the dietary restrictions (foods/rationale).

6.

Start	D/C	

Interventions

Assessment:

1. Monitor and report change from patient baseline:
   a. Temperature, pulse, respirations, apical/radial pulses, peripheral pulses, cardiac rhythm.
   b. BP, pulsus paradoxus.
   c. Heart sounds, murmurs, rubs.
   d. Jugular vein distension.
   e. Pulmonary artery pressure, pulmonary wedge pressure, cardiac output/index.
   f. Skin color, temperature, moisture.
   g. Fluid balance:
      • Presence of peripheral edema
      • Intake and output
      • Lung auscultation
      • Daily weight
      • Electrolyte levels
   h. Mentation.
   i. Pain.
   j. Diagnostic studies:
      1) ECG
      2) ABGs
      3) CBC
      4)
      5)

2. Monitor action and side effects of prescribed medications.

3. Assess patient/family knowledge on condition, treatment, and prognosis.

4.

Treatment:

1. Maintain physical and emotional rest by:
   a. Organizing nursing and medical care to allow rest periods.
   b. Providing for a calm environment.
   c. Restricting activity to reduce oxygen demand.
   d. Progressively increasing patient activity as tolerated.
   e. Monitoring sleep patterns and administering sedative p.r.n.

2. Maintain adequate ventilation/perfusion by:
   a. Maintaining Fowler's position.
   b. Alter oxygen therapy as indicated.

3. Maintain optimal fluid balance by:
   a. Restricting fluids as indicated.
   b. Weigh patient daily.

4. Administer medications as ordered, noting response and observing for side effects and toxicity.

Figure 9-7. (Continued)

5. Monitor ECG for rate, rhythm, ectopy, and change in PR, QRS, QT, interval every _____ hours. If arrhythmia occurs, document patient response and report if significant.

6. Monitor therapeutic aids within prescribed protocol (IABP, pacemaker). Specify: _____

7.

8.

Patient Education/Discharge Planning:

1. Instruct patient/family in action usage, side effects, and administration of prescribed medications.

2. Explain dietary restrictions and their importance to patient and significant others.

3. Explain symptoms and interventions for decreased cardiac output related to etiology.

4. Teach patient energy conservation methods for activities:
   a. Sit rather than stand when performing activities.
   b. Rest every 3–5 minutes when performing activities.
   c. Stop an activity if fatigue and signs of cardiac stress are present (increased pulse, dyspnea, chest pain).

5. Assist patient in identifying stressors (home, work, social).

6. Explain effects of stress on cardiovascular system (increase HR, increase RR, increase BP).

7. Discuss various methods of stress reduction:
   a. Relaxation techniques.
   b. Biofeedback.
   c. Meditation.
   d. Regular exercise.
   e.

8. Discuss the effects of smoking and if patient smokes, refer to a program that can assist in smoking cessation.

9.

Mutual goals: The plan of care has been reviewed with the patient/significant other.
        Registered nurse: _____   Date: _____
        Unable to establish mutual goals due to: _____
        Registered nurse: _____   Date: _____

Nursing Diagnosis: _____
Initiated by: _____
Review/Revision

Date	Initial	Date	Initial	Date	Initial

Signature	Initial	Signature	Initial

Figure 9-8. Preprinted Disease-Specific Care Plan with an Educational Diagnosis Listed as One of Many Problems

Diagnosis: _____ DRG: 209 MDC: 8 Length of Stay: 7 Unit: Grant Joint Implant Center

Problem	Expected Outcome	Time Frame	Physician Process	Nursing Process
Potential complication of surgery/general anesthesia: • Fluid imbalance • Hemodynamic instability • Hypoxia • Atelectasis • Dysrhythmias • Urinary retention • Nausea and vomiting • Wound separation	Patient will: • Maintain fluid balance with + 1000 ml difference between intake and output • Maintain clear breath sounds • Maintain UO – 250 ml/8 hours • Void spontaneously within 8 hours after foley removed • Maintain pulse _____ • Maintain blood pressure _____ • Maintain O$_2$ saturation – 92 • Experience no life-threatening cardiac arrhythmias • Experience no vomiting • Maintain well-approximated surgical wound edges without drainage	24–48 hours post op	Institute individualized preprinted physician orders as follows: Pelvic X-ray Labs (hematology, chemistry) Medications (antiemetic, antipyretic, Urecholine, antibiotics) Respiratory therapy (oximetry, O$_2$ incentive spirometry) Diet Patient care (monitoring, vital signs circ/neuro checks, intake/output, wound care, intravenous therapy, dysrhythmia management)	1. Measure and record intake and output every 8 hours. 2. Assess breath sounds, bowel sounds, postop dressing, and neurocirculatory status of affected extremity/ies every ____ hours. 3. Interpret telemetry strips every shift; document changes in cardiac rhythm and institute protocols p.r.n. 4. Cough and deep-breathe every 2 hours for 24 hours; use incentive spirometry every hour for 24 hours while awake. 5. Assess voiding within 8 hours post-catheter removal.
Alteration in comfort, acute pain R/T ☐ Surgical procedure ☐ Inflammation ☐ Swelling ☐ Muscle spasm ☐ Ischemia/impaired perfusion	Patient will verbalize low to moderate levels of discomfort by rating pain less than 3. Patient will exhibit nonverbal behaviors of increased comfort: ☐ Effective coughing and deep breathing ☐ Relaxed facial expression ☐ Increasing self-care ☐ Increasing mobility Patient will exhibit physiological evidence of increased comfort: ☐ Pulse _____ ☐ Blood pressure _____ ☐ Respirations _____ Patient will state that pain is controlled by oral analgesics.	DHS DHS DHS By discharge	Institute individualized preprinted physician orders as follows: Medications (epidural, PCA, analgesic, sedative)	1. Assess pain intensity p.r.n. by having patient rate level of pain on 0-5 scale. 2. Ask patient to describe pain with each episode: location, character, intensity, frequency, duration, precipitative events, and relief measures. 3. Assess nonverbal behaviors and physiological evidence of pain p.r.n.: restlessness, muscular tension, grimace, elevated pulse, respirations, blood pressure. 4. Instruct patient on other comfort measures: ☐ Repositioning ☐ Distraction ☐ Progressive relaxation ☐ Heat and cold 5. Assist patient to exercise within limits imposed by pain or type of surgery.

Potential complications	Expected outcomes	Timing	Orders	Interventions
Potential complications • Skin breakdown • Deep vein thrombosis • Atelectasis • Constipation R/T impaired mobility	Patient will: • Maintain skin integrity • Remain free from deep-vein thrombosis as evidenced by absence of redness, swelling, tenderness, unilateral prominence of veins • Maintain clear breath sounds and temperature under 99° F. • Have bowel movement	DHS DHS DHS Every other day DHS	Institute individualized preprinted orders as follows: Labs (coags) Medications (laxative, anticoagulants) Respiratory therapy (oximetry, O_2, incentive spirometry) Patient care (activity, exercises, positioning, occupational therapy consult)	6. ☐ Instruct on PCA pump ☐ Instruct on epidural analgesia 7. Evaluate effectiveness of pain relief measures: ☐ Analgesics (pain control and degree of sedation, level of consciousness) ☐ Other comfort measures (heat, cold, repositioning) 8. Provide teaching on pain medications prior to discharge. 1. Assess skin on coccyx, heels, elbows every shift for redness, skin breakdown. 2. Calculate/record every skin breakdown risk score every 24 hours; implement protocols if score exceeds 8. 3. Assist to reposition every 2 hours maintaining alignment within hip/knee precautions. 4. Instruct on use of T-bar, triangles, heel protectors.
	Patient will maintain/regain mobility skills as evidenced by: ☐ Correct body alignment ☐ Performance of postop exercises ☐ Correct use of assistive devices ☐ Use of correct gait/ambulation techniques ☐ Compliance with activity restrictions ☐ Use of safety measures			5. Assess lower extremities for redness, swelling, tenderness, prominent veins, or complaint of heavy sensation in legs when standing every _____. 6. Position with legs elevated (no severe flexion of knees or hips). 7. Increase mobility within limits of activity restrictions: ☐ Range-of-motion every _____ ☐ Ankle pumps every _____ ☐ Quad sets every _____ ☐ Knee slings every _____ ☐ Gluteal tucks every _____ ☐ Up in chair every _____ with legs elevated ☐ Ambulate every _____

(Continued on next page)

185

Figure 9-8. (Continued)

Problem	Expected Outcome	Time Frame	Physician Process	Nursing Process

Knowledge/skill deficit in home care following joint replacement:
• Activity restrictions
• Signs and symptoms of complications
• Safety measures at home
• Medications
• Follow-up plans
 	
R/T
☐ Lack of experience
☐ Cognitive or psycho-motor limitations
☐ Noncompliance
☐ Lack of understanding of previous instruction
	Patient will:
	• Demonstrate safe ambulation, exercises, and proper body mechanics:
	☐ In/out of bed independently
	☐ On/off commode independently
	☐ Ambulate 25 feet with assistive device
	☐ 75° active knee flexion
	☐ Straight leg raise without extension lag
	☐ Ability to dress self with minimal or no assistance
	• Verbalize activity restrictions for first six weeks postop
	• Describe signs and symptoms of complications, how to prevent, and when to call physician
	• Describe home environment modifications to maintain safety
	• Describe home medications, dosages, schedule, side effects
	• Identify plan for follow-up
		By discharge	Institute individualized preprinted physician orders as follows:
			
			Activity, exercises, positioning, occupational therapy consult
				8. Assess breath sounds every _____; monitor temperature trends.
				9. Assess bowel sounds, abdominal distention every shift.
				10. Verify bowel movement every other day.
				11. Consult with physical therapy for activity progression p.r.n.
				
				1. Assess current level of knowledge; correct misperceptions or inaccurate information.
				2. Give booklet *The JIS Guide to Recovery After Total Knee/Hip Replacement.*
				3. Show discharge teaching videotape.
				4. Teach patient/_____ activity limitations;
				  • Elevation of leg when lying down
				  • Sitting for brief periods only
				  • Use of assistive devices
				  • Use of raised toilet seat
				5. Reinforce physical therapy protocol for crutch walking and weight bearing.
				6. Teach patient/_____ signs and symptoms to report to physician:
				  • Temperature over 100° F.
				  • Swelling, tenderness, or pain in calf or upper thigh unrelieved by elevation/ice for 24 hours
				  • Redness, swelling, pain, or drainage in wound area
				7. Teach patient/_____ ways to modify home environment for safety:
				  • Removal of loose rugs, cords
				  • Raised toilet seat
				  • Avoidance of using room furniture to assist in ambulation
				8. Give medication handouts; review schedule, dosage, side effects:
				  ☐ Coumadin
				  ☐ Analgesics _____
				9. Validate knowledge about follow-up appointment.

Figure 9-9. Generic Teaching–Learning Flow Sheet Not Preprinted for a Specific Patient

Page: _____

Date/Contact Time	Teaching Interventions (Learner, content, and materials)	Teaching Methods	Evaluation	Evaluation/Comments	Follow-up	Initials

Signature	Initial

Teaching Methods

E—Explanation
D—Demonstration
R—Role-play
AV—Audiovisual
H—Handout

IC—Individual class
GC—Group class

Evaluation

1. Identifies key points
2. Verbalizes understanding
3. Returns demonstrations
4. Performs skills independently
5. Applies knowledge
6. No evidence of learning

Follow-up

1. Re-teach material
2. Reinforce content
3. Repeat demonstration
4. Assist with skills
5. Other (describe)

Reprinted, with permission, from Grant Medical Center, Columbus, Ohio.

Sandra J. Cornett, Ph.D., R.N.

Figure 9-10. Preprinted Disease-Specific Patient Teaching Record and Progress Notes—Diabetes

Diabetes Patient Education—Level I

Medical Record	Progress Notes

Date	Multidisciplinary Patient Teaching Record
	Educational Assessment (ability to learn, sensory/other limitations, past knowledge of condition, obstacles to following treatment regimen).
	Able to read: _____ Yes _____ No
	Learns best: _____ Visual _____ Hearing _____ Doing
	Barriers: _____ Language _____ Vision _____ Hearing
	Readiness to learn: _____ Yes _____ No
	Educational Needs/Plan/Goals (cite ways to overcome obstacles to adherence, self-care approaches).
	Instruct patient using Diabetes Patient Education Program—Level I

For each entry include: signature/title, outcome code (as listed below), inpatient or outpatient status.

1. Indicates understanding or performs successfully
2. Needs reinforcement or needs to repeat demonstration
3. Unsuccessful
4. Not applicable

Teaching Dates	Patient Objectives (Expected Behavioral Outcomes)	Signature/Title	Code	Inpatient	Outpatient
	Diabetes Patient Education Level I				
	1. Define the individual's type of diabetes.				
	2. Name two common symptoms of high blood sugar.				
	3. Name two common symptoms of low blood sugar and what to do.				
	4. Demonstrate blood sugar testing.				
	5. Demonstrate how to give insulin.				
	6. Describe what to do when you are sick.				

(Continue on reverse side)

Patients Identification (For typed or written entries give: Name-last, first, middle; grade; rank; hospital or medical facility)	Register No.	Ward No.

Department of Veterans Affairs

Progress Notes
Standard Form 509 (Rev. 11-77)
Prescribed by GSA/ICMR
FirmR(41CFR)201-45.505

509-111

Figure 9-10. (Continued)

Progress Notes						
Date		For each entry include: signature/title, outcome code (as listed below), inpatient or outpatient status.				
		1. Indicates understanding or performs successfully 3. Unsuccessful 2. Needs reinforcement or needs to repeat demonstration 4. Not applicable				
Teaching Dates		**Patient Objectives (Expected Behavioral Outcomes)**	**Signature/Title**	**Code**	**Inpatient**	**Outpatient**
	Nutrition					
	7. Name one reason for the diabetic meal plan.					
	8. Describe the individual's diabetic meal plan.					
	a. Name 3 high sugar foods to avoid. b. Name 2 sugar-free foods that can be used.					
	c. Name the 6 food groups and portion sizes. d. Name 1 example of a bedtime snack.					
	9. Plan a menu for 1 day.					
	Medications					
	10. Name the individual's medication for diabetes and dosage.					
	Discharge					
	11. Name the supplies needed on discharge from the hospital.					

PO:1985-0-509-032 Standard Form 509 Back (Rev. 11-77)

Reprinted from the Department of Veterans Affairs, Albuquerque, New Mexico.

Sandra J. Cornett, Ph.D., R.N.

Figure 9-11. Preprinted Disease-Specific Patient Teaching Record and Progress Notes—Ostomy

Ostomy Patient Education

Medical Record	Progress Notes

Date	Multidisciplinary Patient Teaching Record
	Educational Assessment (Patient states knowledge of health status, healthcare needs and self-help or how to get help)
	Able to read: _____ Yes _____ No
	Learns best: _____ Visual _____ Hearing _____ Doing
	Barriers: _____ Language _____ Vision _____ Hearing
	Readiness to learn: _____ Yes _____ No
	Educational Needs/Plan/Goals (cite ways to overcome obstacles to adherence, self-care approaches).
	Instruct patient using Ostomy Patient Education Manual.

For each entry include: signature/title, outcome code (as listed below), inpatient or outpatient status.

1. Indicates understanding or performs successfully   3. Unsuccessful
2. Needs reinforcement or needs to repeat demonstration   4. Not applicable

Teaching Dates	Patient Objectives (Expected Behavioral Outcomes)	Signature/Title	Code	Inpatient	Outpatient
	1. Discuss any fear of surgery.				
	2. State the type of surgery planned.				
	3. State 2 things that will happen before surgery.				
	4. Describe 3 things that will happen after surgery.				
	5. Name the type of ostomy performed.				
	6. Describe a healthy stoma.				
	7. Measure stoma to find the proper size of pouch.				

(Continue on reverse side)

Patients Identification (For typed or written entries give: Name-last, first, middle; grade; rank; hospital or medical facility)	Register No.	Ward No.

Progress Notes
Standard Form 509 (Rev. 11-77)
Prescribed by GSA/ICMR
FirmR(41CFR)201-45.505

509-111
VA-10-509-OP114 (501)
10/91

**Department of
Veterans Affairs**

Figure 9-11. (Continued)

Progress Notes						
Date		For each entry include: signature/title, outcome code (as listed below), inpatient or outpatient status.				
		1. Indicates understanding or performs successfully 3. Unsuccessful 2. Needs reinforcement or needs to repeat demonstration 4. Not applicable				
Teaching Dates	**Patient Objectives (Expected Behavioral Outcomes)**		**Signature/Title**	**Code**	**Inpatient**	**Outpatient**
	8. Clean and protect the skin around the stoma.					
	9. Apply a colostomy pouch or appliance.					
	10. Demonstrate irrigation procedure if patient has a descending or symoid colostomy.					
	11. List patients ostomy supplies.					
	12. Discuss personal lifestyle.					
	13. Describe dietary regime.					
	14. Name 5 situations when the doctor should be called.					
	15. Name 1 available hospital or community resource.					

*U.S.GPO;1985-0-509-032

Standard Form 509 Back (Rev. 11-77)

Reprinted from the Department of Veterans Affairs, Albuquerque, New Mexico.

Sandra J. Cornett, Ph.D., R.N.

Figure 9-12. Form Used to Document Results of Assessment

The Ohio State University
Columbus, Ohio

Nursing Data Base

Name preference _____

Arrival date _____ time _____ to room _____

from _____

walking ☐   wheelchair ☐   cart ☐

accompanied by self ☐   hospital staff ☐   other ☐

Significant other _____

Relationship _____

Nutrition Diet at home/appetite, eating patterns, food allergy/intolerance, dentures, oral cavity, alcohol/caffeine use, weight changes, and physical appearance	Height 5'8"	Weight kg *123* lbs

S: "I've been unable to swallow solid food for about 6 weeks. That's why I'm here, to have a tube put in my stomach so I can feed myself that way. My wife wants to learn, too. I've lost about 25 pounds in the last 3 months."

O: Thin white male. Upper and lower dentures in place. Oral mucosa pink and moist.

Reprinted, with permission, from The Ohio State University Hospitals, Columbus, 1992.

Form Development

This section discusses some of the factors that need to be taken into consideration when developing a patient education documentation form. It should be kept in mind that, in and of itself, creating or revising a form does not ensure successful documentation unless an assessment of the system indicates that the form is the real cause of the documentation deficiency. A good rule of thumb is to create a new form only if current records cannot be revised to adequately reflect all parts of the patient education process. Patient education documentation should be integrated into the current system to ensure that it is implemented as an integral part of the total care.

Flow sheets and checklists are actually progress notes designed to delineate specific patient information according to preestablished parameters. These "abbreviated progress notes" allow variables unique to a patient or a group of patients to be documented with ease, as well as data trends to be recorded. Often flow sheets and checklists are used in conjunction with other record forms, such as a data base, and progress notes. Flow sheets or checklists need to be linked to accompanying progress notes and the data base, regardless of which charting system and method are in place.[8] Figure 9-16 (p. 195) presents some of the advantages and disadvantages of using flow sheets and checklists.

Figure 9-13. Form Used to Document Planning Phase

R/T = Related to
DHS = Duration of hospital stay
DC = Discharge
Tr = Transfer

No.	Educational Diagnoses (include date/initials)	Expected Outcomes (include date/initials)	Time Frame	Educational Interventions (include date/initials)	Time
1	Knowledge/skill deficit in home care of G-tube and administration of tube feeding R/T lack of experience/ instruction. 5/11/92 SC	Patient and/or spouse will be independent with care of gastrostomy tube and administration of tube feeding using bolus method. 5/12/92 SC	by DC	1. Explain purpose and anatomical placement of G-tube.	By 5/12/92 12 N
				2. Demonstrate care of G-tube site: • Change dressing. • Cleanse exit site with H_2O and water. • Apply neosporin ointment (clean technique). • Cover with clean, dry split dressing and tape with nipple in place. • Observe site for redness, drainage, pain, swelling, and/or heat when changing dressing.	5/13/92 7–3 shift
				3. Patient to do dressing change demonstration.	5/13/92 3–11 shift
				4. Continue to have patient do dressing change every day (patient to determine time).	QD
				5. Give patient list of supplies and tell how to obtain them.	5/14/92 7–3 shift
				6. Demonstrate administration of tube feeding using bolus method. Equipment: 250cc Ensure and 125cc H_2O, toomey syringe, umbilical clamp, two measuring containers. Frequency: four times a day Method: gastric residual (do not give if residual is > 100); administer tube feeding with toomey syringe (after removing plunger) by gravity.	
				7. Have patient give tube feeding.	5/14/92 3–11 shift
				8. Instruct about complications of tube feeding and how to prevent them: diarrhea, constipation, gastrointestinal upsets, dehydration. 5/11/92 SC	5/15/92 7–3 shift

Initials	Signature	Initials	Signature	Initials	Signature
S.C.	S. Cornett, RN				

Sandra J. Cornett, Ph.D., R.N.

Figure 9-14. Form Used to Document Intervention, Evaluation, and Revision

The Ohio State University Hospitals
Columbus, Ohio

Teaching—Learning Flow Sheet

Teaching method code* A = audiovisual
R = role play
E = explanation
D = demonstration
H = handout
G = group class

No.	Date and Time	Intervention — Include content taught and identity of learner (if other than the patient)	Teaching Method*	Response/Evaluation — States/ Identifies	Applies Knowledge	Can Return Demonstrate	Routinely Performs	No Evidence of Learning	Other	Revision — Reinforce Content	Re-Teach	Needs Practice	Other	Comments	Initials
1	5/11/92	10 AM Explained purpose and anatomical placement of G-tube to patient/wife.	E	✓	✓										SC
1	5/13/92	9 AM Showed patient how to change G-tube dressing according to nursing order #2.	E/D	✓						✓		✓		Patient stated "that doesn't look too hard."	SC
1	5/13/92	7 PM Patient changed own G-tube dressing with RN supervision.			✓	✓								Patient correctly did dressing but needed help c̄ taping — MF	
1	5/14/92	8 AM Patient changed own G-tube dressing. Wife observed. Explained how to obtain supplies in own community.	D / E	✓ ✓	✓	✓				✓				Required no help from RN. Review how to get supplies in 5/15.	SC
1	5/14/92	12 N Showed patient and wife how to give bolus tube feeding as per nursing order #6. Gave handout on G-tube feedings at home.	E/D H	✓						✓		✓		Both verbalized understanding of method but expressed fear of "doing this myself." —	SC

Initials	Signature and Title	Initials	Signature and Title	Initials	Signature and Title
SC	S. Cornett RN				
MF	M. France RN				

The Ohio State University
Form 10304 HMS #30010

Reprinted, with permission, from The Ohio State University Hospitals, Columbus, 1992.

Figure 9-15. Progress Notes

Date	Hour	Patient Progress Notes
5/11/92	9$\frac{30}{}$ PM	S: "My doctor says he's going to put a tube into my stomach for feeding. My neighbor had one in his nose. His wife blenderized food and put it into the tube. I know I need this; I just don't have the appetite to eat much, and my mouth is sore from the chemo." Wife states she also wants to learn to care for the tube and give feedings. Wife not employed. Available for classes G.D. —————————
		O: Scheduled for G-tube placement 5/12 @ 1 PM. Patient and wife calm when discussing education. Both have adequate manual dexterity. No tremors or abnormal movements. Able to read written handouts. ————————
		A&P: see nursing diagnosis, expected outcomes & orders #1 ————————— S. Cornett RN

Reprinted, with permission, from The Ohio State University Hospitals, Columbus, 1992.

Figure 9-16. Advantages and Disadvantages of Flow Sheets and Checklists

Advantages:

1. Allow a variety of subject areas to be recorded over time.
2. Permit patient and staff to select mutually appropriate goals, especially if a copy of each form is given to the patient.
3. Enhance legibility and accuracy.
4. Increase efficient use of staff time.
5. Fragmentation of data is less.
6. Reminders or cues are provided to include all essential elements of documentation.
7. A concise, quick reference is provided so that patient's status can be seen at a glance.
8. Increase availability of data so trends can be demonstrated over time.
9. Responses to specific interventions are outlined to facilitate patient evaluation.
10. Patient education standards are reinforced.
11. A recording of legally relevant and useful information occurs.

Disadvantages:

1. The volume of records may be increased, creating problems of use and storage.
2. Duplication of documentation may occur.
3. Problems in design and format can result in certain parts of the form left unused. Blanks can be misinterpreted and chart review may give rise to legal questions.
4. Inadequate space for recording unusual events.
5. Problems with individualizing standard, preprinted forms.

Design Components

Although there are no standards for the design of flow sheets and checklists, there are some common components that need to be considered. The form or forms developed need to include all the standard phases of documentation content discussed previously.

Below are listed some elements to consider when the form is being designed so that staff can readily use it:

1. Space for entering the patient's name, identification, month, day, year, time, staff initials, and verifying signatures
2. Columns with spaces for check marks, code letters, or preprinted information to decrease repetitious writing (adequate space should be provided to document unusual events)
3. Predetermined categories or cues that serve as specific reminders for both structured and spontaneous teaching activities
4. Titles that describe the elements of appropriate entries
5. A design that is concise, simple, relevant, and can provide a quick reference so that patient teaching can be seen at a glance
6. Forms that are diverse (core essential information is preestablished and preprinted, but space or ways to individualize the information are available)
7. Incorporation of patient education into forms already used for other purposes (for example, preoperative checklist, discharge planning sheets)
8. Teaching protocols integrated into all patient care plans
9. A pressure-sensitive form so that copies can go to the patient, the physician, and the medical record
10. A form for use in both inpatient and outpatient settings

Process components of forms are related to some of the procedural mechanisms that can enhance the use of flow sheets and checklists. Suggested steps of procedures include the following:

1. Develop a procedure so the educational needs and teaching can be easily updated.
2. Prepare a procedure sheet of instructions and a key on the use of the form, including a definition of terms and approved abbreviations.
3. Verify that the patient education documentation form is consistent with the written standards of care recognized by the various disciplines.
4. Centralize the patient education documentation done by the various disciplines into an interdisciplinary patient care record form.
5. Use a problem-centered format to provide for efficient retrieval of data during an audit.
6. Keep forms in a convenient, accessible location (for example, bedside) so that entries can be made when they occur. (The medical record needs to follow the patient as he or she progresses through the health care delivery system.)
7. Focus on patient outcomes to provide data for evaluating the patient's care according to the standards of care.
8. Integrate patient education and discharge planning documentation together.

Computerized Patient Education Documentation

A substantial increase in the use of computers to automate documentation of patient care is likely to occur in the next decade. Automated information systems will be mandated to improve documentation of patient care as required by legal, financial, and research requirements, as well as to reduce the burden of paperwork. Fischbach[9] describes seven basic features of an ideal automated documentation system, summarized in figure 9-17.

Figure 9-17. Seven Basic Features of an Automated Documentation System

1. *One-Time Data Capture with Automatic Transcription.* Data are only entered once into the system and transcribed to all appropriate records automatically.
2. *Fast Response Time.* The user does not have to wait to process requests for input data.
3. *Integrated Data Base with Interfaced Systems.* The data collected must be integrated so they can be used by many departments. Patient data in all the various computer systems of the hospital interface with the hospital's information system.
4. *Adaptability.* The system must be flexible so that it can be adjusted and tailored to meet multiple needs.
5. *No Duplicate Recording:* The system should not require charting the same data in more than one way. Entering the data where and when they are collected is the ideal.
6. *Detailed Security System.* A security system must be in place to govern who may access what data, so patient confidentiality is a priority.
7. *Fast, Reliable, Well Understood.* The system should be fast for primary entry, highly reliable in terms of accuracy and timeliness, inexpensive in material cost, and well understood.

Adapted, with permission, from F. T. Fischbach. *Documenting Care: Communication, the Nursing Process and Documentation Standards.* Philadelphia: F. A. Davis, 1991, p. 251.

Just as handwritten patient education documentation should be an integral part of the total record-keeping system for patient care, computerized charting needs to reflect the process of patient care, including patient education, from admission to discharge. The systems that offer the most benefits for patient education documentation are those that fully mesh with other computer functions and follow the "established" processes of health care delivery. These processes include all the activities a professional performs: gathering patient information, developing an individually directed plan of care, and evaluating the outcome of the plan. Some computer systems provide complete automation of all patient care applications, including patient assessment, classification, and care planning; diagnostic test reporting; medication and IV; vital signs and intake and output recording; order entry and communications; and progress notes.

Hinson and Bush[10] described a computerized nursing care planning system that integrates hospitalwide standards. A six-step process is used to generate the computerized care plan. In the first step, the nurse identifies the patient's problems by choosing from a list of 17 nursing diagnoses. Among these diagnoses are "knowledge deficit" and "self-care deficit," which specifically reflect patient education needs. In addition, many of the other diagnoses in this list have patient education components; for example, "impaired physical mobility" and "alteration in nutrition." Step 4 of the care plan development is to identify desired outcomes for the patient from a selected list.

Outcomes related to patient education, such as "performs necessary self-care routines," are among the entries in the menu. The fifth and sixth steps of the computerized care plan include selecting from an index categories of actions that address each identified problem and selecting optional actions necessary for a specific patient, thereby ensuring a degree of individualization.

In a recent report on creating and using computerized patient records, the Institute of Medicine identified 12 requisites that a system must possess to meet patient record-keeping needs in the year 2000.[11,12] Its vision of a future computer-based patient record system encompasses a broader view of the patient record than is currently used. In addition to longitudinally recording the systematic measurement and documentation of the patients' health status and outcomes, the future system should be designed to support health care professionals in other ways. Access to aids such as prognostic risk assessments, decision analysis tools that guide problem solving, reminders and alerts to fulfill certain tasks, and links to bodies of medical knowledge will change the way patient care is delivered.[13]

Computer-assisted instruction can provide improved documentation of patient education. The microcomputer, with well-developed educational software, can present learning objectives to the patient that can be individualized to meet specific needs. Records of educational activities completed, as well as an evaluation of patient responses, can be documented through the use of computer-assisted instruction.[14,15] Individualized informed-consent and discharge instruction sheets can be computer generated and printed. If these documents indicate that explanations and answers to questions were given to patients and are signed by patients, they become documented evidence of a hospital's patient education efforts and patient responses.

Educate Staff to Document Patient Education

Another major component in the process of planning and implementing an effective patient education documentation system is the staff training that needs to be done on an ongoing basis. Results from quality improvement record audits will help identify staff education needs about patient education documentation. Staff from various disciplines are usually involved in the planning phase when the policy, procedures, and forms are developed. They provide a rich resource for other staff as changes in the documentation system are pilot-tested and implemented, and formative evaluation takes place.

If the documentation system needs to be totally revised to include patient education, the new system can be implemented in phases. Phase I can be implemented when the data base is revised to include assessment questions for patient education efforts. Phase II includes planning for the patient's expected outcomes and educational interventions. The Teaching–Learning Flow Sheet (figures 9-9 and 9-14), where the teaching that was given and the evaluation of the learning are recorded, can be implemented as the third phase.

Several strategies can be used to teach a large number of health care providers who need to learn how to do the documentation. It is important to start this process by informing the hospital's department managers of the documentation changes. A centralized workshop is usually the best way to do this in order to ensure that the information given is consistent. The managers need to be the first to learn about the changes, even though some of the managers were involved in the planning phase. The knowledge and value managers place on patient education and documentation influences how staff will accept and implement the changes.

If it is unrealistic to put all health care providers from patient care departments through repeated workshops offered by the hospital's education department, educational strategies that can be used by the departments and units need to be developed. A slide and tape program with independent study modules consisting of readings, policies, procedures, forms, samples, question-and-answer sheets, and pretests and posttests is helpful. The legal aspects of documentation and the health care professional's role in risk management as it relates to patient education need to be emphasized. Case studies on specific patient populations can be used during in-services at the department or unit level to help staff apply the information in the workshops and self-learning modules. In-services and workshops on various clinical topics should incorporate both the education of the patient population being discussed and the documentation requirements for that education.

In addition, posters that explain the documentation system changes can be placed in prominent places. Bulletin boards can be used to display standardized forms for a unit's specific patient population. Normal communication channels and opportunities such as a patient education newsletter, department newsletter, department and unit staff meetings, national patient education week activities, patient education committee agendas, and so on can be used to educate staff about documentation.

Structured patient education program staff guidelines should include a preprinted standardized documentation form(s), as defined by hospital policy and procedure. Because structured programs are developed by an ad hoc committee of health care experts for a given patient population, there is more adherence to high-quality standards of care when staff use these forms.

If a staff preceptor program is available, or if there is a patient education resource person responsible at the department or unit level, documentation of patient education can be reinforced periodically. The patient education manager can provide interdisciplinary train-the-trainer workshops on documentation for these resource people.

Obtain Organizational Supports for Patient Education Documentation

Organizational supports are very important in this change process. First and foremost, a feeling of accountability for documentation needs to be fostered by department managers. Staff need to recognize that it is an institutional expectation to appropriately and accurately document all patient care, including patient education. Institutional expectation is not only communicated through staff education, but also in job descriptions, clinical ladder standards, criteria-based performance evaluations, and departmental standards of care.

All health care disciplines with staff from all levels need to be involved in developing the policies, procedures, and forms for documentation and in pilot-testing the changes to the documentation system. In addition to the traditional patient care areas, other functions that need to be involved include risk management, continuity of care, medical records, physicians, administration, and staff development. Interdepartmental collaboration is imperative if the documentation process is to be directed toward interdisciplinary patient care and not fragmented according to the various disciplines involved. In practice, interdisciplinary discharge planning rounds on each unit once or twice a week can help in documenting both patient education and the discharge plans. If a patient classification system is used to help determine acuity levels and staff allocation, the patients' and families' educational requirements and documentation time need to be considered.

Managers need to take definitive actions to correct deficiencies in patient education documentation identified through ongoing auditing of records and other evaluation methods. One criterion used to evaluate a manager's performance could be the status of patient education documentation and the actions taken to improve the process. Frequent feedback about the level of compliance with patient education documentation needs to be directed to the hospitalwide patient education committee and to the appropriate managers and administrators. The PEM may need to provide human and material resources to help managers take actions to correct the deficiencies in their departments.

Evaluate the Patient Education Documentation System

As mentioned in the previous section on staff education, documentation initiatives or revisions can be implemented in stages or phases, depending on how much change is required. Each phase needs to be pilot-tested before hospitalwide implementation is done. Therefore, formative evaluation is an important part of the implementation process.

Record audits need to be ongoing at both the unit and department levels to monitor how effectively the policy, procedures, and forms are meeting patient education documentation standards. Figure 9-18 is an example of a generic auditing tool that can be used to evaluate the use of the teaching–learning flow sheet. An attempt should be made to include some aspect of evaluating patient education documentation in each unit-based quality improvement program. The indicators and tools can be generic to a particular unit's aspect of care, or they can be very specific to the education a certain patient population receives and to what the patient outcomes should be at discharge.

In addition to record audits, it is important to ask staff to identify the strengths and weaknesses of the policies, procedures, and forms that are being used. This can be done through written surveys, focus groups, peer reviews, or self-assessments. Revisions are made in the procedures and forms based on this evaluation.

Figure 9-18. Example of a Quality Assurance Monitor Tool for Evaluating a Teaching–Learning Flow Sheet

Unit: _____
Problem: _____
Date: _____

Directions: Circle the correct response. (Y = yes, N = no, NA = not applicable)

Medical Record Number: _____
Date: _____

Screening Criteria	1	2	3	4	5	6	7	8	9	10
1. Form was stamped with the embosser plate or identified with the patient's name and hospital number?	Y N NA	Y N NA	Y N NA	Y N NA	Y N NA	Y N NA	Y N NA	Y N NA	Y N NA	Y N NA
2. Number of the relevant nursing diagnosis recorded (if applicable)?	Y N NA	Y N NA	Y N NA	Y N NA	Y N NA	Y N NA	Y N NA	Y N NA	Y N NA	Y N NA
3. Date (month and day) recorded?	Y N NA	Y N NA	Y N NA	Y N NA	Y N NA	Y N NA	Y N NA	Y N NA	Y N NA	Y N NA
4. On the first entry of the page, the year was noted.	Y N NA	Y N NA	Y N NA	Y N NA	Y N NA	Y N NA	Y N NA	Y N NA	Y N NA	Y N NA
5. The time (including a.m. or p.m.) recorded?	Y N NA	Y N NA	Y N NA	Y N NA	Y N NA	Y N NA	Y N NA	Y N NA	Y N NA	Y N NA
6. Each entry was identified by the initials of the writer?	Y N NA	Y N NA	Y N NA	Y N NA	Y N NA	Y N NA	Y N NA	Y N NA	Y N NA	Y N NA
7. Each set of initials identified by a signature at the bottom of the page?	Y N NA	Y N NA	Y N NA	Y N NA	Y N NA	Y N NA	Y N NA	Y N NA	Y N NA	Y N NA
8. Each signature includes the first initial, last name, and title?	Y N NA	Y N NA	Y N NA	Y N NA	Y N NA	Y N NA	Y N NA	Y N NA	Y N NA	Y N NA
9. Content of teaching was recorded?	Y N NA	Y N NA	Y N NA	Y N NA	Y N NA	Y N NA	Y N NA	Y N NA	Y N NA	Y N NA
10. Identity of the learner was recorded (if other than patient)?	Y N NA	Y N NA	Y N NA	Y N NA	Y N NA	Y N NA	Y N NA	Y N NA	Y N NA	Y N NA
11. The teaching method(s) was identified using approved code letters?	Y N NA	Y N NA	Y N NA	Y N NA	Y N NA	Y N NA	Y N NA	Y N NA	Y N NA	Y N NA
12. Names of handouts, group classes, or audiovisual aids were recorded?	Y N NA	Y N NA	Y N NA	Y N NA	Y N NA	Y N NA	Y N NA	Y N NA	Y N NA	Y N NA
13. At least one column was checked in the section "response/evaluation"?	Y N NA	Y N NA	Y N NA	Y N NA	Y N NA	Y N NA	Y N NA	Y N NA	Y N NA	Y N NA
14. The evaluation column marked was appropriate in view of the teaching done?	Y N NA	Y N NA	Y N NA	Y N NA	Y N NA	Y N NA	Y N NA	Y N NA	Y N NA	Y N NA

15. If indicated, at least one column of the "revision" section was checked?	Y N NA	Y N NA	Y N NA	Y N NA	Y N NA	Y N NA	Y N NA	Y N NA
16. Additional comments were recorded in the "comments" section (if indicated)?	Y N NA	Y N NA	Y N NA	Y N NA	Y N NA	Y N NA	Y N NA	Y N NA
17. The chart of a patient who had been discharged included the following:								
Medications	Y N NA	Y N NA	Y N NA	Y N NA	Y N NA	Y N NA	Y N NA	Y N NA
Diet	Y N NA	Y N NA	Y N NA	Y N NA	Y N NA	Y N NA	Y N NA	Y N NA
Treatments or procedures	Y N NA	Y N NA	Y N NA	Y N NA	Y N NA	Y N NA	Y N NA	Y N NA
Signs and symptoms of complications	Y N NA	Y N NA	Y N NA	Y N NA	Y N NA	Y N NA	Y N NA	Y N NA
Follow-up care	Y N NA	Y N NA	Y N NA	Y N NA	Y N NA	Y N NA	Y N NA	Y N NA
Activity level	Y N NA	Y N NA	Y N NA	Y N NA	Y N NA	Y N NA	Y N NA	Y N NA
Knowledge of disease or treatment	Y N NA	Y N NA	Y N NA	Y N NA	Y N NA	Y N NA	Y N NA	Y N NA

Evaluation of the patient education documentation system does not stop after it is implemented throughout the hospital. Periodic audits and surveys are done to provide necessary information to improve the system. The system needs to remain dynamic if it is to meet the ever-demanding challenges in patient education influenced by changes in JCAHO criteria, health care delivery systems, reimbursement, professional standards, technology, and other changes and issues unimaginable at this time.

☐ Conclusion

To be most effective, a patient documentation system should be integrated into the hospital's total record-keeping system. Other requirements for an effective system include communication of the institutional expectation that teaching efforts will be correctly documented, ongoing staff training in the system's use, continuous evaluation of the system through medical record audits and examination of the deficiencies, and implementation of improvements.

References

1. Fiesta, J. Informed consent process: whose legal duty? *Nursing Management* 22(1):17, Jan. 1991.

2. Fiesta, J. *The Law and Liability: A Guide for Nurses.* 2nd ed. New York City: John Wiley and Sons, 1988.

3. Barron, S. Documentation of patient education. *Patient Education and Counseling* 9(1):81–90, Feb. 1987.

4. Ohio Hospital Association, Bulletin No. 89-008-A. *Joint Commission Contingencies/Recommendations: Finding in Ohio Hospitals.* Columbus, OH: OHA, 1989.

5. Longo, D. R., Laubenthal, R. M., and Redman, R. Hospital compliance with JCAHO nursing standards: findings from 1982 surveys. *Quality Review Bulletin* 10(8):243–47, Aug. 1984.

6. Fischbach, F. T. *Documenting Care: Communication, the Nursing Process and Documentation Standards.* Philadelphia: F. A. Davis, 1991, pp. 19–24.

7. Joint Commission on Accreditation of Healthcare Organizations. *Accreditation Manual for Hospitals.* Oakbrook Terrace, IL: JCAHO, 1993, p. 103.

8. Fischbach, pp. 233–37.

9. Fischbach, pp. 251–53.

10. Hinson, D. K., and Bush, C. Corporate standards for nursing care: an integral part of a computerized care plan. *Computers in Nursing* 6(4):141–46, July–Aug. 1988.

11. Simpson, R. L. Computer-based patient records, part I: the Institute of Medicine's vision. *Nursing Management* 22(10):24–25, Oct. 1991.

12. Simpson, R. L. Computer-based patient records, part II: IOM's 12 requisites. *Nursing Management* 22(11):26–28, Nov. 1991.

13. Simpson, R. L. Computer-based patient records, part II.

14. Bell, J. A. The role of microcomputer in patient education. *Computers in Nursing* 4(6):255–58, Nov.–Dec. 1986.

15. Vargo, G. Computer assisted patient education in the ambulatory care setting. *Computers in Nursing* 9(5):168–69, Sept.–Oct. 1991.

Bibliography

Allen, S. K. Selection and implementation of an automated care planning system for a health care institution. *Computers in Nursing* 9(2):61–67, Mar.–Apr. 1981.

Barbiasz, J. E., Hunt, V., and Lawenstein, A. Nursing documentation: a format, not a form. *The Journal of Nursing Administration* 11(6):22–26, June 1981.

Boyd, M. D. Policies, guidelines, and legal mandates for health teaching. Chapter 2 in: *Teaching in Nursing Practice: A Professional Model.* N. I. Whitman, B. A. Graham, C. J. Gleit, and M. D. Boyd, editors. Norwalk, CT: Appleton-Century-Crofts, 1986, pp. 17–29.

Brady, M. Bedside nursing/hospital information system integration must include productivity gains for nursing. *Computers in Nursing* 9(2):61–67, July–Aug. 1991.

Burke, L. J., and Murphy, J. *Charting by Exception: A Cost- Effective, Quality Approach.* New York City: John Wiley and Sons, 1988.

Coles, M. D., and Fullenwider, S. D. Documentation: managing the dilemma. *Nursing Management* 19(12):65–72, Dec. 1988.

Comstock, L. G., and Moff, T. E. Cost-effective, time-efficient charting. *Nursing Management* 22(7):44–48, July 1991.

Deane, D., McElroy, M. J., and Alden, S. Documentation: meeting requirements while maximizing productivity. *Nursing Economics* 4(4):174–78, July–Aug. 1986.

Eggland, E. T. Charting: how and why to document your care daily and fully. *Nursing 88* 18(11):76–84, Nov. 1988.

Fox, L., and Woods, P. Nursing process—evaluation of documentation. *Nursing Management* 22(1):57–59, Jan. 1991.

Haggard, A. Documenting patient education. In: *Handbook of Patient Education,* Chapter 10, pp. 143–57. Rockville, MD: Aspen Publishers, 1989.

Iyer, P. W. New trends in charting. *Nursing 91* 21(1):48–50, Jan. 1991.

Kuehnel, C., and Rowe, B. Patient education and the audit. *Supervisor Nurse* 11(12):15–19, Dec. 1980.

Langel, B. C., Brewer, S. G., and Olszewshi, C. Developing quality documentation. *Nursing Management* 22(11):48–52, Nov. 1991.

Laros, P. With this flow sheet, less is more. *Nursing 85* 15(7):25–29, July 1985.

Lower, M. S., and Hauert, L. P. Charting: the impact of bedside computers. *Nursing Management* 23(7):40–44, July 1992.

Montemuro, M. Core documentation: a complete system for charting nursing care. *Nursing Management* 19(8):28–32, Aug. 1988.

Morris, A., and Thomas, S. A med/surg nursing record: convenient, adequate—and accepted. *Nursing Management* 23(5):68–72, May 1992.

Murphy, J., Beglinger, J. E., and Johnson, B. Charting by exception: meeting the challenge of cost containment. *Nursing Management* 19(2):56–72, Feb. 1988.

Schlehofer, G. B. Informatics: managing clinical operations data. *Nursing Management* 23(7):36–38, July 1992.

Worthy, M. K., and Siegrist-Mueller, L. Integrating a "plan of care" into documentation systems. *Nursing Management* 23(10):68–70, Oct. 1992.

Chapter 10

Linking Patient Education with Quality Improvement

Carolyn E. Maller, M.S., C.H.E.S., R.N.,
and Barbara E. Giloth, M.P.H., C.H.E.S.

☐ Objectives

The reader will be able to:

- Define quality improvement terminology as it relates to patient education
- Reference existing standards for patient and family education
- Cite examples of patient education quality improvement activities
- Apply quality improvement concepts in developing and implementing a plan for patient education at the institutional, target population, and case levels

☐ Quality Improvement Issues and Terminology

The primary purpose of this chapter is to review the types of quality of care activities that apply to patient education. The first section assesses the positive and negative forces influencing the priority level assigned to quality improvement for patient education. The second reviews the wide range of standards and guidelines that have particular relevance for patient education. The third section describes the development of quality improvement plans. The fourth section surveys a broad range of specific examples of applicable quality improvement activities. The final section looks at specific ways to implement quality improvement plans for patient education.

An initial challenge to development of quality of care initiatives for patient education is the lack of clarity in defining the parameters of high-quality patient care. Although it is important that each institution decide how narrowly or broadly these terms are to be used in defining scope of service, an American Hospital Association (AHA) management advisory can be used as a basis for such determinations. In 1990, the AHA defined the hospital's responsibility for patient education in terms of the impact of the service that "should enable patients, and their families and friends, when appropriate, to make informed decisions about their health; to manage their illnesses; and to implement follow-up care at home."[1] For the purposes of this chapter, current and emerging terminology is defined to guide the reader in distinguishing current and future directions for quality assessment and continuous quality improvement initiatives.

Carolyn E. Maller, M.S., C.H.E.S., R.N., and Barbara E. Giloth, M.P.H., C.H.E.S.

Patient care quality is defined as "the degree to which patient care services increase the probability of desired patient outcomes and reduce the probability of undesired outcomes, given the current state of knowledge."[2] Characteristics of quality and high-quality care have been addressed by O'Leary,[3] Merry,[4] and a host of others.

Quality assurance (QA) established itself as a standard for achieving quality in the health care environment. In the formative years, QA activities searched for problems to solve rather than for solutions to improve patient care. The trend emerging in QA today focuses on finding a solution to fixing the system using a continuous quality improvement process.

Total quality management (TQM) first surfaced in industry as a management philosophy committed to improving quality by overcoming systems problems. Crosby,[5] Juran,[6,7] and Deming[8] are credited with looking at management systems in America to better quality, productivity, and customer satisfaction. The introduction of TQM to the health care arena is still occurring. Berwick[9] and Gottlieb and others[10] have forged ahead with clinical models in an effort to apply this quality management system to health care settings. In *Curing Health Care*, quality management strategies are applied to clinical practice issues.[11] Similar applications are feverishly appearing in the literature[12-16] as health care systems struggle to contain costs without sacrificing quality.

Continuous quality improvement (CQI) applies total quality management principles to health care institutions to provide better patient care, benefiting patients as well as staff.[17,18] Emphasis is clearly on identifying systemwide solutions to gaps in delivering improved quality of care. CQI is "an approach to quality management that builds upon traditional quality assurance methods by emphasizing the organization and systems (rather than individuals), the need for objective data with which to analyze and improve processes, and the ideal that systems and performance can always improve even when high standards appear to have been met; also called total quality management."[19] In this chapter, the phrase *quality improvement* refers to the contemporary movement toward total quality improvement in patient care.

Selected examples from clinical practice are cited throughout this chapter to begin to address the complexities of measuring and quantifying quality of care as it relates to patient education. Patient educators will need to assess and evaluate clinical examples for relevance and applicability to their particular hospital climates for CQI, as well as the organizational structure for patient education.

☐ Status of Quality Improvement for Patient Education

After reviewing the current extent and depth of quality improvement activities, an inconsistent picture emerges. On the negative side, despite consumer and business interest in patient education, it has remained financially tenuous within hospitals, especially if dedicated staff are to be assigned. Less priority, therefore, has been placed on quality of care issues. Staff resistance to the application of teaching standards has been reported in the literature[20] and anecdotally. This problem may relate to health care professionals' continuing discomfort with the adequacy of their teaching skills and the low priority that teaching may receive in their hospital setting.[21]

The ubiquitous nature of patient education and multiple levels of program development also cause some problems. The delivery of patient education is difficult to isolate from other health care interventions and, because of the critical interpersonal component, is also very difficult to standardize. Although the research base is improving, it remains very difficult to define the relationship between process and outcome. Patient education requires a substantial amount of patient and family/consumer involvement in order to be effective, an involvement that continues to be viewed with skepticism by many health care professionals.[22] Because of their voluntary nature, the success of patient education programs cannot be assessed only in terms of achieving desired compliance rates.

Finally, within the overall quality of care process, patient education is more frequently identified as a major strategy to respond to deficiencies. This may have the unintended effect of reducing the salience of internal assessments of service quality.

On the positive side, however, there is a growing research base that supports the burgeoning field of patient education. For example, a five-year follow-up of hypertensive patients who received one or more educational interventions documented a 57.3 percent reduction in all causes of mortality and a 53.2 percent reduction in hypertension-related mortality compared to the control group.[23] This type of study not only underscores the critical contribution of patient education to important health outcomes, but identifies those specific interventions that are most effective, in this case family support. A meta-analysis of medication instruction research found that in terms of impact on knowledge and drug error outcomes, the choice of educational strategy is somewhat less important than whether educational principles—reinforcement, feedback, individualization, facilitation, and relevance—are used in designing the intervention.[24] (See the section titled Techniques Used in chapter 14 for a description of how meta-analysis works.)

As emphasis in health care continues its dramatic shift from an acute to a chronic focus, the importance of patient behaviors in ensuring desirable health outcomes also increases dramatically.[25] To try to ensure that patients achieve positive health outcomes, patient educators need to look at why patients behave the way they do from a theoretical perspective in order to arrive at a practical educational approach.[26] Whether the disease process is hypertension, diabetes, arthritis, or something else, the ability of the patient and his or her family to problem-solve and incorporate new monitoring behaviors in their life-style is necessary to contain the degenerative potential of the disease as well as to limit its side effects. Participation of both patient and family in care has been identified by the Joint Commission on Accreditation of Healthcare Organizations (JCAHO) as one of the 12 factors that determine quality of patient care.[27]

The Medical Outcomes Study has conceptualized relevant health outcomes to include not only clinical end points, but also functional status, general patient well-being, and satisfaction with care. Additionally, the conceptual framework divides process of care variables into two major categories: technical style and interpersonal style. The latter includes patient participation and counseling as well as aspects of the way clinicians relate to patients.[28] Other researchers more strongly support the notion that health-related quality of life outcomes, especially for chronic disease patients, take precedence over traditional survival and cure outcomes.[29] Continuing research suggests that the involvement of patients in care planning and decision making has a positive impact on health status measures as well as participation and satisfaction variables.[30]

Recent articles detailing the results of the Picker/Commonwealth Patient-Centered Care survey[31,32] bring the patients' view of hospitalization into focus. In this survey, a telephone interview process was used to query patients about specific events that occurred or did not occur while they were in the hospital. Interviewees identified a high percentage of problems related to communication and patient education as well as discharge preparation. Patients wanted clearer instructions prior to going home from the hospital. They asked to be more informed regarding diet, medication use, danger signals to watch for, and other aspects of their recovery. This research supports not only the importance of patient education, but also the usefulness of engaging patients as reporters in improvement initiatives. This makes particular sense with regard to patient education programs, because the essence of the function is patient involvement.

Passage of the Patient Self-Determination Act of 1990 mandated hospitals to educate patients about their right to refuse medical treatment and attests to the power of consumer demand for involvement in decision making.[33] Health care administrators are enlisting patient educators to inform patients about their rights to formulate advance directives such as a living will or a durable power of attorney for health care. A new patient's rights chapter published in the 1993 Accreditation Manual for Hospitals[34] references standards for implementing advance directives and provides the structure for monitoring how well a facility performs.

Carolyn E. Maller, M.S., C.H.E.S., R.N., and Barbara E. Giloth, M.P.H., C.H.E.S.

□ Patient Education Standards

In addition to the growth of a research base and increased understanding of the links between patient behavior and health outcomes, a wide variety of patient education standards have been developed. Most of them have focused on structure and process at institutional, target population, or case levels rather than behavioral or clinical outcomes. At the same time, program evaluation focusing on knowledge or behavioral change outcomes has been emphasized as compared to the traditional medical QA approach based on a structure/process accreditation foundation and focusing on therapeutic outcomes.[35] Baker has suggested that these two approaches are coming together and that this melding of monitoring processes will strengthen the ability of patient educators to track program quality.[36] The proliferation of standards, often introduced and sanctioned by professional associations, will determine future directions for meeting hospital as well as national criteria for the quality of patient care and patient education.

Five different categories of patient education standards are reviewed in the following sections: (1) accreditation standards, (2) clinical practice guidelines, (3) institutional guidelines, (4) target population and disease-specific guidelines, and (5) professional certification programs. Overall, the standards are structure and process focused. Their impacts have not been validated by a research program, although many have been built on previous research findings. Although very different in terms of scope and organizational focus, their elements appear generally consistent, and as such they can serve as a rich source of indicators for quality improvement activities.

Accreditation Standards

Although the JCAHO historically has integrated a substantial number of references to patient education into its standards programs,[37] the commissioners have only recently approved a new patient and family education chapter for the *1993 Accreditation Manual for Hospitals*.[38] (See figures 10-1 and 10-2.) This new chapter consolidates what were heretofore a dispersed set of required characteristics in dietetic services, hospital-sponsored ambulatory care services, medical records services, nursing care, patient rehabilitation services, special care units, and surgical and anesthesia services.

Although there has been concern in the field about the impact of removing specific standards related to patient education from chapters that deal with specific hospital departments, the new survey process is expected to query each department currently reviewed on patient and family education. The patient and family education chapter is also scheduled for further revision in 1994, at which time a more comprehensive set of standards can be considered.[39] In spite of the limitations of this first chapter, it does have the potential to increase the visibility of patient and family education within the JCAHO survey process and therefore within the organization itself. It also represents a further step, in line with the AHA's 1990 management advisory referenced earlier, toward defining hospitalwide responsibility for patient education.

Another JCAHO publication, the *Ambulatory Health Care Standards Manual*, in addition to medical record and rights and responsibilities chapters that reference patient education, has a quality of care standard with at least four of the required characteristics related to patient education (QC.1.1.3, 4, 9, and 12). This standard states that provision of high-quality health care services includes "patient instruction and education" and "reasonable follow-up regarding patient adherence to a plan of care."[40] Although the managed care accreditation program has been discontinued, the *Managed Care Standards Manual* had a unique chapter dedicated to consumer rights and responsibilities that included substantial requirements regarding information that must be provided to the enrolled population. Standard 8 in this chapter required that "Patients [be] given the opportunity to participate in decision-making regarding their health care."[41]

Figure 10-1. 1993 JCAHO Chapter on Patient and Family Education

PF.1
The patient and/or, when appropriate, his/her significant other(s) are provided with education that can enhance their knowledge, skills, and behaviors necessary to fully benefit from the health care interventions provided by the organization.   1 2 3 4 5 NA

PF.1.1 The patient and/or, when appropriate, his/her significant other(s) receive education specific to the patient's relevant health care needs, in ways understandable to the patient and/or his/her significant other(s).   1 2 3 4 5 NA

PF.1.1.1 Such education includes instruction in the specific knowledge and/or skills needed by the patient and/or, when appropriate, his/her significant other(s) to meet the patient's ongoing health care needs, including

PF.1.1.1.1 the safe and effective use of medication, if any;   1 2 3 4 5 NA

PF.1.1.1.2 the safe and effective use of medical equipment, if any;   1 2 3 4 5 NA

PF.1.1.1.3 instruction on potential drug–food interactions and counseling on modified diets, as appropriate; and   1 2 3 4 5 NA

PF.1.1.1.4 when and how to obtain further treatment, if needed.   1 2 3 4 5 NA

PF.1.2 Information about any discharge instructions given to the patient and/or his/her significant other(s) is provided to the individual or organization responsible for the continuing care of the patient.   1 2 3 4 5 NA

Notes and Comments:

Reprinted, with permission, from the Joint Commission on Accreditation of Healthcare Organizations. *1993 Accreditation Manual for Hospitals.* Oakbrook Terrace, IL: JCAHO, 1992.

Clinical Practice Guidelines

Out of a heightened consciousness for quality improvement and cost containment, practice guidelines are being developed as panels of experts convene to draft standards for what should be done in clinical decision making.[42] Although the intent is not meant to regulate clinical practice, such guidelines are intended to reduce variations in practice and ultimately improve the quality of patient care. Practice guidelines are emerging from a variety of sources as pressure mounts to screen out ineffective and costly practices. The Agency for Health Care Policy and Research (AHCPR) is one such source that oversees development of clinical practice guidelines. Through its Forum for Quality and Effectiveness in Health Care, the AHCPR recently released a guideline entitled *Acute Pain Management: Operative or Medical Procedures and Trauma.* Of particular interest to patient educators is the patient education booklet *Pain Control after Surgery,* which enlists the patient in pain management prior to surgery. To date, 16 practice guidelines are being prepared by the AHCPR, with more slated for development.[43] The future of clinical practice guidelines is yet to be determined. Successful implementation requires strong physician commitment and hospital support for quality improvement in practice.

Figure 10-2. Scoring Guidelines for the 1993 JCAHO Patient and Family Education Standard

In addition to the scoring expectations described for each standard in this chapter of scoring guidelines, the following track record requirements will be applied:

Score 1 The organization has substantially complied with the standard for 12 months prior to survey.

Score 2 The organization has substantially complied with the standard for 9–11 months prior to survey.

Score 3 The organization has substantially complied with the standard for 6–8 months prior to survey.

Score 4 The organization has substantially complied with the standard for 5 months or less prior to survey.

Score 5 There is no evidence that the organization complies with the standard.

PF.1 The patient and/or, when appropriate, his/her significant other(s) are provided with education that can enhance their knowledge, skills, and those behaviors necessary to fully benefit from the health care innovations provided by the organization.

INTENT OF PF.1 THROUGH PF.1.2 The education and instruction of the patient and/or, when appropriate, his/her significant other(s) is an integral part of the provision of patient care. Positive outcome of a patient's care is often dependent on, for example, (1) the instructions given to a patient prior to care or treatment (for example, prior to diagnostic testing or surgery), (2) the activities of the patient and/or his/her significant other(s) subsequent to the discharge of the patient from the health care organization, and (3) information given concerning health maintenance. The organization is to assist the patient or his/her significant other(s) in gaining the knowledge and skills needed to meet the patient's ongoing health care needs.

Note: PF.1 is not scored.

PF.1.1 The patient and/or, when appropriate, his/her significant other(s) receive education specific to the patient's relevant health care needs, in ways understandable to the patient and/or his/her significant other(s).

SCORING

Score 1 Evidence in the medical record indicates that the patient's educational needs pertaining to self-care are assessed, identified, and addressed. For example, progress notes, flow sheets, or referral/consultation notes may indicate such assessment and intervention.

AND

Evidence in 91%–100% of the medical records reviewed indicates that the patient's and/or significant other's understanding of any instruction or education for self-care is assessed.

Score 2 The organization has not defined an approach to patient education, but evidence in 91%–100% of the medical records reviewed indicates that such education is provided to patients and/or their significant other(s)

AND

Evidence, as appropriate, in 76%–90% of the medical records reviewed indicates that the patient's and/or his/her significant other's understanding of any instruction or education for self-care is assessed.

Score 3 Evidence, as appropriate, in 51%–75% of the records reviewed indicates that the patient's and/or his/her significant other's understanding of any instruction or education for self-care is assessed.

Score 4 There is evidence in the medical record that the patient's educational needs are assessed and identified but such needs are not addressed in 76%-100% of the medical records reviewed.

Score 5 There is no evidence, as appropriate, that the patient's and/or his/her significant other's understanding of any instruction or education for self-care is assessed.

Figure 10-2. (Continued)

OR

There is no defined approach to patient education and no evidence in the medical records that the patient's educational needs are assessed, identified, and addressed.

PF.1.1.1 Such education includes instruction in the specific knowledge and/or skills needed by the patient and/or, when appropriate, his/her significant other(s) to meet the patient's ongoing health care needs, including

PF.1.1.1.1 the safe and effective use of medication, if any;

Note: PF.1.1.1 is not scored.

Scoring for PF.1.1.1.1

Score 1 Responsibility for instruction regarding provision of safe and effective medication is assigned.

AND

The specific learning needs of the patient and/or his/her significant other(s) concerning the safe use of medications are identified and addressed in 91%–100% of the medical records reviewed in which such instruction is indicated.

Score 2 The specific learning needs of the patient and/or his/her significant other(s) concerning the safe use of medications are identified and addressed in 76%–90% of the records reviewed in which such instruction is indicated.

Score 3 The specific learning needs of the patient and/or his/her significant other(s) concerning the safe use of medications are identified and addressed in 51%–75% of the records reviewed in which such instruction is indicated.

Score 4 The specific learning needs of the patient and/or his/her significant other(s) concerning the safe use of medications are identified and addressed in 26%–50% of the records reviewed in which such instruction is indicated.

Score 5 Responsibility for instruction regarding the provision of safe and effective medication is not assigned.

OR

The specific learning needs of the patient and/or his/her significant other(s) concerning the safe use of medications are identified and addressed in fewer than 26% of the records reviewed in which such instruction is indicated.

PF.1.1.1.2 [Such education includes instruction in the specific knowledge and/or skills needed by the patient and/or, when appropriate, his/her significant other(s) to meet the patient's ongoing health care needs, including] the safe and effective use of medical equipment, if any;

Scoring

Score 1 Responsibility for instruction regarding the provision of safe and effective medical equipment is assigned.

AND

The specific learning needs of the patient and/or his/her significant other(s) concerning the safe and effective use of medical equipment are identified and addressed in 91%–100% of the medical records reviewed in which such instruction is indicated.

Score 2 The specific learning needs of the patient and/or his/her significant other(s) concerning the safe and effective use of medical equipment are identified and addressed in 76%–90% of the medical records reviewed in which such instruction is indicated.

Score 3 The specific learning needs of the patient and/or his/her significant other(s) concerning the safe and effective use of medical equipment are identified and

211

(Continued on next page)

Figure 10-2. (Continued)

addressed in 51%–75% of the medical records reviewed in which such instruction is indicated.

Score 4 The specific learning needs of the patient and/or his/her significant other(s) concerning the safe and effective use of medical equipment are identified and addressed in 26%–50% of the medical records reviewed in which such instruction is indicated.

Score 5 Responsibility for instruction regarding the provision of the safe and effective use of medical equipment is not assigned.

OR

The specific learning needs of the patient and/or his/her significant other(s) concerning the safe and effective use of medical equipment are identified and addressed in fewer than 26% of the medical records reviewed in which such instruction is indicated.

PF.1.1.1.3 [Such education includes instruction in the specific knowledge and/or skills needed by the patient and/or, when appropriate, his/her significant other(s) to meet the patient's ongoing health care needs, including] instruction on potential drug–food interactions and counseling on modified diets, as appropriate; and

Scoring **Score 1** The specific learning needs of the patient and/or his/her significant other(s) regarding dietary and nutritional instruction, including potential food–drug interactions, are identified and addressed in 91%–100% of the medical records reviewed in which such instruction is indicated.

AND

Dietary and nutritional counseling is provided and includes instruction on drug–food interactions.

Score 2 The specific learning needs of the patient and/or his/her significant other(s) are identified and addressed in 76%–90% of the records reviewed in which such instruction is indicated.

Score 3 The specific learning needs of the patient and/or his/her significant other(s) are identified and addressed in 51%–75% of the records reviewed in which such instruction is indicated.

Score 4 The specific dietary and nutritional learning needs of the patient and/or his/her significant other(s) are identified and addressed in 26%–50% of the records reviewed in which such instruction is indicated.

Score 5 The specific learning needs of the patient and/or his/her significant other(s) are identified and addressed in fewer than 26% of the records reviewed in which such instruction is indicated.

PF.1.1.1.4 [Such education includes instruction in the specific knowledge and/or skills needed by the patient and/or, when appropriate, his/her significant other(s) to meet the patient's ongoing health care needs, including] when and how to obtain further treatment, if needed.

Scoring **Score 1** In 91%–100% of the records reviewed for which such instruction is indicated, the patient and/or his/her significant other(s) are given instructions about any follow-up care needed and how to obtain that care.

Score 2 In 76%–90% of the medical records reviewed for which such instruction is indicated, the patient and/or his/her significant other(s) are given instructions about any follow-up care needed and how to obtain that care.

Score 3 In 51%–75% of the medical records reviewed for which such instruction is indicated, the patient and/or his/her significant other(s) are given instructions about any follow-up care needed and how to obtain that care.

Score 4 In 26%–50% of the medical records reviewed for which such instruction is indicated, the patient and/or his/her significant other(s) are given instructions about any follow-up care needed and how to obtain that care.

Figure 10-2. **(Continued)**

Score 5 In fewer than 26% of the medical records reviewed for which such instruction is indicated, the patient and/or his/her significant other(s) are given instructions about any follow-up care needed and how to obtain that care.

PF.1.2. Information about any discharge instructions given to the patient and/or his/her significant other(s) is provided to the individual or organization responsible for the continuing care of the patient.

Scoring **Score 1** 91%–100% of the pertinent medical records reviewed indicate that information regarding any relevant discharge instructions provided to the patient and/or his/her significant other(s) was provided to the individual or organization responsible for the continuing care of the patient.

Score 2 76%–90% of the medical records reviewed indicate that information regarding any relevant discharge instructions provided to the patient and/or his/her significant other(s) was provided to the individual or organization responsible for the continuing care of the patient.

Score 3 51%–75% of the medical records reviewed indicate that information regarding any relevant discharge instructions provided to the patient and/or his/her significant other(s) was provided to the individual or organization responsible for the continuing care of the patient.

Score 4 26%–50% of the medical records reviewed indicate that information regarding any relevant discharge instructions provided to the patient and/or his/her significant other(s) was provided to the individual or organization responsible for the continuing care of the patient.

Score 5 Fewer than 26% of the medical records reviewed indicate that information regarding any relevant discharge instructions provided to the patient and/or his/her significant other(s) was provided to the individual or organization responsible for the continuing care of the patient.

Reprinted, with permission, from the Joint Commission on Accreditation of Healthcare Organizations. *1993 Accreditation Manual for Hospitals.* Oakbrook Terrace, IL: JCAHO, 1992.

Although not of the same high level of sophistication as clinical practice guidelines, patient education practice guidelines are now appearing. As of March 1991, 26 practice guidelines specifically address patient education and counseling. Topics include asthma, cholesterol, nutrition, substance abuse, and exercise counseling.[44] These standards have relevance for developing good clinical indicators to measure performance in patient education practice.

Institutional Guidelines

Several important documents appeared in the late 1970s and early 1980s that laid out guidelines for the development of organized patient education and health education programs in a variety of settings. In 1979, for example, the American Public Health Association (APHA) produced *A Model for Patient Education Programming* that defines three levels of patient education in a hospital or other medical facility—institutional, target population, and patient levels. A detailed planning scheme breaks down each level into program development stages—assessment, planning, implementation, and evaluation.[45] (See table 1-1.)

More recently, the Department of Veterans Affairs (VA) has applied this model to the VA system through the development of the 1988 *Guidelines for the Development of Patient Health Education Programs.*[46] A detailed patient education program review guide provides a checklist of criteria that can be applied to a variety of target population programs as a self-assessment tool for needs assessment, education plan, coordination, implementation, evaluation, and staff training processes.

Standard-setting activities for patient education are emerging as nursing practice integrates patient education within the overall quality improvement plan. At Vancouver

Carolyn E. Maller, M.S., C.H.E.S., R.N., and Barbara E. Giloth, M.P.H., C.H.E.S.

General Hospital, an elaborate set of patient education standards and criteria outlines expected performance for nurses at the institutional, programmatic, and target population levels to meet the overall nursing service standard.[47] Other hospitals have invested in similar initiatives for drafting patient education standards and guidelines.[48]

Target Population and Disease-Specific Guidelines

As individual clinical areas develop practice standards and guidelines that address patient education components of care, the development of quality improvement plans is facilitated.

The diabetes field provides perhaps the most complete example of standards that define the clinical, educational, and professional indicators of high-quality care. In October 1988, the Board of Directors of the American Diabetes Association (ADA) approved standards that define basic medical care for persons with diabetes.[49] The recommended parameters for the initial visit and continuing care address the critical need for extensive patient education as part of the management plan. Although these standards show the integration of patient education into clinical care, the National Standards for Diabetes Patient Education developed in 1983 under the aegis of the National Diabetes Advisory Board specifically outline 10 categories of standards for diabetes patient education at the programmatic and case levels. These standards are currently the basis of a voluntary recognition program run by the ADA that by summer 1992 had recognized 263 programs, primarily outpatient and hospital-based.[50] Although currently specific to diabetes, these standards and the associated detailed criteria[51] to measure their achievement have relevance for most chronic disease concerns.

North Carolina, through its Department of Human Resources, operates a certification process for cardiac rehabilitation programs. In the *Rules Governing the Certification of Cardiac Rehabilitation Programs,*[52] program staff must include a patient educator, among other personnel. A companion volume, written by Wake Forest University cardiac rehabilitation staff, provides guidelines for development of cardiac rehab programs including a chapter outlining key components of effective patient and family education programs and lists of goals for the inpatient, early outpatient, and follow-up phases of treatment.[53]

A variety of other types of guidelines are becoming available in other fields. For example, the article entitled "1988 Report of the Joint National Committee on Detection, Evaluation and Treatment of High Blood Pressure" in *Archives of Internal Medicine* outlines consensus recommendations for patient care regimens that both define the content of patient instruction (always a potential source of conflict) and identify the needs for non-pharmacologic therapy that will require life-style modification.[54] On the other hand, Grueninger and others have developed a model characterizing the process of change that a patient must pass through in order to integrate a new behavior such as weight reduction or medication adherence—awareness, intention, trial, implementation, and maintenance—and the educational interventions that could be used to facilitate each stage of the process.[55]

The Oncology Nursing Society incorporates the concept of change in their *Outcome Standards for Cancer Patient Education,* which identifies a wide range of knowledge and behavioral outcomes that should flow from a patient education program. The five-step nursing process is also applied here to planning patient education interventions.[56]

In the spring of 1991, *Arthritis and Musculoskeletal Patient Education Standards* were developed for formal rheumatic disease patient education programs. Developed by a committee consisting of representatives from a variety of organizations, the purposes of the standards are to: "(1) assure the quality of patient education programs, (2) promote the easy access to education for the patient with rheumatic disease, and (3) secure documentation of outcomes of patient education that can be used to improve care."[57] Although voluntary in nature, such standards and the related review criteria serve as a useful guide for program planning and evaluation.

Professional Certification Programs

Although most licensed or certified health providers see patient education/health education as part of their professional role, a sprinkling of certification programs have emerged that have special relevance. The newest is the National Commission for Health Education Credentialing, Inc., which completed a charter phase for Certified Health Education Specialists (CHESs) in 1989.[58] More than 3,500 health education specialists had been certified by fall 1991. The basic responsibilities and related competencies of these professionals are closely related to the standards defined earlier at the institutional and target population levels. An earlier state project in Michigan, building on the early stages of health education credentialing and the APHA patient education model, produced a list of competencies for a hospitalwide patient education manager (PEM) that clearly define the scope of a hospitalwide position.[59]

Disease-specific certification programs have also been developed, most notably the National Certification Board for Diabetes Educators, a separately incorporated body established by the American Association of Diabetes Educators (AADE). To sit for the examination given twice yearly, candidates must be a licensed or registered health care professional or have a master's degree in a health care profession and have at least two years' experience or 2,000 hours in direct diabetes patient education.[60] Another relevant certification includes childbirth education certification by the American Society for Psychoprophylaxis in Obstetrics (ASPO).[61]

☐ Development of a Hospitalwide Quality Improvement Plan for Patient Education

The way a quality improvement plan is developed depends to a great extent on the way patient education is organized within a given hospital. If the model is very decentralized, patient education would likely be seen as an important aspect of care within a variety of departmental and unit plans. If there is a department of patient education, or a coordinating committee and/or staff, a more comprehensive plan would likely be seen that crosscuts many departments and units as well as components of unit-specific plans.

For many of the reasons cited earlier in this chapter, development of comprehensive quality improvement plans continues to lag. However, as many of those interviewed report, patient educators and PEMs are feeling strong pressure to develop such plans given the renewed emphasis on continuous quality improvement in their hospitals. Although a substantial variety of quality improvement activities are reviewed later in this chapter, the examples immediately following focus on hospitals that have developed institutionwide approaches.

Kaiser Permanente Massachusetts Area Health Education Department

Kaiser Permanente Massachusetts Area Health Education Department developed a quality improvement plan that focused on six areas of study. Two of the areas addressed in the plan were a cholesterol reduction program (CRP) and quality improvement guidelines for patient education materials.

The CRP studied whether matching educational interventions with the level of patients' needs was a cost-effective approach to providing high-quality care. Two patient groups were identified: low-risk and high-risk. Low-risk patients received mailed and written materials as well as group referrals. High-risk patients were given more personal follow-up through phone calls and tracking. In determining the effectiveness of the interventions, data were collected from medical record reviews and staff and patient comments. Success was reflected in several ways: Collaboration with physician groups resulted in setting standards for interpreting cholesterol test results as well as jointly establishing a protocol for patient education; and staff were providing more consistent information to patients. The CRP embraced the concept of CQI because it improved quality of care, was interdepartmental, responded to a systems problem, and resulted in cost savings for the hospital.

A second area of study was development of quality improvement guidelines for patient education materials. The patient education coordinator routinely returns a copy of the guidelines to the developer, along with the proposed draft for any new patient handout, to support recommendations for change. (Included in the guidelines are criteria for titling, readability, inventory, medical review, consistency, pretesting, and graphic presentation.) In this instance, the standards have effectively depersonalized the issue of revision, and developers of patient education materials have written guidelines to follow. Making standards work in practice links the process with outcome.[62]

Department of Patient and Community Education, Kent General Hospital, Dover, Delaware

Although the Department of Patient and Community Education provides a variety of direct inpatient, outpatient, and community services, staff at Kent General Hospital in Dover, Delaware, also consult with other departments about program design and development of clinical indicators. In an eight-page document, Sandra Klima has formalized a comprehensive internal quality improvement plan for her department. From a managerial perspective, such a document has several strengths. First, authority and responsibility within the hospital for such a program are clearly defined with an organizational chart. Second, identifying such parameters as scope of service, aspects of care, indicators and criteria, monitoring processes, reporting mechanisms, and annual reviews is critical to successfully implementing a quality improvement plan.

Attachments to this document include various reporting forms in use. For example, the "Quality of Care/Service Report" is the data collection tool for indicators. Part one of this report documents volume indicators for consultations—inpatient, outpatient, and scheduled community programs, and staff orientation programs. Part two focuses on quality indicators that track medical record reviews, acceptable return demonstrations, satisfaction evaluations, follow-up referrals, telephone follow-up, broken appointments, number of patients refusing services, and follow-up to physicians. A written quarterly report analyzes discrepancies identified by these indicators. Another form in place is a "Quality Assurance Summary/Monitor Sheet" to track each new program and/or a program where a problem has been identified, for example, a drop in attendance. This informal running commentary tracks the stages of program implementation and addresses problems as they arise. A list of specific risk management indicators for patient education (see figure 10-3) is also attached for monitoring, as part of the quality improvement plan.[63]

Clinic Education, Virginia Mason Clinic, Seattle, Washington

At this 240-physician specialty and subspecialty clinic, which is part of the Virginia Mason Medical Center, Kathy Linnell, director, Clinic Education, reports that each specialty section manager is asked to review the clinic's set of quality indicators (divided into three sections—finance, patient care, and operations) in order to identify those with the greatest impact and potential for their own operation. One indicator is specific to patient education—"patient education materials updated and coordinated with others in the Medical Center"—and Ms. Linnell works collaboratively with each section to ensure that issues and problems with materials are identified and resolved quickly. Working proactively, she has also been able to bring patient education strategies to the attention of physician leaders and managers as they address a variety of quality of care indicators, including those related to patient complaints, patient satisfaction, patient waiting time, follow-up phone calls, and use of health screening tools. For example, a problem with pharmacy

Figure 10-3. Risk Management Indicators for Patient Education, Kent General Hospital, Dover, Delaware

603301	Failure to carry through with the Patient Education process (notifying the Patient Education Department within 12 hours after referral).
603302	Failure for adherence to Patient Education Protocols (nursing)/Individual Practice Standards.
603303	Patient given misinformation; patient based health intervention on this information. Monitored by Quality Assurance referrals, Patient Education staff and/or Nursing staff.
603304	Failure to use accepted Patient Education Protocols.
603305	*Failure to communicate newly found clinical information or change in health status.
603306	Breach of patient confidentiality.
603307	*Failure to follow through with referrals (follow-up within 72 hours from Patient Education).
603308	Incomplete referrals for Patient Education.
603309	Failure to initiate referrals for skin evaluation; notice of decubiti (any state).
603310	*Failure to complete questionnaires identifying satisfaction with services.
603311	*Failure by Patient Education staff or Nursing staff to obtain a percentage of acceptable return demonstration of knowledge/skills by patient.
603312	Readmission rate for patients having service.
603313	*Failure to document Diabetes Education.
603314	*Failure to initiate referral for infants discharged with Apnea Monitor to the Patient Education Department within 24 hours.
603315	Failure to accomplish CPR teaching for parents/grandparents and significant other of apnea monitored babies within 24 hours after physical order.

*Indicator included in Quality Assurance Report.

Reprinted, with permission, from Kent General Hospital, Educational Resources, Dover, Delaware.

waiting time can be addressed by decreasing the actual waiting time, but it can also be addressed by providing patient activities that can be viewed as a legitimate part of the visit, such as brochures, displays, and other educational interventions.[64]

These examples offer the perspectives of PEMs who are developing quality of care systems that address the patient education components of the services they provide. This is often done through consultation by the PEM to specialty clinics and departments.

Methodist Hospital of Indiana, Indianapolis

Another hospitalwide approach, although not a formal plan, is from Methodist Hospital of Indiana. Through its publication called *Quality Audit Systems for Primary Care Centers*, by Benson and Van Osdol, this hospital demonstrates a comprehensive approach to examining whether the appropriate patient information is provided. Clinical protocols, including a patient education section, have been developed for a wide range of diagnoses and conditions commonly found in primary care settings. Each section is further evaluated in terms of the most critical elements; for example, "Patient must stop smoking" is the critical patient education element under the chronic obstructive pulmonary disease protocol.[65] Data on the element are assessed during medical record audits as well as overall adequacy of the patient education provided. A "Give Us a Grade" satisfaction survey form can be used to assess patient satisfaction with the patient education provided as well as with the patient's own compliance.

Ambulatory Care Nursing: Policies and Procedures, which has detailed nursing guidelines for dozens of ambulatory care procedures, includes recommended patient education elements and patient information sheets. Although the publication is not a quality

Carolyn E. Maller, M.S., C.H.E.S., R.N., and Barbara E. Giloth, M.P.H., C.H.E.S.

of care manual per se, its guidelines could be used similarly as the basis for quality assessment described in the Benson model. The strength of both these resources is that they help ambulatory care departments to assess the adequacy, appropriateness, and effectiveness of limited patient education interventions that are provided on a daily basis by dozens of clinicians. This assessment can identify problems in the delivery of this information and the need for additional, more in-depth patient education interventions. For example, Benson's clinical protocol for diabetes mellitus includes a substantial list of critical patient education elements. For many patients, acquisition of these skills would require participation in both a diabetes education class and an ongoing support group.

□ Examples of Patient Education Quality Improvement Activities

Although comprehensive quality assessment plans are difficult to find, there currently exists a wide range of assessment, monitoring, and program development activities that, taken together, offer a framework for such a plan. Six different types of common activities are described in the following sections:

- Program review
- Program development
- Clinical indicators
- Documentation
- Instructor evaluation
- Materials review

Program Review

A major way that program development has been streamlined and standardized has been through development of a program review mechanism. Hospital-specific standards are applied by a body, usually a hospitalwide patient education committee, to a new program or one that is up for an annual or biannual review. In some cases, these standards rest within one major department such as nursing;[66] in other cases, they are applicable to all departments and specialties. For example, at Group Health of Puget Sound, the patient education coordinator for the cooperative spearheaded development of a patient education workbook that incorporates program development guidelines into a step-by-step approach for staff to use as they develop a new patient education program.[67] At Sacred Heart Medical Center in Spokane, Washington, the hospitalwide patient education committee has approved a set of guidelines for program development (see figure 10-4). Once a program has been developed, however, it is the responsibility of the individual department or unit using the program to integrate a periodic review into its own quality of care program.[68] A checklist for updating patient education programs, in use at one Department of Veterans Affairs medical center, triggers the review process and documents that the program continues to meet established standards and continues to have physician endorsement (see figure 10-5, p. 220).

In an interesting collaboration that has boosted the opportunity for peer review, the University of Massachusetts Student Health Services (UHS), Health Education Division; and Kaiser Permanente (KP), Northeast Region (Massachusetts Area), Health Education Department, have pilot-tested "Quality Assurance Guidelines for New Program Development or Existing Program Review" that they jointly developed (see figure 10-6, p. 221). These guidelines identify the first step of the process as determining whether the program is comprehensive or brief. A comprehensive program or intervention—that is, one that is ongoing, expensive, labor-intensive, and with complex methodology—requires a more in-depth needs assessment and planning process as well as program review by peers, colleagues, supervisors, and consumers before implementation. A brief program or

Figure 10-4. Patient Education Program Request Form, Sacred Heart Medical Center, Spokane, Washington

---

Program/booklet name or topic _____

_____ New

_____ Major revision

Please complete the following information for the Patient Education Committee.

A. Problem/need identification:
   1. a. What is the problem/need?
      b. How was this need identified? (please check one or more below and describe):
         High patient volume (# /month)
         Patient request:
         Staff request:
         MD suggestion:
         Other:
      c. If a formal needs assessment was conducted, please briefly describe:
   2. Target patient population:
      a. Approximate number of patients per year in target group _____
      b. Average length of stay for these patients _____
   3. Briefly describe expected program outcome:
   4. What changes will this illness/problem necessitate for the patients?
      _____ knowledge   _____ attitude
      _____ behavioral   _____ other (please describe):
   5. Type of program desired:
      _____ informational pamphlet(s) only
      _____ videotape/audiotape only (circle one)
      _____ integrated educational program. If integrated program is desired, what techniques do you
              anticipate using:
              _____ pamphlet, booklet   _____ chart(s)
              _____ videotape/audiotape   _____ other:
              _____ other:
   6. a. Are there similar existing programs?   _____ Yes   _____ No   N/A
      b. If yes, please describe (or attach sample).

Program Development:

   1. a. What staff do you anticipate would be involved in developing the program? (Please include position)
      b. What staff do you anticipate would be involved in teaching the program?
   2. Estimated completion date _____
   3. Estimated development cost:
      a. Staff hours _____
         (approximate hours for development × average salary)
      b. Materials _____
         (purchase price or estimated development cost excluding staff time)

Implementation:

   1. Estimated in-service plan _____
                                    (number of employees × length of service)
   2. Estimated teaching time per patient per hospital stay _____

Evaluation:

   1. Has this program material been piloted?   _____ Yes   _____ No
      If yes, please describe (include length of time).

      If no, should it be?   _____ Yes   _____ No
   2. How do you plan to evaluate the program?

Comments: _____
                                              Signature, Initiator   Date
For cost center manager:
   Has this program been budgeted?   _____ Yes   _____ No
   If not, are there other funds available to produce it?   _____ Yes   _____ No

                                              _____
                                              Signature, Cost Center Manager   Date

---

Reprinted, with permission, from Sacred Heart Medical Center, Spokane, Washington.

Carolyn E. Maller, M.S., C.H.E.S., R.N., and Barbara E. Giloth, M.P.H., C.H.E.S.

Figure 10-5. Checklist for Updating Patient Education Program Manuals, Department of Veterans Affairs, Albuquerque, New Mexico

Title of Program   _____

Date of Release   _____

Concurring Physician   _____

A. Introduction
   1. Does it provide a current program description?
      _____ Yes   _____ No
   Comments: _____

B. Learner Objectives and Content
   1. Is subject matter up-to-date? (Are there statements in the material that are no longer true or about which there is currently debate?)
      _____ Yes   _____ No
   Comments _____

C. Developers
   1. Is there evidence that physicians who are content experts have been involved in the review process?
      _____ Yes   _____ No
   Comments _____

   2. Has the content been developed by the appropriate disciplines (for example, nursing, pharmacy, dietetics, social work, rehab medicine, and so on)?
      _____ Yes   _____ No
   Comments _____

D. Teaching Materials
   1. Is the reading level 8th grade or lower?
      _____ Yes   _____ No
   Comments _____

   2. Do you know of other materials on the same subject that you think are better?
      _____ Yes   _____ No
   Comments _____

E. Documentation
   1. Does the documentation form reflect: _____ educational assessment
                                               _____ educational plan
                                               _____ implementation
                                               _____ evaluation of patient outcomes

      _____ Yes   _____ No

   Comments _____

Your recommendation (*please check one*)

      _____ Manual needs revision
      _____ Manual does not need revision

Comments:

_____
_____
_____
_____
_____
_____
_____
_____

Thank you for your time.   Reviewer Signature/Service/Date

Please return the completed form to _____.

Figure 10-6. Quality Assurance Guidelines for New Program Development or Existing Program Review, Kaiser Permanente, Massachusetts Area

Step I. Determine whether intervention is comprehensive or brief
    a. informal discussion with peers
    b. review program criteria (see a. and b. below)

---

a. Comprehensive Program/Intervention Criteria
  —ongoing
  —highly visible
  —long-term importance
  —expensive
  —labor-intensive
  —focus is on change at the individual, program, and/or system levels
    —methodology is complex
    —objective driven

Step II. Plan Intervention/Program
    1. Conduct a needs assessment.
      a. collect and review existing data based on experience/literature review
      b. consult staff and consumers
      c. consider need for pilot program before large-scale intervention
    2. Write a proposal, including:
      a. summary of needs assessment and rationale
      b. theoretical basis for design
      c. target group(s)
      d. measurable objectives
      e. content/methodologies
      f. evaluation plan that includes:
        1) documentation (i.e. attendance, final costs, medical record entries (if applicable)
        2) informal program review by staff and consumers
        3) instructor effectiveness (see document on instructor standards)
        4) consumer satisfaction measures
        5) measure of at least one outcome objective
        6) design and selection of appropriate instruments/procedures and statistics to measure all of the above
      g. time line/schedule of activities
      h. budget/staff time
      i. publicity/registration procedures and follow-up
      j. community development plan
    3. Review proposal with peers, colleagues, supervisor, and consumers.
    4. Design/collect/pretest program materials.

Step III. Implementation Program
Use proposal and evaluation plan as a guide. Modify based on current climate, availability of resources, etc.

Step IV. Evaluate Program
Collect information according to evaluation plan through surveys, meetings, computer analysis, etc., and summarize findings. Make suggestions for future programming.

Step V. Summary Reports
Write reports for Department, larger organization. Consider publication and/or presentations at professional organization. For ongoing group program, complete Group Program Standards.

---

b. Brief Program/Intervention Criteria
  —emphasis on short-term impact
  —focus on activities
  —low cost and not labor-intensive
  —short time line
  —maybe a one-time intervention and/or piloting of new idea

(Continued on next page)

Figure 10-6. (Continued)

Step II. Program Planning
1. Meet to discuss with requestor, consumers, and/or staff.
2. Write a proposal of program's rationale, activities, time line, cost, and brief evaluation plan.
3. Publicize.

Step III. Implement Program

Step IV. Evaluate Program
1. Informal program review with those involved in planning for strengths and weaknesses and future recommendations.
2. Documentation of completed activities, attendance, cost, materials used and program review.
3. Consider if program should be repeated or expanded (if so, may meet comprehensive program criteria).

Step V. Summary Report
Write a report summarizing program with documentation and plans for the future.

Reprinted, with permission, from Kaiser Permanente, Amherst Medical Center, Boston, 1991.

intervention—one that is short term, low cost, and not labor-intensive, such as a Community Health Lecture Series—requires a much less detailed and more informal planning process.[69]

Program Development

Nearly all versions of standards or guidelines for patient education programs specify basic planning processes including needs assessment, staff/consumer involvement, program development, implementation, and evaluation. Given chronic lack of time and resources, PEMs are continually looking for ways to implement these processes effectively.

A Department of Veterans Affairs Task Force has developed a generic patient education assessment tool to overcome four major problems:[70]

- Lack of existing tools
- Inadequate communication skills among providers
- Exclusion of the patient as an active participant in goal setting
- Lack of assessment of multiple factors related to encouraging adherence to medical regimen

Processes to support the effective implementation of needs assessment include the organization of multidisciplinary committees. The Patient Education Section at M. D. Anderson Cancer Center, in Houston, for example, has supported the development of several dozen working committees to identify needs of specific patient groups and plan appropriate interventions.[71]

At The Ohio State University Hospitals, in Columbus, interviews of first-line managers responsible for patient education on their units or departments identified problems in planning and implementing evaluation activities. In response, a subcommittee of the hospitalwide Patient Education Committee developed an evaluation kit to be used at the unit/department level by staff to enhance their knowledge, skill, and efforts in evaluating the learner(s) and the program. Presented at a series of patient education workshops where interdisciplinary teams participate, the kit answers basic questions about evaluation and provides a set of generic evaluation tools that can be modified to meet the needs of specific areas.[72]

Going to the consumer is increasingly used to find out what patients are looking for in health care and to assess how existing programs and services measure up to their expectations. A focus group, case-level approach invites patients to come together to provide insight into how well the hospital is doing. Basch[73] has described features and processes of the focus group interview as a research tool in health education.

In an effort to "ask the customer" (which is part of the CQI effort) at Virginia Mason Clinic in Seattle, three focus group discussions were held in December 1991. Excellent information was gathered that had direct impact on the quality indicators affecting the delivery of care and patient education. One specific suggestion generated from the focus group format was to "give us something we can use to take notes on and jot down questions on." In response to this patient request, a simple tool was designed for patient note taking at the time of the clinic appointment. The format of the "Doc Talk" form (see figure 10-7) guides patients in identifying their need-to-know concerns and empowers them to be more assertive in their communication with physicians. Based on pilot results in several specialty sections, a decision will be made whether to implement and monitor the process throughout the medical center.[74]

Within the Department of Veterans Affairs, 20 focus groups were conducted at five sites around the country in 1988 and 1989. Group participation ranged from patients and family members to clinicians to health education experts at the local and regional levels. A report on the focus group findings identified themes for administrative as well as patient education interventions.[75] These results will form the basis for future practice and inquiry into improving the quality of patient health education services within the VA system.

The Picker/Commonwealth Patient-Centered Care Program has compiled extensive survey data across the nation from patients and their friends and family members. The intent is to learn from patients themselves how to improve the quality of patient care in the hospital environment. A unique feature of the Picker/Commonwealth survey process involved querying patients about specific aspects of their hospitalization, rather than the more traditional system of rating care. This approach has yielded descriptive data reflecting the patients' view of high-quality care.[76]

Clinical Indicators

Indicators are intended to provide an ongoing monitor of patient care quality.[77] Technical guidelines, including a suggested format for developing clinical indicators, can be found in the *Primer on Clinical Indicator Development and Application*.[78] Patient educators with responsibility for a broad, hospitalwide patient education program may want to consider developing indicators from a multidisciplinary perspective.[79] The important issues in developing an indicator are the rationale for selection and how it relates to the scope of care or types of patients served, to reflect change over time.

In developing clinical indicators, it is important to be cautious and not overzealous in indicator selection. Selection should be limited to "that single datum or set of data which, when used to collect information about the aspect of care, can be used to *indicate* whether care or service is being delivered appropriately."[80] Using this approach, it is possible to avoid voluminous data collection, which may yield unmanageable results.

Of the three categories used to measure quality—structure, process, and outcome—current emphasis is clearly on outcome. Nonetheless, without well-developed program policies (structure) that guide the delivery of actual patient teaching (process), any learning or behavioral change (outcome) will be inconsistent and haphazard, at best. Therefore, attempts must be made to strengthen all three categories to reach high-quality outcomes of patient care. The linkage between process and outcome is clear in a study conducted with diabetic inpatients.[81] Careful attention was given to the structure and process of a formal diabetic patient education program to identify appropriate patient outcomes. Two pilot studies were conducted, and the results indicated that changes in staff education and time allotment needed to occur in order for self-care outcomes to improve.

The following questions should be considered in determining process criteria at the programmatic level:

Carolyn E. Maller, M.S., C.H.E.S., R.N., and Barbara E. Giloth, M.P.H., C.H.E.S.

Figure 10-7. Doc Talk, Virginia Mason Medical Center, Seattle

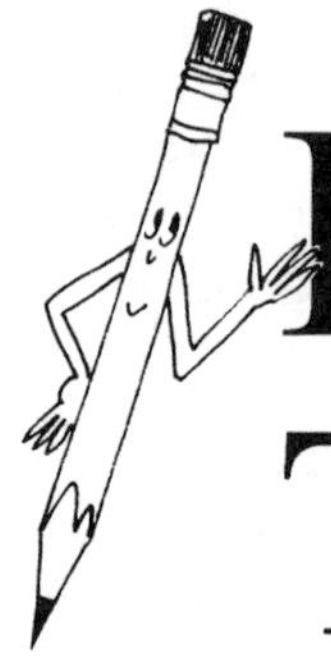

Doc Talk

Use this pad to jot down questions you might want to ask. Feel free to take this with you when you see your doctor.

☐ **Tests.** Please explain any tests I will take. What is the purpose, and how will you act on the results?

☐ **Results.** Please tell me how I'll find out about the results. Will I be told if something is all right, or only if it needs attention?

☐ **Diagnosis.** What's wrong with me, what causes it, and how serious is it?

☐ **Options.** What treatment choices do I have?

☐ **Medications.** If I'm given a prescription, please tell me about its side effects and how this prescription will interact with my other prescriptions or over-the-counter drugs.

☐ **Questions?** Turn this over and jot down things you want to discuss with your doctor. ☞

VIRGINIA MASON Medical Center

My questions _____

_____
_____
_____
_____
_____
_____
_____
_____
_____
_____
_____
_____
_____
_____

Doctor's orders _____

_____
_____
_____
_____
_____
_____
_____
_____
_____
_____

If I have problems, call

_____
_____
_____
_____

Reprinted, with permission, from the Virginia Mason Clinic, Seattle, 1992.

- Have written teaching plans been developed for disease-specific teaching areas?
- Does the content meet stated learner objectives?
- Are learning outcomes documented?
- Do teaching plans meet existing standards (for example, Diabetes Recognition Standards or hospital standards)?
- How has priority for program development been determined?
- Have the top 10 institutional discharge diagnoses been researched to validate program development?
- Is there a standard for the delivery of teaching?
- Are educational assessments made on all inpatients? In other words, are all patients offered disease-specific instruction relevant to their teaching needs?
- Does inpatient teaching link with outpatient teaching?
- What is the referral mechanism for organized outpatient classes?
- Are patients being referred to established classes on discharge?
- Once a referral is made, do patients attend class? If they attend, how do they rate the quality of patient teaching?
- Are follow-up contacts made (for example, either by mail or telephone contact)?

Although a variety of patient education quality indicators have already been described, several additional ones may be cited. One model for a hospitalwide patient education committee structure identifies potential indicators for quality of care review at the hospital level (see figure 10-8). For example, allocation of quarterly funds is the responsibility

Figure 10-8. Patient Health Education Advisory Committee Organizational Chart, Department of Veterans Affairs, Albuquerque

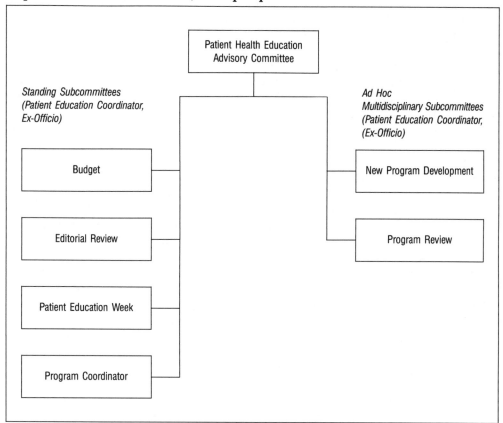

of a standing subcommittee. The editorial review process of developing patient education materials is the responsibility of another standing subcommittee, as is marketing Patient Education Week. A program coordination committee meets quarterly to provide an open forum for continuous improvement in the delivery of group patient education programs. New program development is initiated with an ad hoc multidisciplinary subcommittee structure under the leadership of the PEM. Regular program reviews are conducted in a similar manner to identify areas for problem resolution, such as changes in technology or medical center practice.

Using this committee structure, the following questions might be asked to identify potential indicators:

- Is the existing committee structure working?
- Are members attending and participating in scheduled meetings?
- Are action plans reflected in committee minutes and carried out over time?
- What is the quality of existing patient education programs?
- Are programs well attended?
- How satisfied are patients with the programs?
- How is the need established for new program development?

Sample patient education *program* outcome indicators may be determined by asking: Are patient education materials reaching the client? Are materials sensitive to cross-cultural differences? Are they used by patients after discharge? Are materials at the appropriate literacy level for the population? How is the distribution of materials monitored?

Sample patient education *teaching* outcome indicators should ask what happens to the patient. How well do patients do once they go home? Do they get better or worse? Are they prepared to manage self-care at home? Is there a mechanism for tracking self-care skills (for example, medication taking and adherence)? Do patients have the knowledge and skill and help to safely administer insulin or manage home oxygen?

Tracking systems are being tested to look at patient outcomes (for example, how well patients are managing their care). A unique feature of one such outcome system uses a questionnaire structured to collect patient data prospectively.[82] This systems approach may provide a blueprint for patient educators designing teaching activities for use at any point of entry into a health care system.

Methodist Hospitals of Memphis measured diabetic self-care knowledge outcomes prior to discharge. In a summary QA report of 44 patients taught and interviewed prior to discharge, 34 patients (77 percent) were able to correctly answer "critical information related to diabetic self-care" (explain what diabetes is, list signs and symptoms of low blood sugar, relate the appropriate response to high and low blood sugar, and list the acceptable ranges of high and low blood sugar) with 100 percent accuracy. The content that was consistently missed (appropriate response to high and low blood sugar) was altered as part of the action plan. A subsequent monitor three months later revealed 92 percent compliance. Further monitors are planned to follow this trend.[83]

An example of a fairly complex attempt to assess the quality of an interrelated series of activities in Kaiser Permanente's Cholesterol Reduction Program cited previously considers these questions: Are people being screened appropriately? Are tests being interpreted in terms of the new guidelines? If the interpretation is proper, does it result in the proper nutrition counseling and retesting scenario? How satisfied are patients with both the information received and the process? What behavioral changes do patients report six months after beginning the program? Although the specific patient education pieces are the group nutrition program, access to patient education materials at appropriate times, and phone follow-up, their effective use depends on the entire protocol.[84]

Two innovative approaches for diabetes patient education with applicability to other chronic diseases come from the Capitol Hill Family Health Center, one of the Group

Health Cooperative Clinics in Seattle, Washington. If a person purchases urine test tapes at the pharmacy, this purchase triggers an assessment of whether he or she needs education about home blood glucose monitoring in order to check blood sugar levels. Alice Lake, nursing director at the clinic, also describes the mailing of a Health and Awareness in the Management of Diabetes survey to all clinic members identified by lab values, the pharmacy, and physicians' offices as having diabetes. The survey has the potential to contribute in the following ways to the quality improvement program:[85]

1. It finds out where things are falling through the cracks, for example, discovering whether patients are actually checking blood sugars or whether classes are needed on blood sugar monitoring. Individual questions ask about specific care protocols such as whether a patient has had an eye exam in the past 12 months.
2. It serves as an overall program needs assessment; various questions about appropriate self-management behaviors are included.
3. It permits follow-up to specific subcategories of respondents, such as targeting those who smoke to invite them to a stop-smoking program.

The drug usage evaluation (DUE) standards published in the *1992 Accreditation Manual for Hospitals* offer a CQI opportunity hospitalwide for educating patients about drug use. Clinical DUE examples with patient education applications have been formulated in the Department of Veterans Affairs. A stepped approach identifies efficacious patient education interventions involving drug therapy. After forming a standard of care, patient questionnaires (clinical monitors) regarding theophylline and inhaler use have not only revealed inaccuracies in the way patients administer their medications, but also have identified patient education interventions, such as the need for more explicit handout materials.[86]

Documentation

Probably no other aspect of patient education has provoked more frustration than the problem of adequate documentation. Although some research has found that staff may overreport the amount of patient education that they actually do,[87] it is still probably true that a substantial amount of teaching that is done is not documented. Because the majority of quality assessment studies look at medical record documentation, patient education often comes up wanting.

Although the perfect form has yet to be discovered, analysis of forms from 40 hospitals across the country suggests some commonalities.[88] Overwhelmingly, the use of standardized patient teaching records for individual target populations was cited as the favored method, although the format varied considerably. Some hospitals developed a generic form that was then preprinted with different lists of goals, depending on the target population. Other hospitals developed different forms for different major target populations. In either case, the need for a generic teaching form for those patients who did not fit major teaching target populations was identified. Many reported the use of checklists to cut down on documentation time, and a substantial minority of respondents completed discharge summary forms for both inpatients and outpatients, a copy of which was usually sent home with the patient. (See chapter 9 for a detailed discussion of patient education documentation.)

Using a nursing process approach to documenting patient education, Iyer and Camp[89] cite examples and guidelines for evaluating patient learning outcomes. Telephone follow-up after discharge is suggested as the final step in determining how well patients have managed once they have gone home. Short and Bair[90] describe a documentation system that incorporates nursing standards of care into nursing care plans and identifies patient teaching outcomes. Standard patient teaching guides reference teaching content to streamline medical record keeping and satisfy JCAHO scrutiny.

Carolyn E. Maller, M.S., C.H.E.S., R.N., and Barbara E. Giloth, M.P.H., C.H.E.S.

The benefits of involving staff at a case-level, unit-based approach to quality assessment are well documented.[91-93] Such a plan decentralized to the unit level enlists staff nurses in monitoring the quality of patient care in their particular setting.[94] A unit-based model for patient education can effectively be linked with the patient education documentation format already in place as nursing staff tailor the tool to meet the scope of care for their specific unit.

In determining scope of care, the following questions should be considered: What types of patients are seen on the unit? What types of patient education have the most impact (for example, high volume versus high risk [warfarin therapy] or low volume versus high risk [right atrial catheter, automatic implantable cardioverter defibrillator])?

The Tulsa Health Awareness Center uses patient involvement and a program flow sheet to increase weekly documentation of progress through all of its chronic disease class series. Participants in each class series are asked to complete a Weekly Home Assessment form (see figure 10-9) at the beginning of each class. This form asks participants to assess how well they managed during the previous week, including how well their support network functioned. Problems identified through this mechanism are noted on the program flow sheet, as are additional notes based on instructor observation during class.[95]

Instructor Evaluation

Instructor knowledge, teaching skill, and ability to develop rapport with participants are important quality indicators for ambulatory patient education programs. The extensive use of contract and part-time staff for these services has made monitoring of these indicators particularly important from a liability perspective. However, anecdotal information suggests that internal staff are less used to and more resistant to such monitoring.

Four general categories of instructor monitoring can occur. The first category is evidence of instructor qualifications, for example, diabetes certification or proven teaching ability. A second category focuses on periodic observation. A third category includes participant assessment data; for some this means a basic happiness evaluation form, yet other tools may be more helpful. For example, Group Health of Puget Sound developed and pilot-tested a 27-item participant-completed form assessing two dimensions—technical competency and interpersonal skill.[96] Finally, the fourth category includes participant attendance (percentage of registered participants who complete the class series), performance (average score on posttest), and outcome data (for example, emergency department use for persons with diabetes, infection rate for patients with catheters).

Earlier adult educator performance competencies[97] appearing in the literature focused on the instructor role in staff development. Comparable standards for staff nurses performing their patient education functions are now evolving. Generic standards of nursing practice at Methodist Hospitals of Memphis reference the following patient teaching standard (Generic Standard VI): "Nursing personnel will initiate, participate in and coordinate a patient and family education plan, as a continuous process starting upon admission."[98] By monitoring compliance with Generic Nursing Standard VI as part of the hospitalwide quality assessment process, patient teaching activities (measured through compliance with the standard) could be demonstrated. Nursing units consistently failing to meet the standard could be targeted for further staff training in patient teaching skill development. Of particular interest was the quality improvement trend noted over time from June 1985 (80 percent) to June 1988 (95 percent), in achieving the 90 percent threshold.[99]

Materials Review

As some of the most visible patient education interventions, print, audio, and audiovisual resources must be assessed in terms of accuracy, appropriateness, and availability. In addition, a delivery system that ensures a smooth flow of material from storage to provider to patient must be assessed. An assessment of medication information being distributed in ambulatory care clinics at the University of Virginia Health Sciences Center, in Charlottesville, wanted to determine:[100]

- How consistently written information was given to patients
- Whether this action was documented in the medical record
- The quality of materials distributed from both educational and production perspectives
- The extent to which materials shared a common format and/or were recognizable as products of the medical center

Figure 10-9. Weekly Home Assessment for Diabetes Patient Education Program, Tulsa Health Awareness Center, Tulsa, Oklahoma

Name: _____ Date: _____

1. My weight today on the Health Awareness Scale is _____

2. Were you able to follow your meal plan this week?

| | No | Rarely | Sometimes | Frequently | Always |

3. Were you able to exercise this week?

| | No | Rarely | Sometimes | Frequently | Always |

4. Do you feel sad or blue?

| | No | Rarely | Sometimes | Frequently | Always |

Are you tense, jumpy, or irritable?

| | No | Rarely | Sometimes | Frequently | Always |

Are you worried or anxious?

| | No | Rarely | Sometimes | Frequently | Always |

Are you afraid that you're losing control?

| | No | Rarely | Sometimes | Frequently | Always |

Do you feel hopeful about the coming weeks?

| | No | Rarely | Sometimes | Frequently | Always |

Do you feel good about yourself?

| | No | Rarely | Sometimes | Frequently | Always |

5. What is your blood sugar reading in the   morning _____ before or after breakfast?
                                              afternoon _____ before or after lunch?
                                              evening _____ before or after supper?
                                              at bedtime _____ with or without a snack?

   (Write down your reading by the mealtime you took it, and circle if it was before or after the meal.)

6. How much did your diabetes affect your life this week?

| | None | Little | Some | A good bit | A great deal |

7. Has family been supportive?

| | No | Rarely | Sometimes | Frequently | Always |

Have friends been supportive?

| | No | Rarely | Sometimes | Frequently | Always |

8. List any special discoveries you made this week, or problems and concerns that you have.

_____

_____

Reprinted, with permission, from Tulsa Health Awareness Center, University of Oklahoma, College of Medicine, Tulsa, Oklahoma, copyright 1985.

Carolyn E. Maller, M.S., C.H.E.S., R.N., and Barbara E. Giloth, M.P.H., C.H.E.S.

At the Albuquerque Department of Veterans Affairs Medical Center, a distribution center for patient health education materials is run by volunteers to provide staff with easier access to patient teaching materials. Located within the acute medical–surgical facility, the center houses all patient teaching manuals, approved documentation forms, locally developed audiovisual programs, posters, flyers, and more than 200 titles of print materials authored by local medical center staff. The PEM no longer spends time delivering teaching materials and stocking clinical areas, and nurses save time by placing orders by mail or assigning the task of ordering to the unit secretary. All materials housed in the distribution center have met criteria established by hospital policy for accuracy in medical content, with physician review and concurrence, peer review, low-literacy requirements, and graphic design standards. The center serves as a focal point to manage the quality of materials produced for the patient health education program.

Many hospitals now have routine processes for development of new materials that include format specification and an internal review protocol that includes readability assessment and patient pretesting. With an estimated 20 percent of the U.S. adult population functionally illiterate,[101] mechanisms to purchase or develop written materials for low-literacy populations are important (see chapter 17).

☐ How to Match a Quality Improvement Plan with a Hospital's Organizational Structure

Given the wide range of quality improvement activities and plans already reviewed in this chapter, it may be helpful at this point to consider further the organizational or management structure supporting patient education within a specific setting. Defining the patient educator's place within the organization is a critical step in implementing a quality improvement plan. A stepped approach looks at the organizational level of program management, for example, hospitalwide or institutional, target population (programmatic), or case level.

Three Levels of Program Management

PEMs at the *hospitalwide or institutional* level may actually operate at all three levels. Varying coordinator roles may demand collaborative mechanisms to function at multiple levels within the hospital. Quality improvement plans tend to be more global and interdisciplinary in nature.

Programs managed within a single department or developed for a specific target population *(programmatic)* are limited by the scope of responsibility for that department or population. Examples would be a program under a nursing department or for a disease-related population such as diabetes. A quality improvement plan may tend to focus on the actual delivery of patient teaching.

A patient education program managed at the *case*, or unit, level is necessarily responsive to those specific teaching needs. In this instance, the PEM may in fact be the direct care provider. Quality improvement is often part of a more broad-based initiative.

Next Steps

Once the organizational level is determined, the scope for developing a quality improvement plan becomes clearer. Initially, it is advisable to limit the scope of service to those areas that organizationally are managed by the patient education program. The scope of service for the patient education function varies by institutional setting. Whether a single department exists for patient education, a PEM reports to a separate department such as nursing, or responsibility falls on a committee structure, clearly defining scope of service is a critical step in developing an appropriate plan.

Increasingly, PEMs need to capture support throughout the hospital by working side by side with other departments to achieve mutual goals in the quality of care. Realistically looking at both fiscal and human resources, PEMs may find themselves limiting a quality improvement plan to one aspect of a patient education program, rather than managing many aspects that may not be under their control.

Conceptualizing an umbrella of quality improvement that fits the PEM's organizational structure offers the ability to look at the delivery of patient education from an organizational perspective. Such a model allows for flexibility as administrative changes occur and broaden a patient education program. Multiple quality improvement plans developed for multiple teaching programs or levels where patient education occurs fail to reflect the flow of patient education from department to department. Greater emphasis on quality improvement is being given to the effectiveness of the systemwide delivery of patient education than to isolated teaching episodes. Tracking systems need to reflect the entire spectrum of patient education services, from entry into the health care system throughout the inpatient stay and extending out into the community. This model supports a systems approach toward continuous quality improvement in patient education.

□ Conclusion

Given the research base, the existence of a wide variety of standards, and the breadth of experience with a wide range of quality assessment and improvement activities, the appearance of more comprehensive quality of care plans for patient education programs is certain. A major question is the extent to which unit- or department-based quality assessment and follow-up activities can effectively monitor complex patient education interventions without a coordinated approach that is both multidepartmental and multidisciplinary. A more subtle challenge, yet one that substantially underlies the development of indicators and thresholds, is the extent to which success can ethically be defined principally in terms of professionally defined outcomes, for example, compliance or adherence. The increasing interest in patient/family involvement in all phases of the quality assessment and improvement process and in quality of life outcomes augurs well for meeting this challenge.

References and Notes

1. American Hospital Association. *Management Advisories on Ambulatory Care and Health Promotion.* Chicago: AHA, 1991.

2. Joint Commission on Accreditation of Healthcare Organizations. *1992 Accreditation Manual for Hospitals.* Oakbrook Terrace, IL: JCAHO, 1990, p. 261.

3. O'Leary, D. S. Accreditation in the quality improvement mold—a vision for tomorrow. *Quality Review Bulletin* 17(3):72–77, Mar. 1991.

4. Merry, M. D. What is quality care? A model for measuring health care excellence. *Quality Review Bulletin* 13(9):298–301, Sept. 1987.

5. Crosby, P. B. *Quality Is Free: The Art of Making Quality Certain.* New York City: New American Library, 1979.

6. Juran, J. M. *Juran's Quality Control Handbook.* New York City: McGraw-Hill, 1988.

7. Juran, J. M. *Juran on Leadership for Quality—An Executive Handbook.* New York City: The Free Press, 1989.

8. Deming, W. E. *Out of the Crisis.* Cambridge, MA: MIT Center for Advanced Engineering Study, 1986.

9. Berwick, D. M. Continuous improvement as an ideal in health care. *New England Journal of Medicine* 320(1):53–56, Jan. 5, 1989.

10. Gottlieb, L. K., Margolis, C. Z., and Schoenbaum, S. C. (Harvard Community Health Plan, Boston, MA). Clinical practice guidelines at an HMO: development and implementation in a quality improvement model. *Quality Review Bulletin* 16(2):80–86, Feb. 1990.

11. Berwick, D. M., Godfrey, A. B., and Roessner, J. *Curing Health Care.* San Francisco: Jossey-Bass, 1990.

12. Duncan, R. P., Fleming, E. C., and Gallati, T. G. Implementing a continuous quality improvement program in a community hospital. *Quality Review Bulletin* 17(4):106–12, Apr. 1991.

13. Burda, D. Providers look to industry for quality models. *Modern Healthcare* 18(29):24–32, July 15, 1988.

14. Burda, D. Prospects of quality measurement project excite the participating systems, alliances. *Modern Healthcare* 19(1):40–45, Jan. 6, 1989.

15. Eskildson, L., and Yates, G. R. Lessons from industry: revising organizational structure to improve health care quality assurance. *Quality Review Bulletin* 17(2):38–41, Feb. 1991.

16. Masters, F., and Schmele, J. A. Total quality management: an idea whose time has come. *Journal of Nursing Quality Assurance* 5(4):7–16, July 1991.

17. O'Leary, D. S. CQI—a step beyond QA [editorial]. *Quality Review Bulletin* 17(1):4–5, Jan. 1991.

18. Re, R. N., and Krousel-Wood, M. A. How to use continuous quality improvement theory and statistical quality control tools in a multispecialty clinic. *Quality Review Bulletin* 16(11):391–97, Nov. 1990.

19. Joint Commission on Accreditation of Healthcare Organizations. *Primer on Indicator Development and Application.* Oakbrook Terrace, IL: JCAHO, 1990, p. 110.

20. Richardson, S. A., Gimarc, J. D., Kettinger, L., and others. Health education quality assessment for public health clinics: responding to staff resistance. *Patient Education and Counseling* 12(3):189–98, Dec. 1988.

21. Rivers, R. Staff nurses' perception of responsibility to provide patient education in hospital setting. *Journal of Healthcare Education and Training* 6(2):8–12, Apr. 1991.

22. Giloth, B. E. Promoting patient involvement: educational, organizational, and environmental strategies. *Patient Education and Counseling* 15(1):29–38, Feb. 1990.

23. Morisky, D. E., Levine, D. M., Green, L. W., Shapiro, S., Russell, R. P., and Smith, C. R. Five-year blood pressure control and mortality following health education for hypertensive patients. *American Journal of Public Health* 73(2):153–62, Feb. 1983.

24. Mullen, P. D., and Green, L. W. Meta-analysis points way toward more effective medication teaching. *Promoting Health* 6(6):6–8, Nov.–Dec. 1985.

25. Wilner, S., Winickoff, R. N., Schoenbaum, S. C., and Lolfin, K. L. The role of patient interventions in ambulatory quality assurance programs. *Health Education Quarterly* 9(1):42–54, Spring 1982.

26. Lorig, K. *Patient Education—A Practical Approach.* St. Louis: Mosby-Year Book, 1991.

27. Joint Commission on Accreditation of Healthcare Organizations. Characteristics of clinical indicators. *Quality Review Bulletin* 15(11):330–39, Nov. 1989.

28. Tarlov, A. R., Ware, J. E., Jr., Greenfield, S., and others. The Medical Outcomes Study: an application of methods for monitoring the results of medical care. *JAMA* 262(7):925–30, Aug. 18, 1989.

29. Revicki, D. A. Health-related quality of life in the evaluation of medical therapy for chronic illness. *The Journal of Family Practice* 29(4):377–80, Oct. 1989.

30. Greenfield, S., Kaplan, S., and Ware, J. E. Expanding patient involvement in care: effects on patient outcomes. *Annals of Internal Medicine* 102(4):520–28, Apr. 1985.

31. Cleary, P. D., Edgman-Levitan, S., Roberts, M., Moloney, T. W., McMullen, W., Walker, J. D., and Delbanco, T. L. Patients evaluate their hospital care: a national survey. *Health Affairs* 10(4):254–67, Winter 1991.

32. Cleary, P. D., Edgman-Levitan, S., McMullen, W., and Delbanco, T. L. The relationship between reported problems and patient summary evaluations of hospital care. *Quality Review Bulletin* 18(2):53–59, Feb. 1992.

33. Hudson, T. Hospitals work to provide advance directives information. *Hospitals* 65(3):26–32, Feb. 5, 1991.

34. Joint Commission on Accreditation of Healthcare Organizations. *1993 Accreditation Manual for Hospitals.* Oakbrook Terrace, IL: JCAHO, 1992, pp. 105-7.

35. Inui, S. A common bond: exploring the interface between health education and quality assurance. *Quality Review Bulletin* 4(11):6–7, Oct. 1978.

36. Baker, F. Quality assurance and program evaluation. *Evaluation and the Health Professions* 6(2):149–60, June 1983.

37. American Hospital Association, Division of Ambulatory Care and Health Promotion. *1990 JCAHO Criteria Supporting Patient Education* [resource sheet]. Chicago: AHA, 1989.

38. JCAHO, *1993 Accreditation Manual for Hospitals,* vol. I, p. 103, and vol. II, pp. 1–5.

39. Telephone conversation with Trudy B. Nash, associate director, Department of Standards, Joint Commission on Accreditation of Healthcare Organizations, Veterans Administration Patient Health Education, Apr. 24, 1992.

40. Joint Commission on Accreditation of Healthcare Organizations. *Ambulatory Health Care Standards Manual.* Chicago: JCAHO, 1988, pp. 5–6.

41. Joint Commission on Accreditation of Healthcare Organizations. *Managed Care Standards Manual.* Chicago: JCAHO, 1989, p. 18.

42. Leape, L. L. (Harvard School of Public Health, Boston, Massachusetts). Practice guidelines and standards: an overview. *Quality Review Bulletin* 16(2):42–49, Feb. 1990.

43. American Hospital Association. Clinical practice guidelines: an awareness paper for hospitals. Chicago: AHA, 1992.

44. Bartlett, E. E. Quality improvement, practice guidelines and patient education. *Patient Education and Counseling* 18(1):1–2, Aug. 1991.

45. American Public Health Association. *A Model for Patient Education Programming.* Edited by S. G. Deeds, B. J. Hebert, and J. M. Wolle. Washington, DC: APHA, Special Projects Report, Public Health Education Section, 1979.

46. Bucher, A., Stechman, A. M., and Bazeley, M. *Guidelines for the Development of Patient Health Education Programs* (unpublished). Washington, DC: Veterans Administration, 1988.

47. Wyness, M. A. Devising standards for patient education in a teaching hospital. *Quality Review Bulletin* 15(9):279–85, Sept. 1989.

48. McCarthy, L. Toward quality assurance in patient education. *Promoting Health* 7(1):5–7, Jan.–Feb. 1986.

49. American Diabetes Association Committee on Professional Practice. Standards of medical care for patients with diabetes mellitus. *Diabetes Care* 12(5):365–68, May 1989.

50. Recognition for diabetes patient education programs. Write to the American Diabetes Association, 1660 Duke Street, Alexandria, VA 22314.

51. American Diabetes Association. National standards and review criteria for diabetes patient education programs: quality assurance for diabetes patient education. *The Diabetes Educator* 12(3):286–96, Summer 1986.

52. North Carolina Department of Human Resources. *Rules Governing the Certification of Cardiac Rehabilitation Programs.* Raleigh, NC: NCDHR, 1990.

53. Wake Forest Cardiac Rehabilitation Program. *Organizational Guidelines for Cardiac Rehabilitation Programs in North Carolina.* Winston-Salem, NC: WFCRP, 1990.

54. National High Blood Pressure Education Program, NHLBI. The 1988 report of the joint national committee on detection, evaluation, and treatment of high blood pressure. *Archives of Internal Medicine* 148(5):1023–38, May 1988.

55. Grueninger, U. J., Goldstein, M. G., and Duffy, F. D. Patient education in hypertension: five essential steps. *Journal of Hypertension* 7(suppl. 3):S93–S98, May 1989.

56. Oncology Nursing Society Education Committee. *Outcome Standards for Cancer Patient Education.* Pittsburgh: Oncology Nursing Society, 1982.

57. Arthritis Foundation. *Arthritis and Musculoskeletal Patient Education Standards.* Atlanta: Arthritis Foundation, 1991, p. 1.

58. Wolle, J. M., Cleary, H. P., and Stone, E. J. Initiation of a voluntary certification program for health education specialists. *Public Health Reports* 104(4):396–402, July–Aug. 1989.

59. Young, B., and Johnson, L. The development of hospitalwide patient-education director competencies. *Patient Education and Counseling* 6(1):19–24, 1984.

60. American Association of Diabetes Educators, 500 North Michigan Avenue, Suite 1400, Chicago, IL 60611.

61. American Society for Psychoprophylaxis in Obstetrics, 1840 Wilson Boulevard, Suite 204, Arlington, VA 22201.

62. Personal communication with Maureen Dion-Perry, patient education coordinator, Kaiser Permanente, Boston, Sept. 1991.

63. Personal communication with Sandra Klima, director, Education Resources, Kent General Hospital, Dover, DE, Sept. 1991.

64. Personal communication with Kathy Linnell, director, Clinic Education, Virginia Mason Clinic, Seattle, Nov. 1989.

65. Benson, D. S., and Van Osdol, W. R. *Quality Audit Systems for Primary Care Centers.* Indianapolis: Methodist Hospital of Indiana, 1988.

66. Wyness.

67. McCarthy, L. Toward quality assurance in patient education. *Promoting Health* 7(1):5–7, Jan.–Feb. 1986.

68. Personal communication with Dorothy Ruzicki, director, Department of Educational Services, Sacred Heart Medical Center, Spokane, WA, Jan. 1992.

69. Personal communication with Maureen Dion-Perry, Jan. 1992.

70. Berg, B. K., Eckoff-Biagi, P., Herbert, P., Rodell, D., and Sprafkin, R. Patient education needs assessment: constructing a generic guide. *Patient Education and Counseling* 9(2):199–207, Apr. 1987.

71. Villejo, L. A., Giloth, B. E., and Zerbe, D. A. Patient education services. In: D. Lerman and S. N. Nathanson, editors. *Outpatient Cancer Centers: Implementation and Management.* Chicago: American Hospital Publishing, 1988, pp. 151–67.

72. Personal communication with Sandra Cornett, patient education coordinator, The Ohio State University Hospitals, Columbus, Jan. 1992.

73. Basch, C. E. Focus group interview: an underutilized research technique for improving theory and practice in health education. *Health Education Quarterly* 14(4):411–48, Winter 1987.

74. Personal communication with Kathy Linnell, Mar. 1992.

75. Office of Academic Affairs. Patient Health Education. *Our Customers' Views.* Washington, DC: Department of Veterans Affairs, 1991.

76. Koska, M. T. Patient-centered care: can your hospital afford not to have it? *Hospitals* 64(21):48–54, Nov. 5, 1990.

77. Nadzam, D. M. The agenda for change: update on indicator development and possible implications for the nursing profession. *Journal of Nursing Quality Assurance* 5(2):18–22, Jan. 1991.

78. JCAHO, *Primer on Clinical Indicator Development and Application.*

79. Joint Commission on Accreditation of Healthcare Organizations. Quality improvement applications of standard QA.3: the use of "multidisciplinary indicators." *Joint Commission Perspectives* 11(1):7, Jan.–Feb. 1991.

80. Correspondence from Carole H. Patterson, associate director for interpretation and acting director, Department of Standards, JCAHO, Oakbrook Terrace, IL, Nov. 1990.

81. Baasch, L. A. Assessing the integrated approach to diabetes patient education: a case study. *Patient Education and Counseling* 12(3):199–212, Dec. 1988.

82. Koska, M. T. Clinical quality initiatives: the search for meaningful—and accurate—measures (Defining meaningful indicators of quality is slow, complex work). *Hospitals* 66(5):29–32, Mar. 5, 1992.

83. Personal communication with Carolyn Speros, director, Nursing Education Services, Methodist Hospitals of Memphis, Memphis, TN, Jan. 1992.

84. Personal communication with Maureen Dion-Perry, Jan. 1992.

85. Personal communication with Alice Lake, nursing director, Capitol Hill Family Health Center, Seattle, Dec. 1989.

86. Beauchamp, C. Quality assurance in the VA. Presentation, Salt Lake Regional Medical Education Center annual liaison conference, Park City, UT, May 14–16, 1991.

87. O'Connor, F. W. A research-based program to increase staff nurses' provision of psychoeducational care to surgical patients: development and evaluation. Doctoral dissertation, Northwestern University, 1986. *Dissertation Abstracts International* 47, 3296B, 1987.

88. Division of Ambulatory Care and Health Promotion and the American Society for Healthcare Education and Training. 1988 conversation by mail [unpublished report]. Chicago: American Hospital Association, Mar. 1988.

89. Iyer, P. W., and Camp, N. H. *Nursing Documentation—A Nursing Process Approach.* St. Louis: Mosby-Year Book, 1991.

90. Short, N. M., and Bair, L. Standards of care: practicing what we preach. *Nursing Management* 21(6):32–39, June 1990.

91. Martin, J. P. From implications to reality through a unit-based quality assurance program. *Clinical Nurse Specialist* 3(4):192–96, Winter 1989.

92. Coyne, C., and Killien, M. A system for unit-based monitors of quality of nursing care. *Journal of Nursing Administration* 17(1):26–32, Jan. 1987.

93. Leary, C. B. Use of nursing process to develop unit specific quality assurance plans. *Journal of Nursing Quality Assurance* 4(2):1–6, Feb. 1990.

94. Schroeder, P. S., Maibusch, R. M., Anderson, C. A., and Formella, N. M. A unit-based approach to nursing quality assurance. *Quality Review Bulletin* 8(3):10–12, Mar. 1982.

95. Personal communication with Mary Haynie, director, Tulsa Health Awareness Center, Tulsa Medical College, Tulsa, OK, Jan. 1992.

96. Miller, J. E., and Lewis, F. M. Closing the gap in quality assurance: a tool for evaluating group leaders. *Health Education Quarterly* 9(1):55–66, Spring 1982.

97. Petersen, M. B. H. Adult educator competencies. *Journal of Continuing Education in Nursing* 14(5):22–27, Sept.–Oct. 1983.

98. Division of Nursing. *Generic Standards of Nursing Practice.* Memphis, TN: Methodist Hospital of Memphis, 1982, p. 1.

99. Personal communication with Carolyn Speros.

100. Personal communication with Annette Rykwalder, director, Patient and Community Health Education, University of Virginia Health Sciences Center, Charlottesville, VA, Jan. 1992.

101. Doak, C., Doak, L., and Root, J. *Teaching Patients with Low Literacy Skills.* Philadelphia: J. B. Lippincott Co., 1985.

Chapter 11

Analyzing Patient Education Deficiencies to Identify and Resolve Real Problems

Dorothy A. Ruzicki, Ph.D., R.N.

☐ Objectives

The reader will be able to:

- Identify the real problems underlying patient education deficiencies
- Describe at least two processes for generating solutions that promote commitment, involvement, and ownership among staff involved in patient education efforts
- Describe at least two strategies that could be used to resolve underlying problems in patient education

☐ Analyzing Quality Assessment and Patient Education Deficiencies

Quality assessment, an important initial phase of the quality monitoring and evaluation process, provides measurements of program quality or quality of care as it relates to patient education, and thus identifies existing problems in patient education programs. However, quality assessment may not go far enough in isolating real problems and defining appropriate action to be taken. This chapter focuses on analyzing deficiencies unearthed by quality assessment (QA) monitors and on developing strategies to address them.

Implementation of sound QA practices can help prevent plunging headlong from identified deficiencies to corrective action without first carefully examining the causes of problems or potential obstacles. Careful analysis of problems requires active involvement of stakeholders and use of objective data. By strengthening the assessment phase of the quality process through use of analytical methods, the patient education manager (PEM) can build a foundation for continuous quality improvement in patient education.

Unmasking the Deficiency

For most patient education managers, setting up a QA plan is a major accomplishment, but unmasking the true problems underlying deficiencies that such plans discover also is important. The first part of the QA plan establishes the indicators to be measured (for example, documentation of patient education) and the monitors to measure them. The next phase involves data collection, comparing data against predetermined thresholds for each indicator, and identifying any deficiencies. If a deficiency is found, the PEM's first tendency is to tackle it as though it is the culprit. But that may not be the case.

Documentation provides an example. If patient education is not being charted on a patient's medical record (the deficiency), the PEM's first action may be to change the forms to make documentation easier. However, the inadequacy of current forms may be only a symptom of other underlying problems. Inadequate documentation could be caused by any of the following:

- Staff do not know how to use existing documentation forms.
- Existing documentation forms are too complicated.
- Staff do not understand their role (who and what to teach).
- Staff are apathetic about providing patient education.
- Staff are not teaching because there is no time, no expectation, and no reward.
- Staff may be expecting someone else to teach.

If the form is changed without examining all possible causes of inadequate documentation, the effort expended to change it may not solve the problem. Therefore, it is critical to identify the real problem—the root cause—before doing anything to rectify a given deficiency.

Deficiencies are identified through indicators and show only that something is amiss that affects that specific indicator. And, as seen above, indicators can be affected by a multitude of other issues, any one of which could be causing the deficiency.

Validating the Deficiency Data

Data leading to identification of deficiencies could include information from medical records, observations, material counts, evaluation form summaries, and other sources. These data are frequently collected by others besides the PEM. In fact, the quality assessment plan itself may be developed by either unit-based QA teams or by a QA coordinator. Therefore, before using deficiency data to identify real problems, it is important that the PEM "own" the data, that is, believe the data are accurate.

If there are any suspicions about data validity, not only will it be difficult to identify underlying problems, but the seriousness of an identified deficiency may even be distorted. Perhaps there really is no deficiency—or the deficiency might be greater than initially thought.

Thus, before accepting that the deficiency is truly a problem, it is important to determine if the data that uncovered the deficiency are valid. Like research, the design, data collection, and analysis processes that identify the deficiency must be objective to be valid. Some questions to ask about the data include:

1. Who collected the data? Were they collected by an objective, careful individual or a team? Who determined that the data should be collected? Was it one person or a committee? Were those who collected the data knowledgeable about what indicator would help identify problems?
2. How were the data collected? Were the instruments used to collect the data valid and reliable? (*Reliability* refers to the degree of consistency of measurement reflected by the data, whereas *validity* refers to the degree to which the data accurately measure what they are supposed to measure.)
3. If a sample was used to collect data, was it representative of the population in question?
4. Were the conclusions reasonable? Did the report reflect actual data, or did it contain opinions without sufficient data to back them up?

If the response to any of these questions is no, or if the process was skewed in any way, it may be necessary to repeat the initial quality assessment steps that led to identification of the deficiency being examined. It may even be necessary to suggest different monitors that will more objectively measure the indicators. There is no point in further examining the deficiency if there is any doubt about its validity.

Determining Actual Causes Underlying Deficiencies

Once the deficiency is accepted as "true," the next phase begins—that of looking for underlying, real causes. Finding the real causes of a deficiency is facilitated by categorizing the types of possible problems and then using tools such as flowcharts and diagrams to examine cause and effect.

Ways to Organize the Search

To search for the real causes of a deficiency, it may be helpful to categorize the areas to search and then to carefully examine each area using methods borrowed from continuous quality improvement (CQI) techniques, which are discussed in the following section. Four possible categories of problems to examine are: (1) system problems, (2) training problems, (3) performance problems, and (4) material problems. In figure 11-1, potential problems in each category are suggested for a deficiency in documentation for patients with diabetes.

Methods to Analyze Cause and Effect

Two excellent methods to examine the relationship between the deficiency and the possible causes are the flowchart and the cause-and-effect diagram, or the fishbone technique. Both of these are described widely in CQI literature.[1]

Figure 11-1. Types of Problems in Documenting Patient Education for Diabetes Patients

System Problems

- Nurses' role in teaching is unclear.
- Time to teach is limited.
- Patient acuity is high.
- Staffing is inadequate.
- Families are not included.
- Program is not well defined.
- Expectations are unrealistic.
- Involvement of other disciplines is unclear.
- Materials are not available for use.

Training Problems

- Program is not explained to staff in in-services.
- Nurses lack knowledge of diabetes and its care.

Performance Problems

- Apathy and burnout are common.
- Poor role models are informal leaders.
- Care of patients with diabetes is inadequate.
- Nurse manager does not expect staff to teach and does not reward teaching.

Material Problems

- Current, easy-to-use resource materials are lacking.
- Documentation forms and program protocols are complex and misleading.

Constructing a simple flowchart clarifies the process by providing a step-by-step visualization of what happens during the process in question. For example, if documentation of diabetic education is of concern, the flowchart can show the process from beginning to end (see figure 11-2). Complexities and problem areas in the process are quickly noted as the chart is constructed.

The cause-and-effect diagram, often called the fishbone technique because of its appearance, is an excellent method for hypothesizing, suggesting, and examining possible contributing factors. This approach encourages a very thorough evaluation of likely causes. See figure 11-3 for a description of how to construct a cause-and-effect diagram and a diagram of its major parts. Figure 11-4 (p. 242) provides an example of a completed diagram, albeit abbreviated, for the documentation example given here.

□ Taking Action

Once the real problems are identified, the best course of action to resolve them needs to be determined. This is not as easy as it seems, because one can either sit back and do nothing, handle the problems quickly, or involve other people in their resolution.

When to Wait and Do Nothing

If the problem is something for which some form of resolution is in process, it may be best to do nothing at present. For example, if the chart form was changed six months

Figure 11-2. Constructing a Flowchart for a Patient with Diabetes Admitted to the Hospital

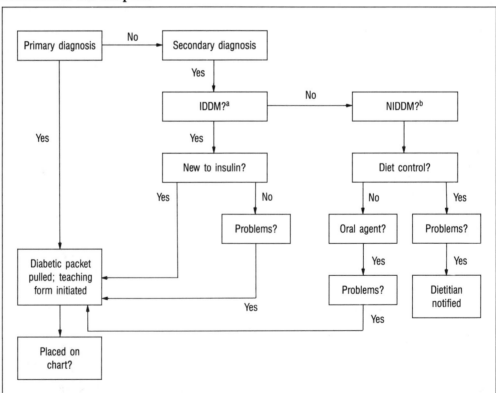

a IDDM means insulin-dependent diabetes mellitus.
b NIDDM means non–insulin-dependent diabetes mellitus.

Figure 11-3. Procedure for Cause-and-Effect Analysis (Fishbone Technique)

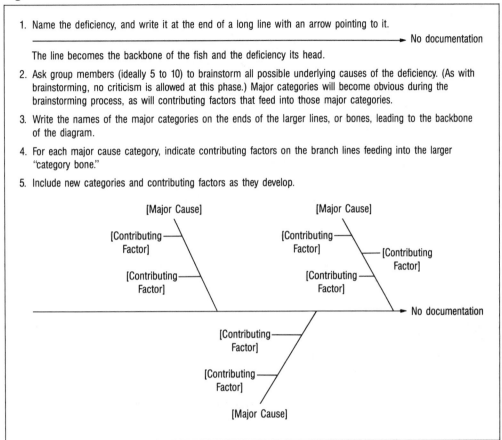

1. Name the deficiency, and write it at the end of a long line with an arrow pointing to it.

   → No documentation

   The line becomes the backbone of the fish and the deficiency its head.

2. Ask group members (ideally 5 to 10) to brainstorm all possible underlying causes of the deficiency. (As with brainstorming, no criticism is allowed at this phase.) Major categories will become obvious during the brainstorming process, as will contributing factors that feed into those major categories.

3. Write the names of the major categories on the ends of the larger lines, or bones, leading to the backbone of the diagram.

4. For each major cause category, indicate contributing factors on the branch lines feeding into the larger "category bone."

5. Include new categories and contributing factors as they develop.

Compiled from information in D. M. Berwick, A. B. Godfrey, and J. Roessner, *Curing Health Care: New Strategies for Quality Improvement.* San Francisco: Jossey-Bass, 1990; and M. LeBoeuf, *The Productivity Challenge.* New York City: McGraw-Hill, 1982.

ago and not enough patients have been admitted to give the current form a good test, it may be too soon to effectively evaluate it. Maybe things are getting better and just need a bit more time.

When to Do Simple Follow-up

Sometimes simple follow-up action on the part of the patient education manager is sufficient to deal with the problem. For example, if, through the cause-and-effect analysis, it is determined that the staff have not had enough in-service training on how to use a documentation form, setting up an education program or encouraging nurse managers to discuss it at a staff meeting may be all that is necessary.

How to Approach Complex Problems

Some problems cannot be resolved by either of the preceding two methods. The rest of this chapter presents ways to address complex patient education deficiencies.

If the problems uncovered involve many people and/or require system changes throughout the organization, it is particularly important to involve all stakeholders—those who are in any way affected by the problem—in the resolution process. There are a number of ways to do this, and the following section focuses on how. It is also important to foster a sense of ownership among the people who generate the solutions.

Figure 11-4. Fishbone Diagram of Documentation Problems

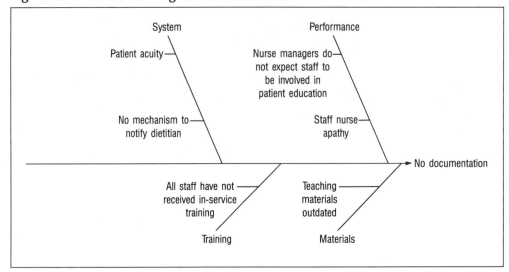

Finding the Stakeholders

A key to finding lasting solutions to complex problems, or at least solutions that will last for a while, is to involve others in working them out. It is critical that the PEM not "lay" a solution to a particular problem on the staff, because if they do not own it—or have the opportunity to contribute to it—they will not implement it. So how does one find the right stakeholders? Begin by asking if the problem is hospitalwide or unit or department based. Does it affect people throughout the institution, or does it affect staff on only one or two nursing units? After this is determined, a task force consisting of appropriate staff members should be formed to generate a solution. If a Patient Education Committee already exists, its members can be helpful in suggesting or even formally designating task force members.

If the problem is hospitalwide, for example, documentation of medication instruction or discharge instruction across the institution, a representative sample of those persons affected by the problem and involved in the patient education program should be determined. Included might be nursing administration, management, staff nurses, a clinical specialist, and perhaps a physician.

If the problem is unit or department based, for example, documentation of pacemaker education on the cardiac unit, the task force is a bit more manageable in terms of size. Very often, all the key people can be included on a task force. If unit quality assessment is practiced, the Quality Assessment Committee should be represented. Manager support is essential. It is very helpful if the staff represented are also informal unit leaders (those who do not have positional authority, but exert influence on staff).

Fostering Ownership of the Problem

As mentioned earlier, members of the task force must agree that the initial deficiency is valid. Involving task force members in these activities ensures their support and acceptance of the identified problem before moving on to determine possible solutions. It is helpful for the PEM to present the deficiency data to them (if they are unfamiliar with it), explain how the data were collected, and answer any questions. Also, even though the underlying problems may be fairly well identified, the task force needs to look at them again and may even identify other issues. The flowchart and cause-and-effect diagram can be used again. It is important to emphasize controllable causes, or the group may go off on tangents for which there can ultimately be no reasonable solution.

☐ Developing Solutions to Complex Problems Using Processes and Strategies

The processes described in the following section are effective in encouraging members of a group to reach consensus on solutions to all kinds of patient education problems. Once consensus is reached, group members can use several strategies to improve the deficiency.

Processes

Any number of creative process techniques can be used to develop recommendations or solutions to patient education problems. And these techniques can even be fun for the participants. Two excellent sources of techniques are the books *Group Power*[2] and *Group Power II.*[3] Four very effective and easy-to-use processes are (1) brainstorming, (2) nominal group technique, (3) Crawford slip writing, and (4) snow cards.

Nearly everyone has used or participated in brainstorming exercises, the purpose of which is to generate ideas. Key to this technique is to be freewheeling and nonjudgmental about the ideas that surface. Participants should be encouraged to let their imaginations go. The person leading the brainstorming exercise explains the process and lists the ideas that participants call out. When no more ideas are generated, the group discusses, categorizes, and prioritizes them.

The nominal group technique[4] is also used to generate ideas and suggestions. It allows opportunity for all participants to share their ideas, and additionally provides for a ranking of priorities. (See figure 11-5 for a description of nominal group technique procedure.)

Crawford slip writing[5] is a type of silent brainstorming. The slips allow for easy categorization of ideas. (See figure 11-6 for a description of this technique.)

Snow cards[6] are very similar to Crawford slip writing. However, Ruzicki added a last step to help prioritize the ideas that surface (see figure 11-7).

Strategies

The processes described in the preceding section are excellent methods to generate solutions to problems. Typically, these solutions fall within a general strategy for implementation.

Figure 11-5. Nominal Group Technique

1. *Purpose.* The group facilitator states the task at hand, which specifies the information desired from the group.
2. *Silent item listing.* The group facilitator asks participants to silently write down as many answers as they can (similar to brainstorming).
3. *Verbal listing.* In round-robin fashion participants contribute their ideas out loud. A recorder lists the ideas on a flip chart or blackboard, and each item is numbered.
4. *Discussion.* The group facilitator asks participants to discuss each item for clarification and understanding. Criticism of items is not allowed.
5. *Preliminary ranking.* The group facilitator asks each participant to silently rank the five (or ten) ideas believed to be best. Votes are then tabulated, and items are written on the flip chart. These are shared with all participants.
6. *Discussion of ranking.* The group facilitator asks the group to discuss ranking of priorities to determine if everyone understands them and if any important priorities have been overlooked.
7. *Reranking.* Participants are then asked to silently rerank the items on the flip chart according to importance. Numeric ratings can be assigned items in order to weight them. For example, the most important on a list of ten items would be ranked "10" and the least important "1." When the facilitator tallies the individual ratings, the weight is reflected in the final score for each item.

Note: For further information, see A. L. Delbecq and A. H. VandeVen. A group process model for problem identification and program planning. *Journal of Applied Behavioral Science* 7(4):466–91, July–Aug. 1971 (or any other description of nominal group technique).

Figure 11-6. Crawford Slip Writing

1. Each participant is given a 3×5-inch notepad.
2. The leader presents a problem in question form. For example: How do we increase staff awareness of the importance of patient education?
3. Participants are then asked to write as many answers as they can on separate slips of paper.
4. When the participants have finished, the leader collects their responses.
5. The responses are categorized and further discussed, which gives rise to additional ideas.

Note: For further information on Crawford slip writing, see M. LeBoeuf. *The Productivity Challenge.* New York City: McGraw-Hill, 1982.

Figure 11-7. Snow Cards

1. Select a facilitator.
2. Focus on a single problem, question, or issue.
3. Silently brainstorm ideas and individually record them on paper.
4. Transfer the five "best" ideas to individual white 5×8-inch cards.
5. Tape cards on the wall; cluster them and give names to similar themes.
6. Discuss, compare, and contrast.
7. Prioritize ideas.
   a. Give group members a limited number of stickers (for example, ten colored dots each).
   b. Ask members to "spend" their stickers on the ideas they like best; placing one or more stickers on any idea.

Note: For further information on the use of snow cards for strategic planning, see M. Bryson. *Strategic Planning for Public and Nonprofit Organizations.* San Francisco: Jossey-Bass, 1988.

Such strategies include (1) integrating solutions into existing systems; (2) developing new policies, procedures, forms, committees, programs, and materials; (3) providing in-service or continuing education programs; and (4) changing systems. However, no matter what strategy is chosen, organizational savvy, or understanding the organizational culture, is critical to its success. (A detailed discussion of organizational savvy can be found in chapter 5.)

Integrating Solutions into Existing Systems

Integrating solutions into existing systems is by far a better strategy than attempting to develop new systems. It takes less time and is less difficult. An example of this would be to include patient education assessment as part of the general nursing assessment or to build documentation into existing documentation forms.

Developing New Policies, Procedures, Forms, Committees, Programs, and Materials

If need be, developing new policies, procedures, forms, committees, programs, and materials is another important strategy that most PEMs use to resolve issues. A new policy procedure or form might clarify a process for staff. A committee or task force might be formed to develop a program and/or teaching materials. A committee might be needed for structure (for example, as part of an official approval process).

Communicating with all the stakeholders, soliciting their suggestions, and letting them know about the resolution is critical for all of these possibilities—so is ease of use. If the policies or forms are complicated, they will not be used or followed by staff. Simplicity is absolutely essential. *Streamline* is an important word in any PEM's vocabulary.

Providing In-Service and Continuing Education

In-servicing newly developed programs is a must, particularly if nursing staff or other disciplines do not know how to implement them. Something as simple as not knowing how to locate the teaching booklets or how to chart what was taught can make or break a program. Continuing education programs can also be developed to help staff nurses integrate patient teaching in daily care delivery. Many staff nurses were taught in their basic educational programs that patient teaching meant developing objectives, content, and teaching materials to provide in-depth instructional sessions; thus, they may not know how to integrate instruction into their daily activities—or even how to recognize instruction they currently provide. Continuing education programs for patient education can consist of seminars devoted to a single topic, or better yet, they can be integrated into clinically focused workshops.

Changing Systems

Changing systems is the most difficult strategy and the one that takes the most time. It should be used when other strategies cannot resolve the root problem; in other words, when the problem is a system problem involving large numbers of people. This strategy is similar to the one on developing new policies and procedures, but differs in that it involves major system changes, such as revising job descriptions or work responsibilities, developing new categories of personnel, or reorganizing entire documentation methods. Because these types of changes take so long to implement and are generally very complex, affecting many people, they should not be considered lightly. However, in some cases systems change may be the only strategy that is effective.

☐ Conclusion

Addressing patient education deficiencies is a critical component of quality assessment. And, as has been seen, it involves more than just identifying the deficiency itself. If the deficiency is not thoughtfully analyzed, it is possible that a great deal of energy and time will be spent on problems that may not be the real causes of it. Strategies will be designed and promoted that cause the entire process to repeat itself—endlessly. Ultimately, patient education will suffer, with its potential benefits lost in a web of irrelevant, cumbersome data.

However, if this step in the quality monitoring and evaluation process is handled carefully and analytically, problems can be effectively resolved. Furthermore, the process of generating solutions, with its necessary teamwork, will go a long way toward building support for patient education and assisting in laying the groundwork for continuing efforts to improve patient education quality.

References

1. Berwick, D. M., Godfrey, A. B., and Roessner, J. *Curing Health Care: New Strategies for Quality Improvement.* San Francisco: Jossey-Bass, 1990.

2. Daniels, W. R. *Group Power: A Manager's Guide to Using Meetings.* San Diego: University Associates, 1986.

3. Daniels, W. R. *Group Power II: A Manager's Guide to Conducting Regular Meetings.* San Diego: University Associates, 1990.

4. Delbecq, A. L., and VandeVen, A. H. A group process model for problem identification and program planning. *Journal of Applied Behavioral Science* 7(4):466–91, July–Aug. 1971.

5. LeBoeuf, M. *The Productivity Challenge.* New York City: McGraw-Hill, 1982.

6. Bryson, M. *Strategic Planning for Public and Nonprofit Organizations.* San Francisco: Jossey-Bass, 1988.

Chapter 12

Managing Staff Development in Patient Education

Rose Mary Monaco Pries, M.S.P.H., C.H.E.S.

☐ Objectives

The reader will be able to:

- Identify the role of staff development in a hospitalwide patient education program
- Utilize appropriate strategies to assess patient education staff development needs
- Design effective patient education staff development programs
- Evaluate the effectiveness of patient education staff development

☐ How Staff Development Supports Patient Education

Staff development is a vital component of a hospitalwide patient education program. It can support patient education functioning at a variety of levels by:

- Ensuring that direct care givers have the necessary skills to serve as effective patient and family educators and counselors
- Assisting teaching teams to develop comprehensive patient education programs for select patient target populations
- Offering an interdisciplinary patient education committee the skills needed to develop a hospitalwide patient education program

This chapter discusses needs assessment, planning and design, implementation, and evaluation of staff development programs for each of these functions, and provides specific examples of needs assessment instruments and programs.

☐ Teaching Effective Patient Education and Counseling Skills

Enhancing the education and counseling skills of direct care givers is a critical focus of staff development in patient education. High-quality patient and family education results when staff can utilize a client-centered approach to integrate effective patient education skills into the limited time available for teaching patients in clinical settings.

Needs Assessment

Like the process of educating patients and family members, staff development begins with needs assessment. In this era of shrinking resources, staff shortages, and decreased lengths of stay, the need for staff development in patient education must be documented. Documenting the need will make it easier to secure the resources needed to conduct the training and the time to permit staff to participate. The need for this type of training can be assessed in a variety of ways.

Conducting focus groups is one specific way of gathering a large amount of relevant information from staff members about their involvement in patient education, barriers to effective teaching, and potential strategies to improve teaching, including staff development. Ideas from such groups can often be used as the basis for broader data collection strategies such as surveys.[1,2]

Often surveys and questionnaires are used as needs assessment tools when input is needed from a large number of staff members. One problem with the use of surveys is that they often have a low rate of return. A higher rate of return can be facilitated in a number of ways. For example, one hospital offers small incentives such as pencils, pens, and pins bearing the patient education logo for the return of surveys. Surveys can also be completed and collected at the conclusion of staff meetings or staff development sessions. They can be used to collect data on a variety of staff development topics or may focus solely on patient education.

Questions on patient education should also be included when querying staff about training needs on any clinical topic. They reinforce the concept that patient education is an integral component of care, not something that is done if "extra" time is available.

If it is impractical to survey a large number of staff, a representative sample may be selected. Surveys can be taken within one discipline, for example, nursing, or within a variety of disciplines. Figures 12-1, 12-2, and 12-3 (p. 250) contain samples of instruments used to survey staff about the need for staff development on patient education. The instrument in figure 12-1 is used specifically with nurses.

The instruments in figures 12-2 and 12-3 are used to survey an interdisciplinary group. The hospital that used the instrument in figure 12-3 has an interdisciplinary

Figure 12-1. Nursing Service Education Needs Assessment, Fiscal Year 1993

The Education Council would like to help you meet your continuing education needs. Please list any educational programs you believe you or any of your coworkers could benefit from in fiscal year 1993 (10/1/92 to 9/30/93). This list must be returned to your service facilitator by April 29, 1992.

Clinical topics (may include disease processes, advanced technology, and so on):

Professional issues (certification preparation, current issues in nursing, politics in nursing, patient/staff teaching, and so on):

Management issues (leadership issues, holding a meeting, managing conflict, scheduling, interpersonal relations, and so on):

Ethical issues:

Other (consider needs from quality assurance monitors, incident reports, and so on):

Thank you for your participation.

Reprinted from the Department of Veterans Affairs, San Diego, California.

Figure 12-2. Learning Needs Assessment Self-Evaluation for Staff

Name: _____ Date of Program: _____

Please check the column or columns that most nearly reflect your learning needs.

Topic	Need to know	Would like to review	Already know
1. Principles of adult learning			
2. How to write behavioral objectives			
3. JCAHO standards for patient health education			
4. How to develop a patient education notebook			
5. How to write patient education materials			
6. Low-literacy teaching skills			

List below any other patient education topics of interest to you.

_____

_____

_____

_____

Thank you for helping to identify topics for program development.

Reprinted from the Department of Veterans Affairs, Albuquerque, New Mexico.

patient education committee. The surveys were distributed to each discipline via its representative on the committee. This strategy can serve several important purposes: It distributes the patient education work load and, by actively involving patient education committee members, it increases their commitment to the hospitalwide patient education program.

Another way to assess needs is to ask managers about the kinds of development needed to enhance their staff's education and counseling skills. Valuable information can be gathered this way, especially if patient education skills are a component of performance appraisal. If clinical staff care for patients for whom patient education standards exist, the standards may mandate either specific skills or participation in continuing education on patient education as a component of practice.

Another source of data on the need for training to enhance the communication and education skills of clinical staff is patient satisfaction or guest relations surveys. Data from this source may be of great significance to management in the allocation of resources and staff time for training. If patients and families, now often referred to as "customers," indicate a hurried or less-than-optimal response to their questions and concerns, staff development in these areas may certainly be considered. However, care must be taken in analyzing data from patient satisfaction surveys. Often the underlying problems are systems issues rather than issues that can be remedied by a staff development intervention.

Quality assurance studies can provide justification for staff development on patient education, and may also support the role that patient education can play in promoting positive patient outcomes. Admission, discharge, and readmission data for a certain group of patients, or from a particular unit, may also identify a need to enhance teaching skills, if effective education plays a role in the patient's or family's ability to manage care at home.

Figure 12-3. Example of a Patient Education Staff Survey

Route to: Patient Education Coordinator

Directions: This survey has been developed to assist us in identifying patient education needs at this medical center. It will also help us to develop programs to meet the educational needs of our patients. Please answer each of the following questions or statements by checking the appropriate response or by filling in the blank(s).

Demographics: Please check the appropriate position.

_____ M.D.   _____ R.N.   _____ D.D.S.   _____ Social worker

_____ Other staff (specify) _____

1. In general, how much do you think patients understand about their health problems?

    _____ a lot   _____ something   _____ very little   _____ nothing

2. How much do you think patients/families understand about tests, procedures, or treatments received while they are in the medical center?

    _____ a lot   _____ something   _____ very little   _____ nothing

3. How much do you think patients understand about their medications and how they are to use them?

    _____ a lot   _____ something   _____ very little   _____ nothing

4. What types of questions do patients ask you? (Check all that apply.)

    About illness or health status   _____
    About procedures performed   _____
    About medications   _____
    About diet   _____
    About what to do upon discharge   _____
    Other (specify) _____   _____

5. Are you usually able to answer patient/family questions to your satisfaction?

    A. _____ most times   _____ sometimes   _____ seldom

    B. If *sometimes* or *seldom*, what prevents you from answering adequately?

    _____

    _____

6. What resources, courses, or areas of instruction would be most helpful to you in the area of patient education? (Use back if more space is needed.)

    _____

    _____

    _____

Thank you for your help!

Reprinted from the Department of Veterans Affairs, Memphis, Tennessee.

Program Planning and Design

Effective staff development for clinicians will model effective patient and family education. In both cases, the educational experience must meet the needs of the intended audience. A well-designed needs assessment and representation on the staff development planning committee will identify those areas of greatest concern and priority for clinicians. The information and skills provided in staff training programs must be readily utilizable in the clinical setting. Skill practice with feedback must be built in, as well as active problem solving with regard to barriers to the integration of information and skills into the clinical setting. The content and skills must also be realistic. For example, it would be futile to teach staff to utilize an effective but lengthy needs assessment form if there is no time to use it in the clinical setting.

Staff development to enhance the patient education and counseling skills of clinical staff can take a variety of formats, such as workshops and minieducational sessions. Workshops, which will be described in the following sections, are advantageous because they provide the opportunity for learners to practice skills and receive feedback. (Minieducational sessions will be described later in the chapter in the section on other alternative staff development designs.)

Workshops may be conducted for one day, or for shorter time periods over several days. Such a staff development program would include a purpose statement, learning objectives, expected outcomes, and an evaluation plan.

This format is beneficial for several reasons. First, it offers time for skill practice. This is critical if staff are expected to integrate the new skills into the patient and family education conducted in their clinical setting. In addition to skill practice, participants usually have an opportunity to actively solve problems concerning barriers to using the information and skills presented.

Second, this format allows participants time to network and share. Networking and sharing reinforces the value placed on patient education efforts in the clinical setting. If staff participate together in staff development on patient education, the importance of this function will be reaffirmed. This will encourage staff to assist and support each other in educating patients and families.

To plan workshops for staff development, it is helpful to form a planning committee. If continuing education units (CEUs) are offered, a planning committee may be required by the accrediting body. In addition to providing needed input into program design and implementation, this committee may serve an important political function. By appropriate selection of planning committee members, support and commitment can be gained not only for the training, but also for the necessary follow-up and evaluation of the training's effectiveness and for patient education in general.

The planning committee should include content experts. These experts may be from within the hospital or the outside, and may also ultimately serve as staff development faculty. Representatives from the audience to be trained should also be included on a planning committee. This ensures that the content and learning activities will support the use of appropriate, acceptable, and readily usable skills in the clinical practice setting. Clinical supervisor representatives on the committee will ensure that the training provides staff with the skills and information needed to enhance their education and counseling responsibilities. These representatives should also facilitate securing staff time to participate in the training and engage in patient education in the clinical setting.

The planning committee should set workshop objectives and provide input on program content and design, appropriate learning activities and handout materials, and evaluation strategies. If the committee is provided with sufficient needs assessment data, this planning can usually be done with minimal meeting time. Information from the needs assessment that should be made available to the planning committee includes: (1) how the need was identified, (2) the information and skills needed, (3) the numbers and type of staff to be trained, and (4) any scheduling specifics that may be important in securing staff attendance.

Depending on the customary management of staff development at the hospital, the workshop planning committee may be involved in securing and allocating staff development program budget and resources. If the hospital has a patient education committee, this committee may be of assistance in validating the need for the training, providing interdisciplinary support for the training, and securing the needed resources to conduct the training. If the training is going to affect the patient education committee's hospital-wide goals or plan, this consideration should be highlighted when securing management approval for the needed resources and time for training.

Several different training design alternatives to workshops can be used to get the needed skills and information to staff. Skills can be learned, but, like teaching a patient skill such as the self-injection of insulin, practice and feedback must be components of the training design. Although it is easier to accommodate skill practice and feedback in the traditional workshop setting, alternative training strategies are possible, and with creative learning activities can provide the necessary skill practice.

Implementation

To accommodate for staff shortages and limited training time, workshops must be flexible in design and scheduling. This may necessitate breaking the training into a number of modules. To ensure maximum attendance, the content and skills covered in any one module cannot depend on mastery of the content and skills of preceding modules. There is usually no guarantee that staff will be able to attend the modules in sequence. Modules whose content and skills are readily utilizable ensure that staff can return to their clinical settings with the tools they need to enhance the patient education they provide.

The Department of Veterans Affairs (VA) has designed a staff development program called "Enhancing Patient Education Skills." This program is designed to teach basic patient education skills to direct care givers. It is offered by VA Regional Medical Education Centers in a train-the-trainers format. A minimum of two staff members is selected as trainers from each hospital electing to participate. The trainers attend a continuing education program that presents the content and skills to them, and assists them in serving as trainers for the program within their own hospitals. Twenty-one total contact-hours are required to train the trainers. In the first 12 contact-hours, the trainers experience the program as clinical staff would. The next nine contact-hours provide them with the information and skills they need to serve as effective trainers.

All training materials for subsequent use by the hospitals are provided by a Regional Medical Education Center. This permits the hospital itself to offer the program whenever the need arises. Hospitals that participate in the train-the-trainers program make the commitment to offer the program to their own staff at least once a year. Staff are selected to participate in the program based on their expertise in patient education and staff development.

The program is offered in four modules with a total of 12 contact-hours. The modules can be compressed within a two-day period, taught one module a week for four weeks, or presented within any other time frame that facilitates staff participation and attendance. The medical centers that have participated in this training report that the most effective way to offer it is in a consecutive two-day period because of the difficulty of scheduling staff for half-day sessions.

The program emphasizes strategies that can be used in brief (10- to 15-minute) encounters with patients, because time for patient education is often limited. It uses a client-centered approach that helps clinical staff empower their patients to take an active role in their own treatment and develop self-care skills. The content and skills presented are drawn from research in health education, communications, and social and behavioral psychology, which was conducted in a variety of patient care settings. Learning activities include demonstrations, individual and group exercises, role-plays, and discussions.

The program's four modules are:

1. *Relationships That Heal* provides the framework for patient education skills in a client-centered approach.
2. *Assessing Patient Education Needs* offers several techniques for assessing individual and/or group learning needs that can be used when time is limited.
3. *Communicating Effectively* presents strategies for analyzing the learning demands of patient education methods and materials, and modifying them to make learning easier for patients.
4. *Facilitating Behavior Change* offers specific techniques to use with patients to help them change health behaviors.

The modules model techniques that clinicians can utilize in interactions with patients. Mirroring the client-centered approach, clinicians become the clients. Their concerns and problems in teaching patients are assessed and dealt with continuously throughout the program.

Figure 12-4 presents the icebreaker activity for trainers to use at the beginning of module I. This activity provides an opportunity for trainers and participants to get acquainted, and permits participants to express their major concerns about educating patients. Lists of helping behaviors remain on the flip charts used during this exercise and are referred to as appropriate, relating program content and skills to participants' needs and concerns. Addressing the participants' needs also models the behavior they should use with their patients.

Evaluation

Because the modules used in the VA workshops stress skill development and practice, there is ample opportunity to integrate the new skills into areas of clinical practice and to actively break down barriers related to patient education. Also built in to these workshops are opportunities for self-assessment as well as feedback from other participants and trainers. Figure 12-5 provides an example of a form that participants use to evaluate their ability to form a helping relationship in a routine attempt to solve a patient problem. Participants also complete similar self-assessments to be used in evaluating both a successful and an unsuccessful encounter, thus identifying the areas in which participants are effective and the skills that require additional work. At the conclusion of each module, participants are able to integrate the information and skills presented into the patient education conducted in their clinical settings.

Other Alternative Staff Development Designs

Although workshops are most effective in enhancing the patient education and counseling skills of clinicians, other options are available when time for staff development is limited. For example, minieducational sessions can be planned for the first 15 to 20 minutes of staff meetings. Research on effective patient education has shown that the most critical components of a teaching session should be covered first, and should include problem solving or discussion on how patients can integrate the information or skills into their life-style. The minieducational session should include a brief discussion of possible barriers and how clinicians can effectively incorporate the information or skills into their clinical practice. Such sessions can focus on a specific skill, such as how to use the Salient Belief Model to assess patient education needs, or introduce how good listening skills can enhance any patient education intervention.

☐ Helping Teaching Teams to Develop Specific Patient and Family Education Programs

A staff development program for teaching teams can assist clinicians in developing formal patient education programs to meet specific hospital needs. Formal patient education interventions can enhance consistency, facilitate appropriate reinforcement of content and skills among health care team members, and ensure survival of a program despite changes in staffing.

The need for development of a formal program may be identified by one or more disciplines. Because many patients require care from a variety of disciplines, the patient education services planned are often interdisciplinary as well and are implemented by teaching teams with members from various departments.

Figure 12-4.   Example of Part of a Staff Development Program: Relationships That Heal

Activity:	Defining a helping relationship
Objective:	To identify personal behaviors that facilitate or hinder a helping relationship
Time:	25 minutes
Supplies:	2 flip charts
Purpose:	This segment of module I is designed to identify the personal behaviors that promote or hinder a helping relationship.
Procedure:	Place two flip charts side by side. Mark off two columns on one flip chart and two columns on the other chart. Place headings in the columns as indicated below.

(Flip charts may be set up in advance.)

Helped	
Attending	Responding

Helper	
Personalizing	Initiating

Procedure:	All of you on the right side of the room individually think about a recent situation when you received help from someone. Identify the specific behaviors associated with being helped.
	Those of you on the left side of the room take about 30 seconds to think about a situation when you helped someone. Identify specific behaviors that enabled you to be perceived as being helpful.
	In this process the participants develop a list of common qualities needed by health care providers to provide effective patient education.
	Ask the participants to state characteristics of a helper. What were those behaviors? Write their responses on the flip chart in the appropriate column of the skill areas (attending, responding, personalizing, initiating).
	Start with a volunteer from the right side of the room. Ask that person to describe the behaviors associated with being helped.
	How would I see it?
	What would it look like?
	Ask for a few more examples.
	Then ask a volunteer from the left side of the room to state the behaviors he or she perceived as being those of the helper.
Key point:	The impact of the patient education process is greatly diminished when these foundation skills are not used—no matter how basic they may seem. These skills are developed over time. They are not personality traits or inherited gifts.
	It takes time to develop these skills, which may seem to be "old hat" for some members of the group and which are chronic challenges to people providing patient education.
Trainer support:	Sample participant responses for Carkhuff skills are in figure 12-5.
	During our discussion we have identified behaviors of people who have been helpful to us and examined our own helping behaviors toward our patients.
	As we place your responses into the appropriate columns, these helping behaviors are being merged into a framework consistent with current research data related to helping relationships.

Note:	Keep this helping skills list in view of participants. It will be used in the next activity.

Reprinted from the Department of Veterans Affairs, St. Louis.

Figure 12-5. Helping Relationships Self-Assessment Questionnaire for Routine Problems with Patients

Directions: Listed are behaviors that are related to effective communication with patients. You are asked to rate yourself for each behavior in a recent routine attempt to help solve a patient's problem. Circle the appropriate number.

Attending/Caring

	Routine Interactions with Patients			
A. Verbal behavior	**All**	**Most**	**Some**	**Seldom**
1. Friendly greeting and introduction. "It's good to see you, Mrs. Jones."	4	3	2	1
2. Positive comments about unique aspects of the patient. "Your hair (skin color and so on) looks good today." "How was your drive here today?"	4	3	2	1
3. Inquiring about unique aspects of the patient. "When did you get that pretty robe?" "What other hobbies do you have?"	4	3	2	1
4. Other (please specify)				
_____	4	3	2	1
_____	4	3	2	1
B. Nonverbal behavior				
1. Making and maintaining eye contact	4	3	2	1
2. Sit/stand facing patient	4	3	2	1
3. Move closer to patient	4	3	2	1
4. Lean toward patient	4	3	2	1
5. Touch patient shoulder, arm	4	3	2	1
Module I				
6. Sit/stand with arms uncrossed	4	3	2	1
7. Nodding head to encourage patient to continue	4	3	2	1
8. Friendly facial expression	4	3	2	1
9. Other (please specify)				
_____	4	3	2	1
_____	4	3	2	1
C. Actions				
1. Change patient's surrounding in response to stated or inferred needs (fluff pillows, fill water pitcher, brighten room)	4	3	2	1
2. Other (please specify)				
_____	4	3	2	1
_____	4	3	2	1

Module I

Scoring: Add up the score for each item under Routine Interactions column. Compare your total score with the score interpretation below.

Score Interpretation:
12–23 You need to consider practicing those behaviors with low scores until they are done automatically.
24–35 You need to identify those few behaviors with low scores and integrate them into your interaction with patients.
36–48 Keep doing the good job that you are doing.

Responding/Communicating

	Routine Interactions with Patients			
Responding to feeling	**All**	**Most**	**Some**	**Seldom**
1. You state patient's feelings in identical terms. "You said you feel . . ."	4	3	2	1
2. You state patient's implicit feelings. "You feel . . ."	4	3	2	1
3. Other (please specify)				
_____	4	3	2	1
_____	4	3	2	1

Score Interpretation:
4–8 You need to practice those behaviors with low scores until you do them more frequently.
9–12 Very good. Try practicing those behaviors with low scores to expand your repertoire of responses.
13–16 Outstanding.

Module I

Reprinted from the Department of Veterans Affairs, St. Louis.

Interdisciplinary involvement in the planning and delivery of patient education programs provides several benefits. Each discipline can contribute to program content, ensuring that all aspects of care are considered. The amount of time any one discipline has to invest in program design will be less than if each developed its own program. Consistency of teaching will also be enhanced because each discipline will be aware of the content to be covered by another.

The concept that there are critical components of patient education programs is becoming more prevalent. In the Department of Veterans Affairs, patient education programs are distinguished from patient education activities. A *patient education program* is a systematically planned, integrated set of activities designed around specific objectives; coordinated, with responsibility assigned to staff; and documented in writing. A *patient education activity* is an effort to bring about behavioral change in ways that are not highly structured. Activities lack one or more of the components of patient education programs.[3]

Many VA medical centers have hospital policies on the review and approval of patient education programs that serve to reinforce their importance to high-quality care. Often the allocation of budget for purchase of print or audiovisual patient teaching materials depends on the use of these resources as a component of a formal program. If teaching resources are designated for use in a formal program, it ensures that the limited resources available will be spent to support patient education services that address hospital needs and priorities.

The American Diabetes Association now recognizes diabetes patient education programs.[4] Meeting the standards required for recognition often results in improvements in the overall quality of diabetes patient education programs, and has become a prerequisite in obtaining third-party reimbursement. The recognition standards demand that certain criteria for diabetes patient education programs be met. These criteria address program description and policy, the target audience, administrative structure, public awareness, the advisory committee, and the patient education process. The patient education process includes patient involvement in needs assessment and objective setting; written behavioral, skill, and knowledge objectives (along with measurable means of determining outcomes) for each patient; and documentation and a follow-up plan.

Needs Assessment

The need to develop formal education programs for patients and families may be identified in a number of ways. If the hospital has a patient education committee that is responsible for establishing an annual or strategic hospitalwide plan for patient education services, one of its goals may be establishment of programs to serve patients with a specific disease or condition. Based on the strategic needs identified, the hospitalwide patient education plan includes goals for the development of programs to serve patients with a specific disease (for example, if the hospital has as one of its goals to open an ambulatory surgery center, the patient education strategic plan might identify the development of a formal patient education program for patients who will undergo an ambulatory surgical procedure). The need for program development may be identified in a less formal way, by the clinicians providing care for those ambulatory surgery patients.

Program Planning and Design

The focus of staff development programs may be determined by many factors. These include needs assessment techniques, selection of appropriate target populations, development of measurable behavioral and informational objectives, selection of appropriate learning activities, selection of teaching resources for special populations (low literacy, visually impaired, elderly patients, and so forth), teaching skills, logistical considerations, marketing strategies, program evaluation, and documentation.

If time permits, an additional component can be team building and team functioning. Too often, it is assumed that because staff work together in the delivery of patient care, they have the skills that are required of all team members to maintain communication, solve problems, and prevent burnout. These issues can be critical in forming and maintaining a functioning patient education team.

Other topics that may be important to include are institutional issues/management focus. This can help participants understand the political climate of the hospital in which their program will exist, and enhance the communication needed to gain administrative support and resources for their program. Additional topics might also include public relations and marketing for patient education programs, as well as such logistical considerations as the scheduling of meeting rooms, the reproduction of teaching resources, and the arrangement of transport services.

In the overall design of a staff development program such as this, it is critical to include time for the team to meet to work on needs assessment, program objectives, and content and selection of learning activities. The team should leave the program with the least possible amount of developmental work to be done. This may necessitate scheduling the staff development program over a period of time.

Implementation

Participants in the kinds of staff development programs just described would be members of the teaching teams responsible for design and implementation of formal patient education programs. Such staff development programs have been offered to VA medical center staff. Program evaluation always includes comments on the value of giving the team uninterrupted time to plan, and what team members learn about each other and their working relationships; these factors are useful to consider during the implementation stage.

An additional component that is helpful, but more complex to build into the program design, is time for the teaching teams to preview audiovisuals they may wish to use in their patient education programs. Additional time is needed to complete the advance work of obtaining information on available audiovisuals and deciding which ones to preview. Previews need to be budgeted for and audiovisual equipment needs to be available.

In VA medical centers the library service is instrumental in helping clinicians locate audiovisuals for use in patient education programs and securing preview copies. If tight budgets restrict ability to rent audiovisuals for preview, a copy can sometimes be borrowed from another hospital via interlibrary loan. Additionally, some distributors will waive preview charges if a hospital has previously purchased audiovisuals. The hospital's medical library should be contacted to determine what support and assistance it can provide and what time line is needed to incorporate the preview of audiovisuals into staff development program design.

The effectiveness of staff development to support planning and implementation of formal patient education programs can be tracked in several ways. One member of each team should be designated as the contact person. Periodic surveys can be sent to each contact person to determine the status of program development. If the staff development program has included components on team building and function, anonymous surveys can be sent out to determine areas in which teams are experiencing difficulty. If the hospital has a procedure for patient education program approval, the entry of programs into the approval process can be monitored.

Evaluation

The desired outcome of staff development efforts is the implementation of formal patient education programs. If the hospital identified the need for these patient education programs as a part of a strategic or annual plan for patient education, a tracking mechanism will be part of the plan. Also, if there is a formal review or approval process for patient education programs, the development of new programs will be easier to monitor.

Hospitals may have patient education policies that include a review and approval process for patient education programs. Such policies often delineate the necessary components of a high-quality patient education program and also mechanisms by which the reviewing and approving body track the patient education program through the planning phase. Tracking by the approving body can assist the tracking team. By monitoring the planning process for a formal patient education program, the approving body can offer assistance and consultation to the tracking team developing the program.

□ Establishing a Hospitalwide Patient Education Program through a Patient Education Committee

Staff development can also offer an interdisciplinary patient education committee the skills needed to develop a hospitalwide patient education program. Many hospitals coordinate the patient education function via an interdisciplinary committee. A patient education committee is often composed of members of the disciplines responsible for delivery of patient education services. The following are possible committee functions:

- To identify and prioritize patient education needs
- To develop and implement policies and procedures
- To set hospital patient education goals
- To establish criteria and guidelines for patient education program development
- To develop patient education programs or establish teaching teams that will develop programs
- To monitor, evaluate, and determine program effectiveness
- To identify need for staff training and development related to patient education
- To clarify and delineate roles in the patient education process
- To encourage and coordinate staff participation
- To provide consultation to staff
- To identify, secure, and allocate resources for patient education
- To review, purchase, or produce patient education teaching resources
- To establish standards and forms for documentation
- To increase awareness and visibility of patient education within the hospital

Not all of these possible functions of a patient education committee will be applicable within any one hospital. However, given their range and breadth, it is easy to imagine that the patient education committee charged with carrying out these functions must have substantial organizational skills. Staff development can offer a patient education committee the skills needed to enhance these functions.

Needs Assessment

Assessing the needs of a patient education committee in establishing a hospitalwide program can be accomplished in a variety of ways. A nominal group process can identify and prioritize topics. A written questionnaire can also be used. Any needs assessment strategy used should identify priorities facing the committee and the skills needed by members to carry out committee functions. Topics may include hospitalwide needs assessment techniques, development of a strategic or annual plan, program evaluation methodologies, organizational development skills, or group process skills (because much of the work of the committee and teaching teams is done in groups).

Focus groups can provide valuable qualitative needs assessment data from a patient education committee. Focus groups uncover the reasons underlying people's behavior by interviewing them in small groups. Although questions are designed for focus groups, they are not asked in a predetermined order; but they are used to guide and stimulate discussion. The unique characteristic of the focus group is the free-form discussion it generates. Focus groups provide qualitative information on people's perceptions of services and needs.

Patient education committee members can also be interviewed regarding staff development needs. Using interviews to assess the patient education committee's needs for staff development can accomplish several objectives. By enlisting the assistance of committee members to help conduct the interviews, commitment to both committee membership and patient education can be promoted.

It is important to design an interview form that can be used by everyone conducting the interviews. This ensures consistent data collection. One step to consider is that of sending committee members a list of topics to be covered. This enables them to consider the topics in advance. However, they should not be sent the interview form in advance, because doing so may encourage them to fill it in and send it back. This would defeat the purpose of a face-to-face meeting about their needs.

Interviews are better conducted in the office of the person being interviewed than in the office of the interviewer. If several committee members are conducting the interviews, they should interview committee members with whom they do not have close working relationships. This will facilitate understanding and communication among members.

Program Planning and Design

To understand planning and design for a hospitalwide program, it is helpful to consider an example of a successful program. The Department of Veterans Affairs developed a series of three sessions to assist patient education committees at VA medical centers in developing hospitalwide strategic plans for patient education. The need to develop hospitalwide strategic plans for patient education was identified by a focused needs assessment conducted with staff in patient education leadership roles (patient education coordinators, patient education committee chairs) in VA medical centers across the country.

The program was initially offered as a three-part teleconference series on strategic planning for patient education. The audience for this series consisted of members of patient education committees in several regions of the country. Using this format, a number of VA medical centers could be reached quickly. In addition to offering this program as a teleconference for several VA medical centers simultaneously, it has also been conducted for the patient education committee from one VA Medical Center via a consultation visit by the patient education coordinator from the Regional Medical Education Center. Figure 12-6 describes the purpose of the teleconference series and gives the learning objectives for each of the three sessions.

Implementation

The sessions were conducted one month apart in order to give the committees time to work in the interim on each component of their medical center's strategic plan. When conducted in the consultation format for one VA medical center's patient education committee, the content remained the same; however, the time frame and design were adjusted accordingly. The important design consideration, whether offered through a teleconference or a face-to-face consultation, was to allow the committee time between the sessions for the actual development of their hospital's strategic plan for patient education.

Figure 12-6. Example of Training Material for a Patient Education Committee Doing Strategic Planning for Patient Education

---

Purpose: This series will address major issues in the development of a hospitalwide strategic plan for patient education. It will feature examples of successful planning approaches and considerations for tailoring the planning process for hospital priorities. In each session, participants will have opportunities to share concerns and strategies, and to receive consultation from faculty and other participants.

Session 1

Organizational Diagnosis

By the end of this session, participants will be able to:

1. Identify major concepts of strategic planning and their application to patient education
2. Describe the American Public Health Association Model for Patient Education Programming as a framework for hospitalwide planning for patient education
3. List the steps in conducting an organizational diagnosis, and the sources of information that can be used to complete each step

Session 2

Perspectives on Planning: Putting the Pieces Together

By the end of this session, participants will be able to:

1. Identify the characteristics of a good plan
2. Describe the steps in developing a plan
3. Describe the ways in which decision makers and the Patient Education Committee can be involved in the planning process

Session 3

Making the Planning Process Work

By the end of this session, participants will be able to:

1. Develop creative methods to maintain support for a plan
2. Develop methods and alternative strategies for implementing a plan
3. Identify potential problem areas or "hot spots" that may occur in implementation
4. Specify ways to monitor implementation plans and update them to reflect organizational and environmental changes

---

Reprinted from the Department of Veterans Affairs, St. Louis.

Evaluation

The expected outcome of the VA program was development of a hospitalwide strategic plan for patient education. Because patient education coordinators from the Regional Medical Education Centers serve as consultants to the medical centers in their regions, they were able to monitor and assist with strategic plan development. Because the development of a strategic plan contains time frames and staff responsible for its components, a hospital can track strategic plan development and implementation.

☐ Conclusion

Staff development for patient education serves a variety of functions. It provides clinicians with the information and skills they need to become more effective patient and family educators. It also facilitates development of high-quality patient education programs for specific populations. And it provides staff the organizational skills needed to develop and manage hospitalwide patient education.

Whatever function staff development for patient education is attempting to fulfill, it is important that the educational intervention address the priorities and concerns of the staff for whom it is designed. This includes content and skills, scheduling, learning activities, and an opportunity to problem-solve and address possible barriers. Networking and sharing patient education concerns with colleagues and coworkers increases the base of support, involvement, and commitment to patient education hospitalwide.

References

1. Basch, C. E. Focus group interview: an underutilized research technique for improving theory and practice in health education. *Health Education Quarterly* 14(4):411–48, Fall 1987.

2. Krueger, R. A. *Focus Groups: A Practical Guide for Applied Research.* Newbury Park, CA: Sage Publications, 1988.

3. Patient Health Education Profile in VA Medical Centers. Washington, DC: Veterans Administration, Office of Academic Affairs, 1987.

4. American Diabetes Association. *Meeting the Standards.* Chicago: ADA, 1988, p. iv.

Part Two

Program Development

Chapter 13

Designing Patient Education Programs for Target Populations

Louise A. Villejo, M.P.H., C.H.E.S.

☐ Objectives

The reader will be able to:

- Define, describe, and integrate the components of program development
- Assess the needs of specific populations for patient education
- Plan and design patient education interventions
- Implement patient education programs
- Evaluate the quality and effectiveness of patient education programs

☐ Understanding the Increasing Importance of Patient Education

Changes in the health care system and provision of care in hospitals are mandating that attention be refocused on empowering patients to function at home, outside the hospital and other clinical settings. This refocusing has been occurring since the early 1980s, when prospective pricing for diagnosis-related groups required that hospitals implement stringent guidelines for patient care. These guidelines pressured hospitals to furnish services in the least intensive care setting possible, which decreased hospital admissions and length of stay and increased ambulatory or outpatient services. The implications for patient education are increased responsibilities for the health care provider to design and deliver needed information to patients in a shorter time frame, providing continuity of care from inpatient or outpatient to community settings. The patients and family members also have increased responsibilities in regaining functional independence at an earlier stage in their illness or injury and learning self-care and home care.

Other trends that are going to change and strain the health care system in this country are the aging of the large population of baby boomers, whose risk of chronic disease

Material from an earlier draft prepared by Sharon Dorfman, Sc.M., C.H.E.S., now president, SPECTRA, Ponce Inlet, Florida, was used in this chapter.

will increase as they get older, and the growing number of individuals and families who are uninsured or underinsured. Educationally centered care will benefit these two groups by focusing on health and not disease, encouraging them to participate in their care. Because patient education often has been found to be cost-effective, extending health education services may allow scarce medical resources to be conserved by reducing preventable illness or unnecessary health care utilization.[1]

These and other trends discussed in this book are necessitating that patients become active partners in their care. For example, patients who are discharged sooner from the hospital or are treated as outpatients often need to take personal responsibility for their wellness and become more knowledgeable about their own care. Thus, patient education, which enables patients to learn about and manage their condition, will be an increasingly important component of patient care in the near future.

Although many observers agree on the importance of patient education programs, not everyone realizes how influential the developmental process is in ensuring their effectiveness. A state-of-the-art, streamlined patient education program development process will enhance the likelihood that the provision of patient education is available, appropriate, efficient, and effective. Such a process should be applicable not only to disease- or treatment-specific populations but also to those targeted by age, ethnicity, language, and literacy. In examining this process, this chapter provides a framework for developing patient education programs for defined target populations.

☐ Designing Patient Education Programs for Target Populations and Individual Patients or Families

Patient education programs are planned at a number of levels. Whereas a previous chapter addressed the institutional level, this chapter focuses on designing patient education programs at the target population level and individual patient/family (case) levels. Sometimes such programs are developed after institutional planning has taken place; at other times, programs for specific populations are designed first and become the foundation upon which hospitalwide planning is built.

Population-oriented programs can be directed toward a categorical health or medical problem. They can be specific to disease or treatment modalities or to an aspect of the regimen such as medication adherence. Additionally, as mentioned previously, target populations can be related to age, ethnicity, language, literacy, or any combination of these. It is also common for patients to have more than one diagnosis that may require changes in knowledge, attitude, and behavior.

Developing targeted programs is a very dynamic process. The goal is to provide patients with the information they need to change their behavior or learn self-care skills. To design a patient education program for a specific target population, the patient education manager (PEM) must know as much as possible about learning needs, learning styles, barriers to learning and teaching, and resources available to meet defined needs.

Comprehensive patient education programs should be developed to meet the needs of patients and family members throughout the disease process, from diagnosis to treatment to rehabilitation. In addition, programs need to include prevention and health promotion activities as well as activities addressing terminal stages of illness and grieving. Patient education is no longer just for inpatients; it must also begin or continue in the outpatient and community settings. As more and more people use the emergency department as their first contact with the health care system, this setting must also be included in patient education program planning. Patient education programs developed specifically for emergency rooms include programs to reduce avoidable emergency room visits through improved patient education,[2,3] match readability of patient education materials to literacy levels of patients,[4] and use community health workers to supplement providers' routine efforts in high blood pressure detection, treatment, and follow-up among high-risk African-American men.[5]

Developers of patient education programs sometimes consider the patient and family as one unit, but family members may have separate and unique needs at various stages of the patient's disease. Family members need information about the disease and its treatment, hospital policies and routines, financial resources, and potential outcomes of the treatment; but they also need information about how to physically comfort or psychologically support the patient. Families of patients also need information about coping strategies as the patient's illness affects their own well-being.[6-8] (See chapter 18 for a in-depth treatment of family involvement.)

Despite the many variables involved in designing patient education programs for specific populations, the components of the program development cycle are generic: assessment, planning and design, implementation, and evaluation. These components can be applied to any identified population or problem and adapted to the characteristics of a particular hospital, clinic, physician's office, and community setting to develop a comprehensive patient education program.

To illustrate key points and provide guidance in applying these principles of patient education program design to various settings, examples and work sheets have been included in the figures at the end of this chapter. Selected references for each step in the program design process also are listed for more in-depth study at the end of this chapter.

☐ Assessing the Patient Education Needs of a Specific Population

In an ideal situation, the PEM coordinates, plans, implements, and evaluates patient education programs. He or she has conducted a hospitalwide assessment of resources and has identified specific populations for which patient education programs need to be developed. With the input of the hospital's patient education committee or advisory group, the PEM can prioritize programs according to several criteria:

1. The results of a needs assessment
2. The incidence or prevalence of the problem
3. Visible needs
4. The value of the program to community relations or patient recruitment
5. Current or impending regulations (hospital, government, or legal)
6. The production of revenue
7. The potential for cost savings

Though initially time-consuming, careful consideration of those criteria will prevent future roadblocks in developing effective programs.

Understanding What a Needs Assessment Is

At the programmatic level, a needs assessment is used to identify and prioritize the needs and interests of patients, families, and relevant individuals in the hospital and community. This information is then used to set objectives and plan appropriate, effective programs. A needs assessment is a vital step in patient education program development for several reasons:

• It further defines the patient population.
• It makes it possible to begin education at a point appropriate to the learner rather than from "scratch." Thus patients learn best that which is most important and of immediate interest to them.

- It helps target the patient education program to the population (or patient) and the problem. For instance, cultural factors that affect certain eating behaviors or language barriers may make the use of particular written materials inappropriate if they encourage eating foods foreign to that culture.
- It helps identify all opportunities and channels for patient education. The needs assessment should provide clues about the most efficient and effective interventions.
- It helps prevent duplication of teaching; avoid contradictions by comparing the patient's understanding and behaviors with the expectations of various health care providers, who may be conveying mixed messages; and fill gaps that have been identified.
- It provides insight into factors that will facilitate and those that will impede program planning, implementation, and evaluation. The ability to identify such factors makes it possible to take advantage of and incorporate facilitating factors and to anticipate and address barriers.

Understanding the Process of a Needs Assessment

The first step in a needs assessment is to define the target population. Is the target population healthy or specific to disease or therapy? What are the demographics? Does the target population consist of children, adolescents, adults, parents, spouses, children, or significant others of the patient, or all of the above? The target population's needs must be established in a number of areas:

- *Cognitive.* What is and should be known and understood
- *Affective.* Existing and important attitudes and beliefs
- *Psychomotor.* Existing and important skills and abilities

A number of patient education and health promotion programs use the PRECEDE/ PROCEED model developed by Dr. Lawrence Green and colleagues as a basic framework for community analysis and program development.[9] (See chapter 16 under the section Research on the Current Reality of CCTV to find out how this model can be used in planning a CCTV system.)

PRECEDE is an acronym for predisposing, reinforcing, and enabling factors in educational and environmental diagnosis and evaluation. Needs assessment data on these variables can be gathered through surveys, interviews, or focus groups of the target population (see figure 13-1).

To assess the predisposing factors, the variables that increase the likelihood of individuals to implement new health behaviors or skills or to change attitudes and beliefs must be identified. Enabling factors are the means individuals have available to realize a motivation or aspiration. They include age, sex, race, marital status, education, literacy, English language proficiency, and occupation. They also include personal resources such as family support, family income, health insurance, and available health services, as well as community resources such as transportation to those services and affordable health services. Reinforcing factors follow appropriate behavior and provide a reward, incentive, or punishment that contributes to behavior being repeated or discarded. Reinforcing factors include tangible as well as social benefits. Figure 13-2 (p. 270) provides an example of how the PRECEDE stage of this model can be used to assess the behavioral and educational needs of a specific patient population.

The formulation of priorities, targets, objectives, timetables, and budgets completes the PRECEDE process. This phase of the model includes assessment of administrative and organizational resources and capabilities for implementation and development of a program. Identifying priorities and setting objectives in the PRECEDE phases provides the objectives and criteria for implementation, evaluation, and policy in the PROCEED phases.

Figure 13-1. Cystic Fibrosis Interview Needs Assessment (Parent)

Interview #: _____   Persons Present: _____

Background
1. Child's age _____
2. Sex _____ M _____ F
3. Age when child diagnosed _____
4. How often has your child been hospitalized? _____
5. How often is your child seen by the doctor for cystic fibrosis? _____

Respiratory
1. Does your child do breathing treatments at home? When (and how often) does your child do breathing treatments?
2. Please describe what breathing treatments do for the lungs.

Chest PT
1. Does your child do chest PT at home? When (and how often) does your child do chest PT?
2. Please describe what chest PT does for the lungs.

Nutrition
1. Has your child ever seen a dietitian?
2. Please describe your child's diet. Is it different from that of other children?

Confidence
Rate your level of confidence in doing the following procedures if required for treatment of your child's cystic fibrosis.

	Very Confident	Confident	Somewhat Confident	Not Very Confident	Not Confident
1. Properly giving enzymes	5	4	3	2	1
2. Measuring medications for respiratory therapy treatments	Very Confident 5	Confident 4	Somewhat Confident 3	Not Very Confident 2	Not Confident 1

General
1. What would you tell other parents about caring for a child with cystic fibrosis?
2. What do you wish you had been told when your child was first diagnosed (during the first week)?

Coping
1. Does your child talk about or "worry" about dying from cystic fibrosis?
2. How did he or she learn that people die of cystic fibrosis?

Questions
1. Do you get a chance to ask the doctors your questions? If no, why not?
_____ Visit too short or rushed
_____ They use too many medical terms I can't understand
_____ I'm afraid to ask
_____ They don't really answer a question if I ask
_____ Other—specify
2. How often have you received information that is needed and helpful to you without asking?

Very often	Often	Sometimes	Rarely	Never
5	4	3	2	1

Interviewer's Notes

Instrument has been condensed to provide a sample needs assessment targeting parents. Those desiring a copy of the complete instrument may contact Texas Children's Hospital, Office of Educational Resources (713) 770-2048.

Figure 13-2. PRECEDE Framework Applied to Cystic Fibrosis Model

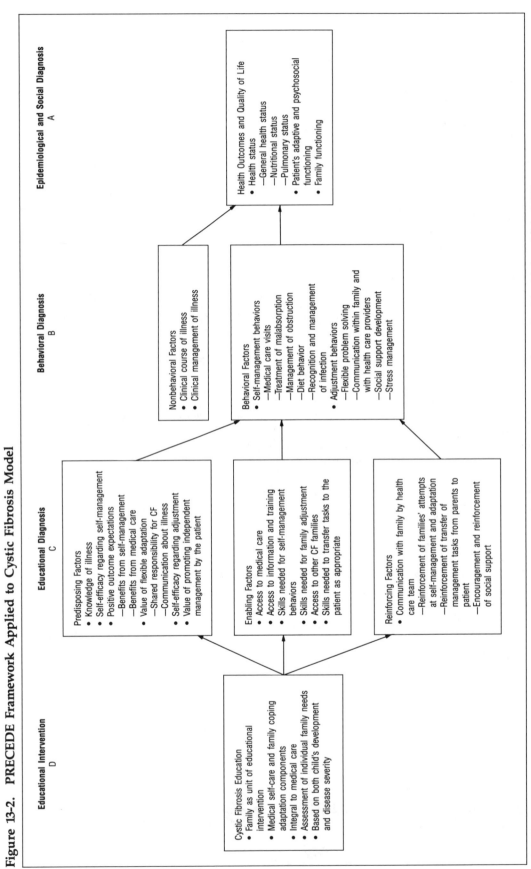

Adapted, with permission, from Green and others. *Patient Education and Counseling*, vol. 13, pp. 57–68, 1988. Elsevier Science Publishers Ltd., copyright ©1988.

PROCEED incorporates environmental factors that examine what resources, barriers, policies, regulations, and organizational factors need to be adjusted to make a program work. The PROCEED model includes implementation and process, impact, and outcome evaluation phases.

This educational and environmental approach calls for greater emphasis on self-care and patient-centered authority and responsibility for planning and controlling the health care regimen. Patients in this model are active in gathering information and in decision making from the earliest stages of seeking diagnosis and treatment information to the posttreatment self-monitoring and self-care stage. Patients are also active in rehabilitation and the appropriate maintenance of or changes in their life-style and environment.

Obtaining Sources of Information for the Needs Assessment

Another important step in the needs assessment process is to review the scientific literature. The five most utilized data bases for nurses and health educators are the Combined Health Information Database (CHID), the Educational Resources Information Center (ERIC), the Nurse and Allied Health Database (NAHD), Medline, and Physician Data Query (PDQ). (See the appendix to chapter 17 for a description of CHID and its address). Reference books include *Index Medicus, Hospital Literature Index,* and *Cumulative Index to Nursing and Allied Health Literature.* These sources may provide data relevant to the patient population and health problems of interest.

If conducted in comparable settings, the projects of others can be a secondary source of needs assessment information, either substituting for or validating the PEM's own data collection activities. If the PEM is planning to gather needs assessment information, published reports can provide ideas on other data sources and specific questions to ask. A literature search can also assist in identifying program content and educational strategies. Model patient education programs can be adapted or adopted.

Additionally, all hospitals have appropriate data available (for example, admissions/readmissions statistics, numbers of procedures, medical records, costs, billing information). These data summarize hospitalizations and services rendered, length of stay, patient demographics, and other information that can assist in focusing patient education efforts and identifying patterns of care that offer patient education opportunities.

Allied health care personnel and volunteers can provide a wealth of information through their contact with and care of the patient. These personnel can provide insight into perceived needs, responsiveness to education and instruction, and retrospective suggestions about valuable or ineffective approaches.

Working with a multidisciplinary patient education committee of health care providers and representatives from the target population will also help the PEM to identify and shape content and educational strategies and will assist in identifying barriers to the teaching–learning process (see figures 13-3 and 13-4, p. 274). Patients, their families, and their significant others (friends, neighbors, coworkers, and so on) are perhaps the most important source of needs assessment data. Use of informal conversations, structured group discussions (focus groups), telephone interviews, or self-administered questionnaires can help encourage members of the target population to articulate their needs, the issues important to them, and the barriers they may perceive in developing the knowledge, attitudes, and skills they need.

In developing several patient education programs, materials, and initiatives, patient educators in the Patient Education Office at The University of Texas M. D. Anderson Cancer Center, in Houston, have used several strategies to ensure patient input. These include:

- Accompanying patients through the registration and admitting process and clinical appointments to assess their educational and informational needs at different stages
- Conducting focus groups, personal interviews, and mail-out and self-administered questionnaires

Figure 13-3. Patient Assessment Questionnaire to Identify Teaching–Learning Barriers

Information Sought	Examples of Provider Questions or Observations
I. Client Priorities A. Key client concerns and expectations for visit	"What would you most like to have us cover today?" "Is there anything you're concerned about right now?" "How have things been going? Any questions come up?" (At end of visit:) "Is there anything else we should cover today? Is there something you'd like me to go into (or think about) for next time?"
B. Client fears	"Are there any (worst) fears that you have about _____?" "You mentioned that your mother had a stroke. Does this worry you at all?"
II. Client Self-Management Level A. Client readiness	• Prior pattern of seeking information • Current pattern of monitoring condition • Energy level • Pattern of responding to crises (actively, passively) • Pattern of language (exhibiting internal versus external control)
B. Client ability to concentrate and to integrate new information	• Loss of eye contact • Vague responses • Frequent confusion • Directing provider to others (e.g., "I think my wife knows about that.")
C. Sense of loss	"What has changed most in your life since you have _____?"
D. Current stressors	"What other stresses are you or your family under right now?"
E. Client need for self-management	• Living alone • Single head of household • Complex life-style precludes frequent health care visits • Pride or fear of dependence • Distrust of medical setting/provider • Distance from clinic
III. Tailoring the Regimen A. Life-style	"Describe a typical day. When do you get up, eat your meals?" "What do you do for fun?" "When during the week are you most likely to get together with other people?" "For what things are you likely to go out of the house?" "What is a typical day of work like?"
B. Sense of loss	"How has your life changed since having _____?" "What has been important to keep the same?"
C. Client prior experience with other regimens	"People often say they have trouble with remembering to take their medications, or sometimes trouble with side effects. Was this true for you then, at all? Did you discover any special way of keeping track?" "How often did you find you took your pills—some of the time, most of the time, not too often? What tended to interfere? What helped you to remember?" "Did you discover any special way of keeping track?" "Have you tried to lose weight before? What happened then?" "What seemed to help you the most to stay on your diet? What got in the way? What was the hardest about staying on? Is there anything you'd do differently this time?"
IV. The Client's Model A. Client model of the condition and its management	"When did you first notice _____?" "What do you think caused it?" "Are there times it gets worse or better? How do you tell? Does anything seem to make it better or worse?"

Figure 13-3. (Continued)

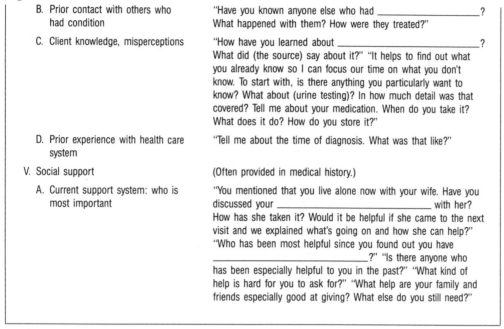

B. Prior contact with others who had condition	"Have you known anyone else who had _____? What happened with them? How were they treated?"
C. Client knowledge, misperceptions	"How have you learned about _____? What did (the source) say about it?" "It helps to find out what you already know so I can focus our time on what you don't know. To start with, is there anything you particularly want to know? What about (urine testing)? In how much detail was that covered? Tell me about your medication. When do you take it? What does it do? How do you store it?"
D. Prior experience with health care system	"Tell me about the time of diagnosis. What was that like?"
V. Social support	(Often provided in medical history.)
A. Current support system: who is most important	"You mentioned that you live alone now with your wife. Have you discussed your _____ with her? How has she taken it? Would it be helpful if she came to the next visit and we explained what's going on and how she can help?" "Who has been most helpful since you found out you have _____?" "Is there anyone who has been especially helpful to you in the past?" "What kind of help is hard for you to ask for?" "What help are your family and friends especially good at giving? What else do you still need?"

Reprinted, with permission, from *Managing Cardiac Patient Education*, copyright ©1983 by the American Hospital Association.

To identify patient needs and pretest materials, office staff have also worked closely with organized patient groups such as the Anderson Network, the U.T. M. D. Anderson Cancer Center's patient-to-patient organization, and the local American Cancer Society's Reach to Recovery groups.

Networking with colleagues who have already developed programs for the same or similar target populations can be extremely helpful and save a tremendous amount of time. Professional organizations such as the International Patient Education Council, the American Nurses Association, the Oncology Nursing Society, the Cardiac Nursing Association, the Critical Care Nursing Association, American Diabetes Association, the Society for Public Health Education, and many others either have been formed to provide patient education resources or have a special interest group dedicated to patient education.

Data from federal, state, or community health agencies can also be used. For example, the American Cancer Society has developed proceedings from many of its national workshops. These proceedings may contain data regarding the knowledge, behavior, or skills that the PEM needs to develop his or her patient education program. Establishing a cooperative relationship with such an organization can make it possible to integrate its resources into the patient education plan, which offers several advantages: (1) the program is extended into the community in a coordinated manner, (2) the community agency may reach and assist an additional population, and (3) the patient has access to a more comprehensive range of patient education options.

Using the Findings in Developing or Enhancing Patient Education Program Planning

Once a needs assessment has been conducted (see figure 13-5, p. 276, for an example), the data should be applied to developing or enhancing the patient education programs. After the PEM reviews the results carefully, he or she may want to draft a summary report for the patient education committee to review, accept, and use in prioritizing the next steps (see figure 13-6, p. 277). A thorough needs assessment will provide a solid foundation for subsequent

Figure 13-4. Chemotherapy Education Program Assessment for Health Care Providers

We need your help! Numerous resources for patients and families have been developed by the Chemotherapy Patient Education Committee. In a continuous effort to keep our programs up-to-date and meet the learning needs of patients and families we would appreciate your candid and thorough responses to our survey. Please return this questionnaire to Patient Education, Box 21. Thank you for your assistance.

Section I. Chemotherapy Patient/Family Educational Program

A. General Information

1. How would you rate the overall quality of the chemotherapy patient education provided in your designated area?

    Excellent _____   Fair _____
    Good   _____   Poor_____
    Why? _____

2. Do you think that the multidisciplinary patient teaching plans are a useful way of coordinating the content for patient teaching?

    Yes _____   No _____
    If not, can you suggest a more useful format?

B. Teaching Strategies

4. What format do you use most often for teaching?

    One-on-one _____   Videotape _____
    Group _____   Other, specify _____

5. Please indicate which of the following chemotherapy patient education resources you are familiar with by checking the first column; if you distribute or promote the materials, check the second column as well.

	Yes—Familiar	Promote or Distribute
National Cancer Institute Pamphlets		
Chemotherapy & You: A Guide to Self Help During Treatment	_____	_____
M. D. Anderson Printed Materials		
Amphotericin	_____	_____
Calcium Leucovorin & Methotrexate	_____	_____
Chemotherapy: A Patient Guide		
M. D. Anderson Produced-Videotapes		
Food for Thought: Nutritional Information for Chemotherapy Patients	_____	_____

C. Needed Resources

7. Are you aware of existing literature/educational material that covers psychological/emotional aspects of chemotherapy treatment?

    _____ Yes   _____ No
    Please list the materials you use _____.

8. Which topics are not covered by the chemotherapy patient education program, but in your opinion need to be?

    Nausea and vomiting _____   Sexuality _____
    Body image   _____   Pain   _____
    Anger   _____   Fear   _____
    Grief and loss   _____   Other   _____

Section II. Chemotherapy Class

A. Referral and Quality of Class

9. How many of your patients do you specifically refer to the Chemotherapy class, encouraging them to attend? Approximately,

    100% _____   75% _____   50% _____   25% _____   1–24% _____   None _____

10. Which of the following are reasons for making the referral? I have noticed that after attending the class the patient

    is less apprehensive.   _____
    is more relaxed.   _____
    is more cooperative.   _____
    has a better understanding.   _____
    needs less teaching time from me. _____
    other _____

Figure 13-4. (Continued)

B. Patient and Family Attendance

    11. Do you think that 12 noon and 1:00 p.m. class time is convenient for patients and families?

        _____ Yes   _____ No

        For staff? _____ Yes   _____ No

        If not, when would be convenient? _____

C. Class Content (For class instructors only)

    14. Which aspects of chemotherapy are adequately covered in the class?

        How chemotherapy works   _____

        Side effects of chemotherapy   _____

        Mouthcare   _____

        Temperature taking   _____

        Nutritional guidelines   _____

        Other (specify)   _____

Instrument has been condensed to provide a sample needs assessment targeting health care providers. Those desiring a copy of the complete instrument may contact Louise Villejo, Patient Education Office, U.T. M. D. Anderson Cancer Center (713) 792-7128.

Reprinted, with permission, from the U.T. M. D. Anderson Cancer Center, Houston.

planning, implementation, and evaluation activities. Goals and objectives for developing program components can be developed as a one-year or multiyear plan.

Questions the needs assessment should have answered include:

- What specific needs have been identified?
- To what extent is there agreement or disagreement about those needs? (Disagreement may exist within the target population, within the provider group, or between providers and patients.) Where there is disagreement, does it need to be resolved or reconciled, or does it represent a range of views that should be addressed in any patient education program?
- What activities currently address the needs that have been identified, in both the hospital and the community? This is important to both avoid duplication of effort and ensure coordination and continuity from setting to setting. A more comprehensive promotion of available resources can ensure that staff, patients, and families are aware of existing resources.
- What untapped opportunities exist for meeting unmet needs?
- What constraints exist that must be changed or accommodated? Conversely, what facilitators have been identified who can be utilized? Many of these may be features of the way care is organized and delivered, shaping the evolution of patient education programs. For example, the opportunity to provide preoperative education the night before surgery is not as great now that same-day morning admissions and one-day procedures have become more common. Thus many hospitals incorporate their presurgery patient education into the admissions process.
- What resources are currently being used to address these needs, and what additional resources might be mobilized?

Needs assessments are also conducted to update existing programs. Important questions at this phase include:

- What parts of the program were acceptable to the target audience? Which resources were utilized most? Which were least utilized?

- Which teaching strategy was preferred? Did patients want more written material? Did they prefer to watch a videotape and have a nurse review the information afterward?
- If a class was not well attended, was the scheduled time appropriate? Does the hospital strongly support staff by providing the requisite time and resources?
- Is the content appropriate? Are the teachers effective?
- Is the classroom space conducive to learning?
- Are resources easily accessible and easy to use?
- Is the program comprehensively and routinely promoted to staff as well as patients and their family members?

Figure 13-5. Surgery Patient Education Needs Assessment

Clinic Sta: _____ / _____ /   Study I.D. / _____ / _____ / _____ /

We need your help! The results of this survey will help us to develop surgery patient education materials and plan future education programs. It is important that all questions are answered completely. Your answers will be kept confidential.

This is not a test, so there are no right or wrong answers. Questions should be answered by circling the number next to the answer you choose. Some questions will have more than one answer, circle all that apply. If you do not find an answer that fits exactly, circle the one that comes closest. If the question does not apply to you or you do not know the answer, circle the number for the answer "not applicable" or "don't know." For fill-in-the-blank questions, please write your answer clearly.

Part I: General Information

1. How old are you? _____

2. What is your sex?
   1 Male   2 Female

Part II: Medical Information

8. How long have you been coming to M. D. Anderson?

   _____

9. What type of cancer do you have?

   _____

Part III: Material Use

11. Which of the following printed patient education materials have you received? (Circle all you have received.)
    1 About Anesthesia
    2 Cryosurgery
    3 Donating Your Own Blood Before Surgery
    4 Laser Surgery

Part IV: Learning Preference

15. Did you find the printed material helpful?
    1 Yes
    2 No
    89 Don't Know
    98 Not Applicable

Instrument has been condensed to provide a needs assessment targeting patients/family members. Those desiring a copy of the complete instrument may contact Louise Villejo, Patient Education Office, U.T. M. D. Anderson Cancer Center (713) 792-7128.

Figure 13-6. Surgery Patient Education Needs Assessment: Summary of Results

Introduction/Background: The Surgery Patient Needs Assessment was administered to approximately 70 patients in several clinic stations and areas (clinic stations 82, 54, 85, 42, 80, SICU & OR) throughout the hospital. Of the 70 questionnaires, 52 were returned to the Patient Education Office, for a 70% return rate.

The questionnaire was initially designed to be analyzed with the statistical package SPSS. However, multiple answer questions proved difficult to analyze with this particular package and only frequencies and cross-tabulations were generated with the data.

Interpretation of Data: Several interesting findings were revealed by the survey.

I. Demographics

1. Age. This was a relatively young patient population with approximately 59% of the patients surveyed 55 years of age or younger. 68% of the patients surveyed were from 35 to 65 years of age.
2. Gender. 65% of the patients surveyed were women. This is perhaps due to the fact that two of the stations surveyed, 82 and 54 (breast reconstruction), as well as breast surgery patients, are composed primarily of women.
3. Employment. The majority (65%) of patients surveyed were employed in professional, service and clerical jobs OR were homemakers. This probably reflects the slanted gender ratio of the survey.
4. Marital Status. A great majority (75%) of the patients surveyed were married.
5. Ethnic Group. Approximately 84.6% of the patients surveyed were Anglo, 9.6% African-American and 5.8% Hispanic.
6. Education. 88% of the patients surveyed had a high school or higher level education.
7. Residence. 75% of the patients surveyed live in Texas.

The demographics reveal survey respondents to be generally under 55 years of age, white, female, working in professional, service or clerical jobs OR as homemakers. They are also a relatively well-educated group who primarily live in Texas.

Although the ethnic breakdown for Anglo and African-American in this survey is comparable to the actual breakdown of patients registered at MDA in 1991, Hispanics and Asians were notably underrepresented.

II. Medical History

Persons with breast, gynecological, hematological and genitourinary (GU) cancers were the most frequent respondents. Approximately 81% of the respondents had already had surgery before answering the survey.

III. Material Use

10. Due to the fact that surgery is often a complex and multidisciplinary process, it is reasonable to assume that patients will need more than just the Surgery Patient Guide to prepare for surgery and its aftermath. For this reason, the proportion (65%) of respondents receiving 3 or more pieces of material may hopefully be an indicator of comprehensive patient education.
11. Most (65%) of the respondents were given the material by the nurse. This reinforces the observational evidence that nurses are of primary importance to the patient education process.

    Due to the fact that the main surgery video is outdated due to department restructuring, the low number of patients watching videos pertaining to surgery is not surprising.

IV. Learning Preference

12. Printed Material Helpful. All of the persons receiving printed educational materials felt that they were helpful. All types of information, print, video and verbal instructions, were considered helpful. However, one-to-one teaching and print materials appear to be the preferred educational methods. This is probably due to the fact that personalized instruction allows for patient participation and printed materials can be referred to repeatedly.

    A cross-tabulation of age versus number of materials received did not reveal any particular association. It appeared as if patients with lower educational levels were just as likely to receive multiple pieces of information as patients with higher education.

V. Recommendations:

1. Although printed materials appear to be a well-established patient education routine in surgery, all surgery patients should be receiving a variety of printed materials. The health care provider should be familiar with the surgery materials available and keep the area well-stocked. Physicians, in particular, need to increase their knowledge of available materials.

(Continued on next page)

Figure 13-6. (Continued)

2. Even though videos are often an effective educational supplement, this survey does not identify them as a preferred mode for receiving information. Of all the methods preferred, video was the only one that received any negative response (11%) to "helpfulness" (although this could be due to the quality of the video and not necessarily the medium). Nevertheless, a general surgery video might be useful in orienting patients to MDA procedure. However, this should be a supplement and not replace the one-to-one teaching and printed materials people prefer.

3. More information on post-operative care is needed. Patients requested greater knowledge of post-op procedures and warning signs of possible problems following surgery. The committee should investigate common surgical procedures and explore the possibility of developing print material and/or teaching plans for post-operative care.

4. Due to the fact that physicians are closely involved with the one-to-one patient teaching, their increased input and participation in the Surgery Patient Education Committee and materials development is essential.

5. Surgery patients' needs vary across areas. For this reason, surveys designed specifically for a particular area might be more revealing. The fact that a good portion of the respondents were from breast, gynecology, hematology and GU might indicate greater concern about educational issues and give the committee a place to start.

This summary report has been condensed to provide a sample format of a needs assessment summary report. Those desiring a copy of the complete summary report may contact Louise Villejo, Patient Education Office at the University of Texas M. D. Anderson Cancer Center, (713) 792-7128.

Reprinted, with permission, from the U.T. M. D. Anderson Cancer Center, Houston.

☐ Planning and Designing Patient Education Interventions

A patient education program consists of a series of planned educational activities. Under the umbrella of a particular patient education program, there might be informal bedside patient teaching, instruction via closed-circuit television, participation in a support group sponsored by a community agency, or coordination with a visiting nurse. The program provides a framework for this series of educational activities, ties them together to achieve continuity of care, ensures the consistency of messages from one provider and setting to another, and offers options from which a patient education plan can be developed that is tailored to the needs of individuals.

Planning a patient education program requires time, patience, perseverance, and skill. The hospital's multidisciplinary patient education committee must agree on educational strategies; identify teachers; and determine content, time, location, and effectiveness evaluation methods.

The successful program provides patient satisfaction, improved patient outcomes, greater self-efficacy, decreased complications, and better utilization of hospital resources. It also allows health care providers to meet their professional standards and increase both their communication and satisfaction.

Understanding What a Patient Education Plan Is

A *patient education plan* spells out in great detail both the content and process of the patient education program. The plan:

- Guides the most effective use of scarce time and resources, based on a thorough needs assessment
- Provides a focus for delivery of patient education services through development of objectives as a framework for implementation and evaluation
- Ensures the relevance and accuracy of content through a logical process of development, review, and revision
- Increases staff participation in the delivery of patient education services by providing a detailed description of program process and content

- Enhances standardization and quality control in the delivery of patient education services, especially when many individuals are involved in patient teaching
- Serves as the vehicle for hospital review and approval, as a model for the development of similar programs or for adaptation to meet special needs, and as a training tool for staff, helping to increase knowledge and skill in patient education

Even if the patient education plan is developed primarily for use in a formal program or class, it can be extremely useful in informal teaching as an outline that can be easily adapted when opportunities suddenly arise, as material that can be shared with interested patients, or as a review of what patients might have already learned. The plan can help a health care provider or volunteer know what to convey, demonstrate, or reinforce in a given situation.

Understanding the Components of a Patient Education Plan

There is no single correct approach to organizing an educational plan. However, there are elements that are important to include whenever possible:

- A specific description of the target population (this should be done during the needs assessment phase)
- Goals and objectives
- Content, including what is currently being taught effectively to the target population, what the target population wants to learn, what health care providers view as important, and what other investigations indicate is necessary and appropriate (this, too, should emerge from the needs assessment)
- Educational strategies and their sequencing (that is, creating change, then maintaining change)
- Responsibility for coordinating the program and providing the education (the same person is frequently not responsible for both)
- Evaluation (discussed later in this chapter) of the quality, efficiency, and appropriateness of the program, as well as its impact and outcome (that is, effectiveness)
- A detailed time line
- Protocols/procedures for preparation, presentation, documentation, evaluation, and follow-up
- A schedule for and approach to periodic program review and update (discussed in the evaluation section of this chapter)
- Promotional plans for staff and patients
- Resources needed, such as space, equipment, educational materials, and refreshments
- A budget displaying both projected expenses and projected income

There is no set order in which a patient education plan is developed. In practice, its development is a reiterative process during which, for example, overall objectives are defined, content and strategies are chosen, objectives are then redefined, content and strategies are refined, and so on. Even when the plan is approved, adjustments continue to be made as implementation experience accumulates (unless a research study is under way; if so, the program must be kept constant).

Setting Goals and Objectives

Statements of goals, purposes, or aims are general expressions of intention. They explain why a program is being developed. Although objectives are sometimes written in the same way as goals, they should be presented in a different, more specific form and have a very important role in program planning and evaluation. When correctly developed, objectives:

- Guide the process of program planning and design (that is, the selection of strategies, content, and materials).
- Serve as the basis for determining whether the program is successful (that is, the standard against which results are compared in evaluation).
- Communicate, when shared with a patient, what is expected so that mutually acceptable objectives can be negotiated. One major difference between goals and objectives is that objectives must be measurable. To be measurable, objectives must state:
  - The specific change or action that will occur
  - The amount of change expected
  - The target population
  - The schedule

Objectives should be set upon completion and summarization of the needs assessment. Because objectives specify what will be accomplished—rather than how—(the "how" of change is decided during program design) they are developed before the selection of program strategies. Two major categories and two types of objectives within each category are differentiated in the following paragraphs.

Program objectives articulate what a particular patient education program should be able to accomplish for the target population. In contrast, *patient objectives* are developed at the case level, and tailored to the specific status and need of individual patients and their families. Program objectives are established by the PEM in conjunction with the planning team for a specific patient education program and serve as a basis for evaluating the status, from an educational perspective, of a defined group of patients over a discrete period of time. Patient objectives should be codeveloped by individual patients and their health care providers. Because individual patients are so different, their objectives are likely to differ within the same patient education program area; collectively, however, these individual sets of patient objectives should be consistent with the program objectives established by the planning team. As with the program objectives, patient objectives must be measurable so that the patient's status over time can be measured against the objectives that were negotiated when his or her learning needs were initially assessed.

Both program and patient objectives should encompass two types: process and outcome. *Process objectives* describe the educational activities: who will be involved, how they will be delivered, and so on. Whether written at the program level to describe how the overall patient education program is intended to be implemented or at the patient level to describe the specific educational activities that are recommended, process objectives make it possible to assess whether the program or activities are implemented in the way that was intended to reach the target population or a specific patient/family. *Outcome objectives* relate to the effect of the patient education program on the target population as a whole or on a particular patient. What happened as a result of the educational intervention(s)? Did learning occur? Did behaviors change? Were health improvements observed?

The following questions can serve as a checklist for the adequacy of the objectives:

- Do they specifically state staff, patient, or family member responsibilities and a time line for a given program or activity?
- If they are accomplished as stated, will they result in the desired benefit(s) to the patient/family, health provider, hospital, and/or community?
- Are they acceptable to the patients/families as well as to members of the health care team?
- Are they realistic with regard to:
  - The status, capabilities, and limitations of the patients
  - Recommendations in current literature regarding reasonable increments of change

—The kind of change that can be expected (cognitive, affective, psychomotor, skill, behavioral, health status) from the type and intensity of intervention being considered

—The policies, procedures, and resources of the hospital/community

Identifying Program Content

Again, a thorough needs assessment should have already established the parameters of the content for the PEM's program. The PEM will already have considered the patients' needs and interests and the providers' judgment of importance in several domains. These include the cognitive (knowledge, awareness, understanding), affective (attitudes, beliefs, feelings), psychomotor (skills), and behavioral domains. Other factors to consider include support (from family, significant others, health care providers) and resources (money, equipment, access to medication or special foods, and so on).

Because of the multifaceted and complex nature of many health problems and medical procedures, multidisciplinary input into program planning, particularly with regard to content, is usually essential. Also, advantage should be taken of the work already done by others to identify important content in similar situations. With the originators' permission, the PEM may be able to adopt or adapt their outlines or materials. After setting highest priority on those factors that are essential to accomplishing his or her objectives, the PEM will find that the elements of the content outline are already in hand.

Conveying information is the most concrete and most common task in patient education, so it is not surprising that this aspect is frequently overemphasized. Overloading the patient with information results in limited recall, inability to differentiate what is important, confusion, and misunderstanding. The pioneer in memory research, Hermann Ebbinghaus, found that one forgets over 60 percent of new information in an hour and 90 percent in 30 days. Additionally, information giving alone is rarely sufficient to have impact beyond increases in knowledge. If the desired impact includes behavioral change, strategies that have been demonstrated to be more effective in that arena must be utilized.

Determining Patient Education Program Design

There is no simple formula for determining the best design for any patient education program. The type of strategies selected is certainly a major variable, but so are such variables as expected outcomes, size and nature of the target population, skills of those who will be teaching, and available resources. A common error made in program planning is the premature choice of one or more educational methods before other factors are recognized and considered. Thus, before any discussion of types of educational strategies, it is important to articulate several basic principles of program design and strategy selection.

- In trying to accomplish a complex change, it is important to ensure that multiple, sequenced, mutually reinforcing strategies are planned: *multiple* because a single intervention is rarely sufficient to accomplish a significant, lasting change; *sequenced* because patients' needs and capacity for education change in type and quantity over time; *mutually reinforcing* because each intervention should be consistent with and build on the previous one for greater cumulative effect.
- The trap should be avoided of using the same educational strategy for every program, such as closed-circuit television or classes. No one method is inherently better than another in all situations. Rather, the effectiveness of a strategy depends on the appropriateness of the selected methods for a specific target population or patient and for the problem being addressed.
- Design strategies should be sufficiently flexible to make programs useful with groups of patients, individual patients and their families, and patients who may have special learning needs.

- Participation of patients in the educational process should be maximized through the use of interactive strategies. Patient involvement is a critical factor in learning, as is discussed later in this chapter in the section on learning styles under Sequencing Educational Strategies into a Program.
- The strategy should match the objectives. For example, if there is a cognitive objective, written or audiovisual instruction with an opportunity for discussion of the materials may be appropriate; but a behavioral objective is likely to require a more behavioral approach, such as demonstration and practice of a new skill.
- Problem-solving skills should be included in the program design if patient self-management is among the objectives. Such skills will be vital after patients leave the clinic or inpatient setting. They should be helped to anticipate common situations, and solutions should be identified that might include increasing their participation in physical activity, adjusting medication, monitoring medical devices, returning to work, or determining when to return for follow-up care or call a provider for advice.
- Because repetition is a proven principle of learning, key information and skills should be repeated at planned points in the educational process to ensure that they have been learned and retained. (Again, the section on learning styles later in this chapter provides a framework for mutually organizing reinforcement and repetition of information.)
- Whenever possible, options for learning should be offered. These choices are important for:
  - Considering learning styles and physical or mental limitations that preclude certain methods (for example, a hearing impairment that precludes listening to a closed-circuit television program; or computer anxiety)
  - Staff's teaching of patients who may feel more comfortable with one approach than another
  - Situational factors that may make use of a particular strategy difficult or impossible (for example, lack of space, time, or privacy)

Figure 13-7 (p. 284–285) provides a patient/parent education program description and figure 13-8 (p. 286) provides a matrix to assess the possibilities or evaluate the components of a patient education program.

Determining Educational Methods and Strategies

The choice of method or teaching strategy used depends on a number of factors such as the skill and preference of the patient educator; the length of stay of the patient; the resources of the hospital or clinic; the number of patients seen; and the size and diversity of the target population in terms of age, language, sociodemographics, and literacy level.

Numerous educational and instructional methods and strategies can be utilized in patient education, and there are myriad ways to combine them into a program. Green organizes teaching strategies within the following areas:[10]

- *Communication methods* such as lecture and discussion; individual counseling; materials such as books, pamphlets, written instructions, picture books with an audiotape, slides, films, filmstrips, recordings, flip charts, videotapes, and educational television; programmed learning such as computer-assisted education and interactive video; and mass media including newspapers, radio, magazines, and commercial television. Print and audiovisual aids are not in themselves the patient education program as some might think; they should be used only to supplement and reinforce one-to-one or group teaching.

- *Training methods* including skills development, simulations, games, role-playing, inquiry learning, demonstrations, practice and feedback, small group discussion, modeling, and behavior modification. Because these methods are interactive and more easily tailored than are prepared materials, they have generally been shown to be more effective than communication strategies in behavioral change and maintenance when well designed and skillfully implemented.
- *Organizational methods* including community development, social action, social planning, and organizational development. These methods are utilized less often than other educational methods. Additionally, they are not implemented directly with patients; rather, they are directed toward others who may be able to make changes that will in turn facilitate changes important for patients to undertake. If swimming is important in a rehabilitation program but an accessible place to swim does not exist for a group of patients, locating and making available community swimming facilities is more effective than simply trying to persuade the patients to swim. If patients must change their eating habits but others in their families are responsible for food selection and preparation, these family members must also be educated. If a group of hospitalized patients needs a particular kind of educational resource, it might be more productive to encourage the hospital to provide it than to encourage patients to seek it elsewhere.

These approaches have the potential to be highly effective because, except for family involvement, the changes that can be brought about usually affect many patients. They are also important because they avoid "victim blaming," the implication that patients are fully responsible for their health and its improvement. Change is more likely to occur and be maintained when a patient's environment is facilitative and supportive. (See chapter 3 for a broader discussion of creating an educational environment.)

The number and type of patients seen daily may also play a role in the educational strategy chosen. Does the target population comprise chemotherapy patients, of whom 500 come for treatment each day, or does it comprise low-literacy patients, who cannot be easily identified or quantified? For large target populations, organizing a comprehensive program with multiple interventions and sequenced, mutually reinforcing strategies is important to ensure that the population receives the education it needs, both as a group and individually. For chemotherapy patients, it is also important to look at the psychosocial and brain function changes they may be experiencing because of the disease and treatment; it would certainly be beneficial to involve family members in programs for these patients.

Clearly, there is a sufficiently wide range of methods to enable PEMs to define what is appropriate for their target population and feasible for their setting. Once this is done, they can select several cumulative, mutually reinforcing, and sequenced educational options.

Sequencing Educational Strategies into a Program

Program content must be divided, organized, and appropriately sequenced so that planned interventions provide continuity over a variety of settings and "teachable moments." Matching a component of the educational program to the appropriate stage of care is important. Emphasis at each stage should be on *survival skills*—what patients need to know, believe, and do at a particular point in time. Chronic conditions present a special challenge because they can last a lifetime and often move through recurring phases of requiring inpatient care, outpatient care, and minimal professional monitoring of patient and family self-management.

Several models have been developed to improve teaching effectiveness in clinical practice utilizing stages of illness. Fredette[11] utilizes a progression of psychosocial stages of adjustment to serious illness during which specific behaviors are exhibited and coping

Figure 13-7. Patient/Parent Education Program Description

Interview #: _____
Program #: _____

Target Population

1. Target
   ___ Parents (___)
   Age
   ___ Children 0 to 2 (___)
   ___ Children 3 to 10 (___)
   ___ Adolescents (___)

2. Target reached (per year)
   ___ Parents (___)
   Age
   ___ Children 0 to 2 (___)
   ___ Children 3 to 10 (___)
   ___ Adolescents (___)

3. How do patients become involved in the program?
   ___ as a part of routine care?
   ___ physician's orders
   ___ patient/request
   ___ other

Implementation

4. Written goals?
   yes ___ no ___ (___)

5. Measurable written objectives?
   yes ___ no ___ (___)

6. Uniform teaching plans or protocols?
   yes ___ no ___ (___)

7. Who developed the program?
   (Name/Title): _____

8. Was the program developed with multidisciplinary (team) input?
   yes ___ no ___ (___)

9. What staff perform the education tasks?
   Title _____ Hours/Week _____

10. Where is the program held? _____

11. How many units of contact with the patient are required to provide the service? Describe:
    _____
    _____

Materials

12. Materials used in instruction:
    ___ Book(s)
    ___ Pamphlet(s)
    ___ Teaching plans
    ___ Contract
    ___ Medical record
    ___ Written patient instruction(s)
    ___ Videotape
    ___ Slide/tape
    ___ Film
    ___ Models
    ___ Pictures
    ___ Flip charts
    ___ Other: _____

    (___) (___) (___)
    (___) (___) (___)

    Please list all materials by title and type:

    Please attach copies of all printed materials.

Methods

13. Instructional methods:
    Lecture: ___ individual
             ___ group
    Discussion: ___ individual
                ___ group
    ___ Patient/individual study:
    ___ Simulation
    ___ Games
    ___ Peer teaching
    ___ Programmed instruction
    ___ Contracting
    ___ Contingency management
    ___ Other: _____

    (___) (___) (___)
           (___) (___)
           (___) (___)

14. Please list all equipment used in this program:

Documentation

15. Do you record that a patient education activity has occurred?
    yes ___ no ___ (___)

16. If yes, where?
    In patient's chart:
    ___ Nurse's notes
    ___ Physician's notes
    ___ Patient education protocol or progress notes
    ___ Other: _____

17. Do you make use of the problem oriented medical record for recording patient education?
    yes ___ no ___

18. Are you comfortable with the POMR format?
    yes ___ no ___

19. Do you find that the SOAP NOTES (a form of chart notes) contribute to educational planning for your patients?
    yes ___ no ___

Interview #: _____
Program #: _____

Evaluation	Staff Training	Costs/Reimbursement	Barriers
20. Has a program evaluation been conducted? yes ___ no ___ (___)	27. Do the staff who teach patients have academic preparation in patient education? yes ___ no ___	30. Please list costs of the program. Staff time: Equipment: Space: Software: Cost: (___) Cost/patient: (___)	33. What are the obstacles you have encountered in the implementation, documentation, and evaluation of this program? (in order of importance) a. _____ b. _____ c. _____ d. _____ e. _____ (___) (___) (___)
21. If yes, how often? (___)	28. Is there need for staff development in this area? yes ___ no ___		
22. Date of last evaluation (___)	29. Please list training needs: (in order of priority) a. _____ b. _____ c. _____ d. _____ e. _____ (___) (___) (___) (___)	31. Does your department/service receive reimbursement for this project? yes ___ no ___	
23. Please describe the evaluation method:		32. If yes, by what mechanism? (___) (___) (___) (___)	
24. Please describe the evaluation findings:		**Interviewer's Notes**	
25. Do you recommend program changes? yes ___ no ___			
26. If yes, what are they in order of priority? a. _____ b. _____ c. _____ d. _____ e. _____ (___) (___) (___)			

Reprinted, with permission, from Texas Children's Hospital, Houston.

Louise A. Villejo, M.P.H., C.H.E.S.

Figure 13-8. Patient Education Needs and Priorities

Interview #: _____ (___)
EED #: _____ (___)
Program #: _____ (___)

Disease/Problem	Target (per year)	Documentation of need	Resources	Points of service contact	Barriers
Describe the disease process including aspects of clinical course and guidelines for medical/nursing care that would affect patient education planning: _____ _____ _____ _____ Pathology ___ Chronic ___ Acute Multiple hospitalizations: ___ yes ___ no Self management aspects: ___ many ___ few (___) ___ complex ___ simple (___) Physical limitations: ___ yes ___ no (___) Learning limitation: ___ yes ___ no (___)	Estimated numbers of patients and parents needing this service: ___ Parents (___) ___ Age ___ Children 0 to 2 ___ Children 2 to 4 ___ Children 4 to 7 ___ Children 7 to 10 ___ Preadolescents 10 to 12 ___ Adolescents 12 to 16 ___ Adolescents 16+ 8. List characteristics of the population that may be relevant to a patient education program:	9. Discuss examples of patient/parent need for information.	10. What resources are available within your department (service for the production and implementation of this program)? Planning Staff: (___) Hardware: (___) Materials: (___) Funds: (___) Teaching Staff: (___) 11. Resource notes:	12. List services provided/points of education contact —parents and children. (This department) a. _____ b. _____ c. _____ Other Departments a. _____ b. _____ c. _____ Suggested Methods/Materials Describe educational methods and materials that would be appropriate for the content and target group of this program. Methods: a. _____ b. _____ c. (___)(___)(___) Materials: a. _____ b. _____ c. _____	13. List potential barriers to the production, implementation or evaluation of this program: a. _____ b. _____ c. _____ d. _____ e. _____ (___) (___) (___) (___) (___)

Reprinted, with permission, from Texas Children's Hospital, Houston.

286

mechanisms utilized. She integrates the theories of Weisman, Crate, Engle, and Kubler-Ross into an educational model for the cancer patient, consisting of six periods. The model in figure 13-9 suggests nursing approaches, educational topics, and teaching strategies based on the patient's behavioral responses. The health care provider can then determine what the patient is ready to learn prior to teaching and can use appropriate teaching strategies. For example, Fredette maintains that during the diagnosis (Educational Period 1), the patient may feel numb, dazed, or highly anxious and unable to concentrate. She suggests that teaching strategies at this time should be simple, short, frequent one-on-one sessions that may be augmented by concise, easy-to-read pamphlets.

It is not until Educational Period 3 that she suggests the use of more varied teaching strategies as the patient moves toward adaptation and joins family and friends who mutually share the loss of health and assist in meeting the needs. Educational strategies at this stage can include information group sessions, print and audiovisual materials, self-learning packages, or programmed instruction.

When considering the most appropriate educational strategies for stage of disease, the patient's learning style must be assessed. Learning style theories recognize the fact that people learn in different ways, that they perceive and process information differently. For example, people who are left-brain dominant process in a more linear sequential fashion and those who are more right-brain dominant process information globally.

Figure 13-10 is based on a part of Dr. Bernice McCarthy's 4MAT System® that focuses on the teacher's (patient educator's) role and the student's (patient's) role. She combined major findings of the learning style research and right/left brain research findings and identified four major learning styles: Type One, Type Two, Type Three, and Type Four. Individual learning styles may be identified by self-reporting instruments, but McCarthy postulates that for every group of learners, approximately 25 percent fall into each of the four diverse styles. Therefore, a patient educator providing information in only one style ignores 75 percent of the patients she or he is trying to reach.

Type One learners ask why: "Why am I learning this?" The patient educator must answer the question and give them a reason. For example, a patient needing a catheter must be told what a catheter is and why it has been recommended for treatment. The appropriate educational strategy to use is one-to-one discussion.

Type Two learners often ask what: "What am I supposed to be learning?" The patient educator should concentrate on providing factual information. The catheter patient must learn proper catheter care before being discharged from the hospital. Appropriate educational strategies include one-on-one teaching, class instruction, videotape, and print materials. The ideal teaching program uses a combination of all these.

A variety of teaching strategies provides reinforcement and building blocks for additional information for all kinds of learners. The strategies also incorporate kinesthetic, audio, and visual learners. Patient educators must remember that from the patient's perspective, learning is complicated by his or her anxiety of diagnosis or treatment and extensive need for information and education.

Type Three learners ask how: "How does this work? Let me try it." Because these learners move into a more active role, educational strategies might include skill development, simulation, and opportunities for hands-on practice of the technique using the equipment.

Type Four learners ask: "If I learn this, what can I do with it? How can I apply it?" The educational strategy would include a return demonstration where patients and family members teach the patient educator or each other.

The learning process is a natural sequence from Type One to Type Four. By teaching in sequence, patient educators can address all four learning styles as different stages of learning. If patient educators tend to teach in just one style, their own style, or the style they were taught in, they need to be aware of other styles. The 4MAT System® provides a model for addressing those styles and learning as a process.

Figure 13-9. The Fredette Model for Improving Cancer Patient Education: A Summary

Period	Adaptation Stage	Content	Strategies
1	Existential plight: impact distress, disbelief, shock	Talk about the cancer as it relates to: harms, threats, resources. Discuss disease: personal aspects, family, social concerns.	Be present whenever diagnosis and treatment discussed by physician. Move out of denial/avoidance. Use one-on-one approach, pamphlets, discussion—short frequent sessions; provide what is asked for.
2	Existential plight proper, developing awareness	Correct misinformation. Expand knowledge base. Re-explain concepts formerly blocked. Explain treatment plan. Teach self-care. Teach about coping strategies, especially information-seeking.	Continue one-on-one. Be accepting of anger and crying. Watch for a "teachable moment." Have short frequent sessions. Toward end of period, use simple audio-visuals always followed by discussion.
3	Mitigation, reorganization, restitution	Strengthen coping. Introduce new ideas and options about disease, treatment, side effects, and treatment for side effects. Reteach facts presented in earlier period. Teach anxiety reduction methods. Model expression of feelings. Use "I Can Cope" program.	Use pamphlets, videotapes, films, self-learning packages, longer sessions, group education. Continue to reserve time for questions/discussion. Include family.
4	Accommodation, resolution and identity change	Discuss new identity, further Rx, Rx of side effects, second opinions, work, sexuality, interpersonal issues, fear of recurrences, coping with a chronic illness, living as a cancer survivor. Teach stress reduction. Use "Living with Cancer" program.	Use group teaching, support groups, all other methods. Encourage all free expression.
5	Decline and deterioration, states of dying	Answer questions asked. Interpret what is happening in the illness. Explain/discuss options. Validate patient's right of choice. Stress hope for comfort rather than cure.	Use one-on-one. Take clues from patient as to when and what to teach. Family may need more attention regarding education and coping.
6	Preterminality and terminality, stages of dying	The dying process The grieving process Spiritual-existential concerns Physical symptom management Psychological symptom management Interpersonal/communication problems Need for open, honest communication	Use one-on-one. Include family. Use short verbal explanations. Use periods of acceptance and physical comfort. Take clues from patient. Have patience with "middle knowledge phenomenon."

Reprinted, with permission, from Sheila Fredette, Ed.D., O.C.N., Professor of Nursing, Fitchburg State College, Fitchburg, Massachusetts. Appeared in *Cancer Nursing* 13(4):209, 1990.

Figure 13-10. The Patient Educator's Role: A Recapitulation

The patient educator's role changes as s/he moves
through the cycle of learning: from Motivator/Witness
to Educator/Information Giver to
Facilitator/Coach to
Evaluator/Remediator and Resource.

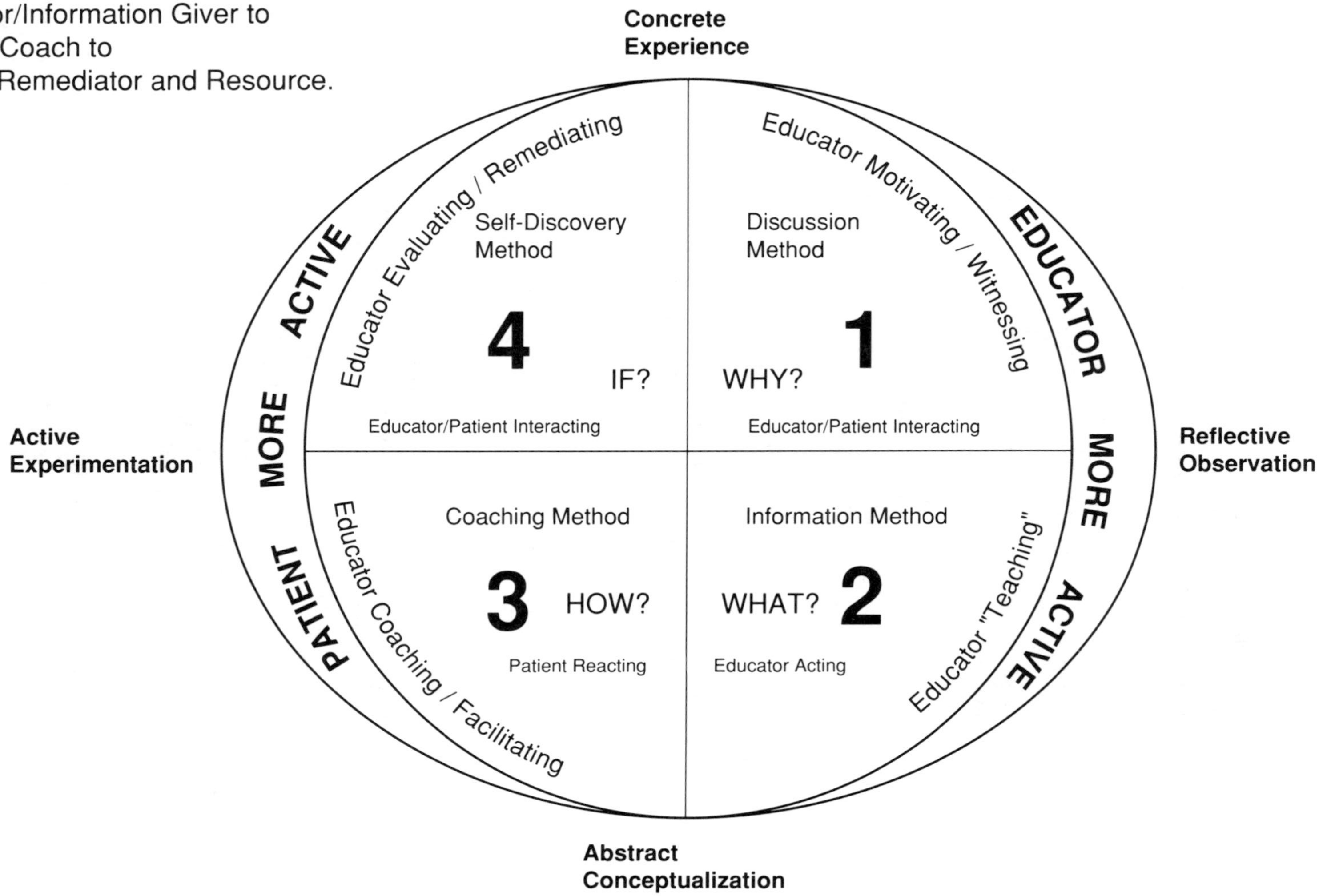

Adapted, with permission, from the *4 MAT® System: Teaching to Learning Styles with Right/Left Mode Techniques*, by Bernice McCarthy, copyright ©1980, 1987, by Excel, Inc. Used by permission.

Determining Staff Responsibility for Patient Education

Three major staff functions must be fulfilled with respect to a hospital's patient education program: program planning, coordination, and teaching. (The first two are considered together here because they overlap). The key here is in understanding the responsibilities that must be assumed, analyzing the organizational environment to learn what kinds of structures are accepted and supported, and then developing an approach that is both appropriate and effective in getting the job done.

Handling Planning and Coordination

Whether or not there is a hospitalwide patient education committee, some sort of committee, task force, team, or work group is usually the mechanism through which population-specific patient education programs are planned and coordinated. The committee's composition varies according to the hospital and the type of program being developed. In most hospitals nurses, pharmacists, physical therapists, dietitians, social workers, or other allied health care professionals are actively involved. Physician involvement is more often in an advisory capacity unless an individual is particularly interested in a specific initiative. Whether team members are appointees or volunteers, supervisor approval of their time recognizes the importance of patient education. It also makes committee members responsible for representing their areas and ensuring that their colleagues are up-to-date on patient education initiatives. Enthusiasm for patient education and the program being developed is also critical to the productivity and success of the effort.

Some hospitals have developed a generic approach to patient education program planning that provides a framework within which these teams function. This also ensures comparability in content and process among all of a hospital's programs, even if different teams are responsible for each one.

Team members serve several functions: In addition to doing much of the program and materials development and review work, they communicate information and feedback from the team to their units and supervisors, and vice versa. The frequency with which they meet depends on the hospital and the task at hand, but work frequently goes on in between team meetings. This leaves meeting time for the review of "homework" assigned during meetings and for decision making. Coordination of programs is also highly variable from hospital to hospital.

In a small hospital with a manageable number of programs, coordination may be a function of the PEM. In some cases, the planning team does not disband once implementation occurs, retaining the responsibility for coordinating the program, monitoring it on an ongoing basis, making changes as needed, and so on. In others, a planning team member might become the PEM. The amount of time and expertise required to be a PEM depends on the complexity of the program.

Some hospitals place primary responsibility for program coordination, not just program delivery, at the unit level. The PEM becomes a resource to these responsible individuals and teams, providing the level of assistance and support that is required and ensuring that hospitalwide program standards are maintained.

Doing the Teaching

Responsibility for patient teaching is shared by everyone in the hospital and, increasingly, with members of the community in which patients live and work. Within the hospital, registrars, appointment clerks, physicians, nurses, dietitians, physical therapists, pharmacists, and others who interact with patients spend some portion of their time teaching patients and families. Depending on the program, the population, and the setting(s) for patient education, any combination of these individuals may share teaching responsibility.

Indeed, team teaching is viewed as desirable, albeit challenging, to orchestrate. It involves linking the notion of sequencing discussed earlier (that is, what needs to be learned by patients at a particular point in time) with the learning opportunities that might exist at that time (that is, at preregistration or admission, in the clinic waiting room or hospital room, or at home while being taught self-care techniques) and the individuals who have, or could develop, the desire and skills to be patient educators.

Thus, within a single educational plan that spans a period of time and many settings, a number of patient educators must function as a team, conveying messages that are timely and consistent and that reinforce those previously delivered. To achieve continuity of care, the members of this team must be involved in reviewing the overall patient education plan, understand their role and responsibility as they relate to the rest of the team, and communicate their experiences, concerns, and suggestions on an ongoing basis so that adjustments can be made as needed (see figure 13-11 for a multidisciplinary teaching plan).

Figure 13-11. Multidisciplinary Teaching Plan for Anticoagulants

Teaching Plan	Teaching Completed (date and initial)
Nurse	
1. Pretest.	_____
2. Name of anticoagulant and its purpose as it relates to patient's diagnosis.	_____
3. Explain protime and its relationship to dosage.	_____
4. Audiovisual shown.	_____
5. Notify pharmacy to visit patient. Relate learning obstacles and anticipated discharge date.	
Pharmacist	
6. Factors which may alter the action of an anticoagulant.	_____
7. Symptoms and side effects warranting doctor's attention.	_____
8. Take-home instruction sheet given to patient.	
Nurse and pharmacist	
9. Evaluate patient's needs for assistance after discharge.	_____
10. Medic Alert card completed and given to patient.	_____
Nurse	
11. Posttest.	_____
12. Name and home dosage of anticoagulant.	_____
13. Protime card and doctor's appointment.	_____
Learning obstacles:	
Family included in patient teaching? Yes No	
Who? _____	
Comments:	

Reprinted, with permission, from St. Luke's Hospital, Fargo, North Dakota.

Other teaching roles include:

- *Specialized instructors.* These are qualified individuals whose primary function is to provide patient education in a particular program area. They may be hospital staff who have other responsibilities in another role or persons hired for some portion of time to fulfill an educational function.
- *Peers.* Many models of programs are led by peer educators, people who have experienced an illness or injury and are willing to educate others facing a similar situation. Although these persons often do not have the same professional credentials as health care providers, they actually may have more credibility because they can communicate the message: "I've been where you are, and I got through it." This approach may be especially valuable in the affective and support domains, when patients and families may need hope and encouragement more than clinical information. Peer educators can function either in groups (for example, self-help associations), in one-on-one situations with patients and families, or incorporated into videotapes as "expert" interviews.
- *Volunteers and patient education interns.* These individuals can be peer educators. Volunteers and student interns can extend the services of an overextended patient education function tremendously (see figures 13-12 and 13-13). This can be done by staffing patient and family libraries or learning resource centers, setting up audiovisual equipment, delivering educational materials, stocking literature racks, putting up bulletin board displays promoting patient education activities, transporting patients to classes, welcoming them, taking attendance, or passing out materials. Sometimes the willingness of volunteers and interns to simply listen to and relay the concerns of patients and families to designated staff members can uncover educational needs or desires that patients have not had the time or comfort to convey to their care providers.

Overall, the composition of the patient teaching team and division of specific teaching responsibilities depends on some of the following considerations:

- In what setting(s) are there patient/family contacts that might provide educational opportunities?
- Who has the content knowledge to convey clinical information and skills?
- Who has or is willing to develop skills as an effective teacher? In addition to whatever ongoing staff development activities might be in place to enhance patient education skills, there may be a need for additional orientation, training, or reinforcement in targeted areas to ensure that staff are competent and confident in fulfilling their teaching responsibilities. For example, at one hospital a local Toastmaster's trainer was used successfully to enhance class instructors' public speaking skills.
- Who can provide support and encouragement to patients and their families?
- Who has or can make time available, has enthusiasm, and has supervisor support for patient teaching?

Establishing a Time Line

There is no avoiding the reality of the time it takes to plan a patient education program. Although skilled staff, organizational support, sufficient budget, prior experience in patient education program planning, simple objectives, and other factors might streamline the process somewhat, the many steps in the planning process must be taken patiently and in turn. The payoff in the long run, however, is substantial: a well-planned program that is implemented efficiently, proven effective, and accepted by both patients and staff.

Figure 13-12. Duties of Patient Education Volunteers

Hours: Flexible, any 3 hours between 8:00 a.m. and 5:00 p.m. Monday–Friday

Job Description:

Volunteers assist the Patient Education Office staff on a variety of levels, involving the distribution, promotion, and translation of patient education materials. There are a variety of activities which a volunteer may be involved in while working with the Patient Education Office, as listed below. A volunteer may be assigned to one or several of these positions:

Bilingual (English/Spanish) Aide: Assists in the translation of patient education materials into Spanish and helps coordinate other Spanish language patient education activities.

Class Aide: Stocks patient education classroom with materials for chemotherapy; welcomes participants to class; prepares materials to be placed in the classroom; keeps monthly attendance logs.

Clearinghouse Assistant: Assists staff in filling orders for patient education materials and putting together packets for classes.

Patient/Family Learning Center: Assists patient/family members in finding information and resources to meet their informational and educational needs.

Literature Rack Stocker: Fills literature racks in inpatient and clinic areas with brochures from the American Cancer Society and the National Cancer Institute.

Patient Education Mobile Assistant: Stocks mobile with patient education pamphlets and brings it to various hospital and clinic waiting areas.

Promotion Aide: Puts together bulletin board displays promoting patient education classes and health information to be placed in waiting areas and lobbies at U.T. M. D. Anderson Cancer Center.

Research Aide: Collates results of patient education surveys and assists in the proofing of revised patient information sheets. Assists with a variety of patient education projects.

Additional Information:

Little or no patient contact

Reprinted, with permission, from the U.T. M. D. Anderson Cancer Center, Houston.

Figure 13-13. Duties of the Health Education Intern in the Patient Education Office

Job Description:

Assist patient education staff in the planning, implementation, promotion, and evaluation of patient education programs. Works under the direct supervision of Patient Education staff.

Potential Internship Projects:

Assist patient education staff in assessing, developing, and coordinating patient education programs for hospital and clinic patients and families

Design, administer learner verification need assessment instruments

Do data entry and perform tally survey results

Draft summary report

Publish and promote semi-monthly newsletter

Assist in the management of patient education volunteers

Assist in the preparation and facilitation of patient education committee meetings

Computer projects utilizing word processing, spreadsheet, and on-line data base literature research software

Assist in planning and implementation of Patient Education Week

Develop evaluation instruments for class instructors

Reprinted, with permission, from the U.T. M. D. Anderson Cancer Center, Houston.

Included in the tasks of assessment, planning, implementation, and evaluation are such time-consuming tasks as clearing multiple levels of review and revision, acquiring or developing educational materials, pilot-testing, training staff and volunteers, and promoting the program. Thus it is essential that the time line developed during program planning reflect realistic deadlines for completion of these tasks, because delays in the promised date of program implementation can result in a loss of enthusiasm, participation, organizational support, and budget allotments.

The easiest and most understandable way to present a time line is in chart form, specifying tasks, the periods during which they will take place, and the person(s) responsible for their completion (see figure 13-14). This format also makes it possible to see how tasks relate to each other and how the program will take shape as time goes on. The program is relatively simple to revise if unexpected circumstances push the time line back.

Developing the Educational Protocol or Procedures Manual

When the planning process reaches a sufficient level of detail, it is necessary to develop a step-by-step, specific protocol that can be used by patient educators without extensive training or instruction. This protocol or procedures manual should be a comprehensive guide to program implementation, starting with any preparation necessary before providing education and moving through presentation, record-keeping, evaluation, and follow-up.

Figure 13-14. Project Time Line

Year 1: September 1992 to August 1993												
Task/Responsible Person	S	O	N	D	J	F	M	A	M	J	J	A
Patient education committee meeting/Coordinator	X											
Draft needs assessment survey for staff/Coordinator	X											
Draft needs assessment survey for patients and family members/Coordinator, intern	X											
Incorporate patient education committee comments and get final approval of surveys/Coordinator and committee		X	X									
Train interns to conduct needs assessment surveys/ Coordinator				X								
Implement survey/Coordinator, Intern					X							
Input data from surveys or collate findings/Intern					X	X						
Write summary report/Intern, Coordinator						X	X					
Present findings to patient education committee/Coordinator							X	X				
Develop patient education program goals and objectives and prioritize needs identified/Committee, Coordinator								X	X			
Develop patient teaching plan/Committee, Coordinator										X	X	X

In addition to guiding program implementation as it is intended to occur, the protocol is valuable to anticipate problems or dilemmas that might arise during implementation and to suggest appropriate actions. If at all possible, the name and telephone number of someone who can be called during an urgent situation should be provided as part of the protocol.

This protocol or manual should be distributed to everyone involved in program implementation and should be stored for reference in accessible locations. As computerization becomes more widespread, more protocols can be stored on-line, providing immediate access, facilitating rapid adjustments, and requiring less storage space.

Planning Promotion Efforts

Sometimes called marketing, the promotion of patient education programs and other hospital services has assumed increasing importance as what used to be a captive population spends less time in the hospital and more time in the community making choices about involvement in any sort of health intervention. What is generally an encouraging trend toward greater availability of health education in hospitals, other medical care facilities, and the community also creates competition in some areas, and patients may find it difficult to make informed choices about which program will best meet their needs and is of high quality. Strategies are needed to:

- Reach patients to promote awareness of and participation in patient education to which self-referral is encouraged
- Encourage referrals to patient education programs by hospital staff
- Encourage referrals to patient education programs by community health care providers

Like effective education, effective promotion generally requires that more than one approach to the target population be utilized. Some approaches may be direct to the patient, either through hospital channels during an inpatient stay or through mailings and local media. Others are designed to reach the target population through intermediaries, such as health care providers and agencies in the community. Although most promotional techniques are inexpensive, much planning, coordination, and monitoring time is necessary to be certain that informative, persuasive, and up-to-date messages reach the target population.

At The University of Texas M. D. Anderson Cancer Center, the promotional effort is multifaceted and targets patients, family members, and staff. Promotion of patient education begins during registration and admission, when the patient receives a patient packet. This packet contains a patient handbook, which includes information on the policies and procedures of the hospital, the multidisciplinary staff, and the enormous array of special services from the concierge desk staffed by volunteer services to the patient education office's Patient/Family Learning Center. The patient packet also contains the patient guide, which includes facts about patient education classes, the in-house cable television system, educational videotapes, telephone numbers, and other resources. The goal of these materials is not merely to inform patients of the specific educational opportunities available to them, but also to create an awareness of patient education, an appreciation of the educational services provided by the hospital, and a positive sense of anticipation and expectation of what the hospital has to offer them on an inpatient and outpatient basis.

Additional efforts used to promote patient education activities include the *MDA Times*, a monthly patient/family newsletter written by patient education office staff; and *In Touch, A Forum for Breast Cancer Patients*, a monthly patient-to-patient newsletter written by patients and edited by patient education office staff. Literature racks in the clinic and inpatient areas are also used to distribute patient/public education materials.

Promotional efforts at M. D. Anderson Cancer Center that target hospital and clinic patient/family members and staff include:

- A health information fair is held quarterly in the hospital cafeteria to promote materials available for patients and families in the library.
- MDA-TV Channel 10 Information offers continuous rolling messages on patient education events and classes, and videotape information.
- Class posters and flyers.
- Patient/Family Learning Centers.
- Twenty-five patient education bulletin boards throughout the inpatient and clinical areas.

Many times office reports, departmental orientations, or in-services can turn into opportunities to promote patient education programs. These can include items such as the following:

- *News You Can Use.* A one-page update of programs, announcements, and new and revised materials distributed monthly to patient education committee members and management-level care providers
- Monthly activity report. A vice-president-level, one-page monthly synopsis
- Quarterly report. A department head, management-level, several-page quarterly synopsis of activities
- Institutional electronic mail. Used to announce patient education programs, classes, and new materials on an ongoing basis
- Patient education orientation. Conducted with all patient care departments on an as-needed basis
- Patient Education Week. An annual fair with exhibits, entertainment, and speakers
- Promotion done by in-service head nurses, clinical nurse specialists, clinic administration services, and hospital administration services staff regarding utilization of patient education resources

A patient education office in Illinois creates bridges between inpatient and outpatient settings to enhance the possibility that patients will continue the educational process after discharge. A calendar of outpatient programs is distributed with the mail and inserted in newspapers that reach a third of the target community. Outreach is designed for specific programs as well: invitations to diabetic individuals based on a registry kept by the hospital, and self-mailers for the high blood pressure patient education program. Contacts are maintained with local media, resulting in occasional newspaper articles, the airing of public service announcements, and a monthly radio talk show.

In addition to these low-cost promotional techniques, the PEM of the Illinois program has a marketing budget that is used for such channels as paid newspaper advertising. The chief advantage is control over content, which is difficult to negotiate when time or space is being donated. The budget also allows for purchases of sufficient advertising space to include not only program scheduling information, but also a description of the program's benefits.

A local health maintenance organization (HMO) agreed to include brochures about the programs on its pamphlet rack. Bundles of 25 brochures are initially delivered, with a postage prepaid inventory card to be returned to the hospital when the supply needs to be replenished.

Relationships with physicians are important in promotion efforts and can be valuable, but require patience and perseverance. Often other intermediaries, that is, a physician's office staff, become involved with the approval of the physician. These relationships require a commitment to collaboration toward a common goal, respect for each other's needs and constraints, and ongoing opportunities to work together that interfere minimally with other responsibilities. Assessing whether these relationships should be nurtured or continued depends on a number of factors, such as the number of physicians with whom such linkages must be maintained, their relationship to the hospital, and their attitude toward and support for patient education. The role of physicians is important not only with respect to promoting hospital patient education programs, but also in providing ongoing support for their patients and reinforcement for the education their patients receive.

Considering Resources Needed

As a labor-intensive activity, patient education first and foremost requires human resources: The functions that must be fulfilled and the options for who assumes those responsibilities have already been discussed. Depending on the particular program, additional human resources may be needed in such areas as communications, graphics, public relations, and so on. Additionally, the extension of services that interns and volunteers provide should not be overlooked.

There are also material resources necessary to program implementation. It is important that the PEM anticipate accessibility and affordability of these resources as he or she designs a program. Some examples of material resources are:

- *Space.* Some of the considerations are:
  - Accessibility to the location of patients, including any need for transportation, barrier-free facilities, and so on
  - The size, comfort, privacy, and appropriateness of the space for interacting with staff/volunteers and utilizing audiovisual materials
  - Locations in which there is regular contact with the target population and families that provide a natural setting for patient education
- *Equipment.* Depending on the program, this may include medical devices, audiovisual equipment, closed-circuit television, computer terminals, furniture adapted to special uses, and so on. It is important to consider the options of purchasing, leasing or renting, costs and time involved in maintenance, availability of backup equipment, and storage when not in use.
- *Educational materials.* If acquired or purchased from an existing source, materials must be reviewed for appropriateness, quantity must be estimated, mailing time must be allowed for, and a system for taking inventory and restocking must be devised. If the material is developed in-house, plans should be made for research and development, review and approval, graphics, and production time. Whatever the source of materials, a system for periodic review and revision or replacement when necessitated by new knowledge or materials must also be planned.
- *Miscellaneous resources.* Particular programs may require special resources that would not be needed in most others. For example, it may be desirable to offer refreshments at training sessions or group meetings, certificates for course completion, and so on.

Planning the Budget

Every program and service consumes resources, even when there is no specific budget identified. In the current climate of cost containment and continual reassessment of expenditures, it is important that PEMs develop a budget for their programs even if the programs are not expected to produce revenue, or in some other way monitor what is being spent (see figure 13-15). Documentation that justifies staff positions and other line items can be crucial to have in hand if questions arise that could threaten the program's resources.

Figure 13-15. Budget Proposal

This budget is to develop a videotape and printed material for X patient education program. Focus groups will be conducted to evaluate the content of the patient education booklet. Assuming the overall Patient Education Office provides the staff, space, equipment, telephone and general office maintenance, the cost and time line are listed below:

Project Administration Costs

Photocopying 24 pages × .05 × 12 people	$	14.40
(For review by Patient Education Committee)		

Office Supplies:

Bond paper	2 reams @ $ 6.75	13.50
Diskettes	@ $13.10	13.10
Staples	@ $ 2.89	2.89
Pens	@ $11.76	11.76
Dictating tapes	14 @ $ 6.35	88.90
	Total	$ 144.58

Logistics for Focus Groups

Six focus groups will be held with ten people in each group at a rate of $20.00 per person. Patient Education Office staff will conduct the focus groups. The snack amount is used by the catering department at the institution.

$36.00 × 6 focus groups	$ 216.00
60 participants × $20.00	1,200.00
Snacks for 12 people per focus group for a total of 72 people × $4.25/person (1 coordinator, 1 assistant and 10 participants)	306.00
Total	$1,722.00

Printed Matter—The pricing is based on an estimate from in-house Medical Illustration and Graphic Design and Print Shop.

Patient Guide (booklet)

8½ × 5½, 6 page, 2 color, 2 sides	$ 350.00
Printing 500 booklets	423.00
Spanish translation	80.00
Total	$ 853.00

Videotape—The pricing is based on an estimate from in-house Video Production Services on a 10-minute videotape.

Services and facilities

Scripting	$1,400.00
Graphics	2,720.00
Field Production	4,400.00
Off-line post production	2,800.00
On-line post production	2,640.00
Videotape duplication	120.00
Audio production	130.00
Freelance producer	5,000.00

Materials

One-inch videotape master	75.00
Video duplications, ¾ inch	50.00
Video duplications, VHS	60.00
Tapes used on location	600.00
Music license fee	130.00
Audio tape stock	50.00
Narration	875.00
Talent fee	1,875.00
Spanish translation	470.00
Computer art storage disks	100.00
Contingency (10%)	2,302.50
Total	$25,797.50

Often a patient education program budget encompasses funds from a variety of sources. Examples are existing hospital budgets, third-party reimbursement, program fees, grants and contracts, the donated time of volunteers, and producers of materials provided at no charge (for example, the government, community agencies, pharmaceutical companies). It is helpful to identify the following categories of costs:

- *Direct costs.* Charges for resources used specifically for the program, such as the salary of specialized instructors or the cost of audiovisual materials
- *Indirect costs.* Utilization of resources that also serve other purposes, such as hospital space, heat and lights, janitorial service
- *In-kind contributions.* Resources that have monetary value but are available at no charge through a donation to the program from another agency or individual

Such information is necessary to itemize if the cost-effectiveness of the patient education program is to be calculated.

In budgeting for the future, it is vital to consider predictable cost increases such as higher salaries, the effects of inflation on goods and services, and so on. A frequent error made by people preparing budgets is underestimating resource needs. Unanticipated cost overruns sometimes can be handled through other mechanisms, but the care with which a budget is developed can ensure a program's financial viability, eliminating the need to seek supplemental funds.

All programs utilize resources, but many also generate resources. Depending on whether the goal is to cover costs or make money, it is important to develop expertise in pricing programs and products so that a profit margin can be added to their cost and they can remain competitive in the marketplace for comparable goods or services.

Finally, attention to budgetary matters does not end with finalization and approval of the budget. A system must be devised for monitoring both expenditures and income so that corrections can be made for overspending, underspending, or errors that can occur when billing, payment, and other accounting functions are handled by another department. Just as program objectives serve as a standard against which results can be measured, a budget should serve as a guide against which actual income and expenditures can be compared to be sure a program is meeting its financial obligations and goals.

Gaining Approval and Support

Although gaining approval and support is a process that in most hospitals begins before planning is initiated and continues throughout program development, a final stamp of approval should be obtained prior to program implementation. In addition to the reviewers whose approval is mandated by the hospital's patient education policies and procedures, it is advisable to include any other individuals (for example, medical staff, other hospital staff, patients or families in the target population, key community contacts) whose review and support might be a strategic asset to program implementation and continuation.

☐ Implementing Patient Education Programs

Patient teaching is only one component of the implementation process. Pretesting or pilot-testing is important to ensure program quality and consistency. Providing orientation and training of instructors, monitoring their activities, documenting the process of patient education, and gathering data needed for program evaluation are all major components of the implementation process.

Pretesting Program Strategies and Materials

Pretesting program strategies is a type of formative evaluation to ensure fine tuning and acceptability for target audiences. Testing a program on a small scale to determine whether it is appropriate and ready for full implementation can save a lot of resources and heartache in the long run. For instance, pretesting may:

- Save the expense of producing or purchasing materials that may later prove ineffective or inappropriate for the target population.
- Prevent any "political" damage to the larger patient education effort. One unsuccessful full-scale program may adversely affect the opinions of key decision makers.
- Ease later full-blown implementation. Introducing the program on a small scale is one way to win staff and patient support.
- Uncover unforeseen problems, the resolution of which can strengthen the overall program.

Pretesting program strategies and materials is very important. Pretesting a program includes training a select sample of staff to conduct the program and then evaluating the staff after the program has been presented. Staff should be asked how effective they felt the program was, and what knowledge and skills they felt patients and family members gained. Patient and family members should also take a written pretest and posttest or perform a posttest return demonstration. Patients should be asked about the quality of the teaching and what they feel they learned. They should also be encouraged to comment on any aspect of the program.

Print materials must also be evaluated. (Development of patient education materials is addressed in chapter 17.) Having the materials reviewed by the multidisciplinary patient education committee not only ensures that the information is as comprehensive and succinct as possible, but also ensures that committee members know what materials are being developed or purchased for their area so that they will be sure to alert their colleagues and use the materials appropriately. It is also important to include the target population in the evaluation of materials. A simple one-page evaluation form that nurses can give patients as they do the teaching can provide the opportunity for patient review and evaluation (see figure 13-16).

To target messages to specific populations (for example, breast cancer patients, patients with low-literacy skills, or patients from different cultural backgrounds), focus groups, which provide a more dynamic feedback loop for participants and staff, may be most effective. Figures 13-17 and 13-18 (p. 302) are examples of evaluations that can be used with low-literacy materials individually or in groups.

Providing Orientation and Training of Patient Educators

The number and nature of individuals to do the direct patient teaching will vary according to such factors as the program's size and complexity, frequency of presentation/delivery, relevant disciplines involved, the size and accessibility of the population to be reached, and the need for resource people at multiple locations. Both general and specific issues need to be addressed in the orientation and training of a diverse group of patient educators:

- Patient educators must have the necessary expertise and must supplement, as needed, their mastery of content and skills in patient/family assessment, interpersonal communication and group dynamics, the setting of educational priorities, and the tailoring and delivery of educational interventions.
- Patient educators must be familiar with every aspect of the particular patient education program, including content, procedures, materials, equipment, and record-keeping.

Figure 13-16. Patient Evaluation of a Patient Information Card

Thank you for agreeing to help us evaluate the _____ (name of procedure, medication, etc.) _____ Patient Information Card. The card is designed to reinforce the patient teaching that you have received from all members of the health care team.

1. Please read the attached card and underline any words that you do not understand.

2. Was the information easy to understand?

   _____ Yes   _____ No

   If no, please tell us below which part(s) you did not understand:

   _____

   _____

   _____

3. Do you have any important questions about the (specify name of card) _____
   that were not covered in the card?

   _____ Yes   _____ No

   If yes, please comment: _____

   _____

   _____

4. Do you have any additional comments or suggestions for improving this card?

   _____

   _____

   _____

Please return this form to the nurse.

Thank you very much for your assistance.

Reprinted, with permission, from the U.T. M. D. Anderson Cancer Center, Houston.

Figure 13-17. Low-Literacy Learner Verification for Radiotherapy Booklet

We've been rewriting some of our instructions booklets. Now we need to know if the message is clear. After you have read the radiotherapy booklet, please complete the following without looking at the book. Thank you.

Check the blanks for statements you read in this booklet.

_____ Radiotherapy is much like taking an x-ray.
_____ The radiotherapy will kill cancer cells and normal cells.
_____ The radiotherapy you receive will not hurt your family and friends.
_____ On your first visit, you will have to put on a hospital gown.
_____ You can wash the colored lines off after your first visit.
_____ When you are placed on the treatment table, you should not change the way you have been placed.
_____ You will never have to wait to see the doctor.
_____ You will get a rest from radiotherapy on Saturday and Sunday.
_____ Radiotherapy can cause side effects that do not last long.
_____ It's OK to wash the colored lines with soap.
_____ If your skin itches in the treatment area, don't scratch it.
_____ You should not use birth control while you are getting radiotherapy.
_____ If you are a woman, you should not get pregnant while you are getting radiotherapy.
_____ While you are getting radiotherapy, you should only eat meats and fruits.
_____ While you are getting radiotherapy, you should get some exercise.
_____ Tell your doctor if you are taking any medicines.
_____ If you have other questions, you can talk to a social worker.

Reprinted, with permission, from the U.T. M. D. Anderson Cancer Center, Houston.

Louise A. Villejo, M.P.H., C.H.E.S.

Figure 13-18. Pretest Questionnaire for Low-Literacy Fact Sheets

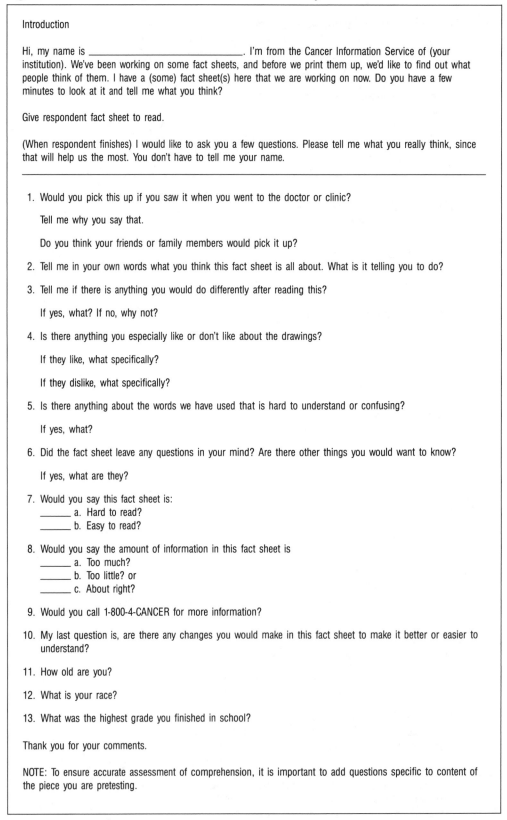

Introduction

Hi, my name is _____. I'm from the Cancer Information Service of (your institution). We've been working on some fact sheets, and before we print them up, we'd like to find out what people think of them. I have a (some) fact sheet(s) here that we are working on now. Do you have a few minutes to look at it and tell me what you think?

Give respondent fact sheet to read.

(When respondent finishes) I would like to ask you a few questions. Please tell me what you really think, since that will help us the most. You don't have to tell me your name.

1. Would you pick this up if you saw it when you went to the doctor or clinic?

   Tell me why you say that.

   Do you think your friends or family members would pick it up?

2. Tell me in your own words what you think this fact sheet is all about. What is it telling you to do?

3. Tell me if there is anything you would do differently after reading this?

   If yes, what? If no, why not?

4. Is there anything you especially like or don't like about the drawings?

   If they like, what specifically?

   If they dislike, what specifically?

5. Is there anything about the words we have used that is hard to understand or confusing?

   If yes, what?

6. Did the fact sheet leave any questions in your mind? Are there other things you would want to know?

   If yes, what are they?

7. Would you say this fact sheet is:
   _____ a. Hard to read?
   _____ b. Easy to read?

8. Would you say the amount of information in this fact sheet is
   _____ a. Too much?
   _____ b. Too little? or
   _____ c. About right?

9. Would you call 1-800-4-CANCER for more information?

10. My last question is, are there any changes you would make in this fact sheet to make it better or easier to understand?

11. How old are you?

12. What is your race?

13. What was the highest grade you finished in school?

Thank you for your comments.

NOTE: To ensure accurate assessment of comprehension, it is important to add questions specific to content of the piece you are pretesting.

Used, with permission, from Cancer Information Services, Mary Babb Randolph Cancer Center, U.T. M. D. Anderson Cancer Center, Houston.

Although nursing staff often conduct the bulk of patient education, the premise here is that all health care team members are patient educators and should be involved in planning, development, and implementation. Basic guidelines for the orientation and training of teaching staff are similar to the principles of program design previously discussed with regard to patients:

- Content should be based on an assessment of the needs and interests of those who will teach.
- Strategies should be as interactive as possible. Opportunities should be included to practice such approaches as role-playing, demonstration, or videotaping with trainer feedback. (See figure 13-19 for an in-service guide that includes a variety of strategies.)
- A single training session is rarely sufficient. Patient teaching skills must be learned, practiced, and then retained and enhanced through periodic monitoring and feedback. The best way to monitor is direct observation (when feasible) combined with the feedback of patients in the population reached. Once the PEM is assured that skilled, confident, effective teaching is occurring consistently, reinforcement and rewards that recognize a challenging job well done are usually all that is needed.

It is important to make program resources accessible to the teaching staff at all times; an updated protocol manual, materials, and a resource person should be conveniently located for all who may need them. (Several models of continuing education, orientation, and mentoring for staff development are provided in chapter 12.)

Providing Effective Documentation

For quality and continuity of care, monitoring, compliance with legal requirements, and evaluative purposes, keeping records of the process and outcome of patient education is essential. As length of stay becomes shorter and patient care encompasses multiple settings, record-keeping assumes a central role in ensuring communication from time A to time B, site A to site B, and provider A to provider B. Documentation, primarily in the form of medical records, is an established part of the health care process. However, it is clear from many quality assurance studies that there are problems with the completeness, accuracy, clarity, and usefulness of provider documentation. (Documentation issues are addressed in more detail in chapter 9.)

The medical record is a vital, though not the only, mechanism for patient education record-keeping. Many hospitals have developed patient education documentation forms to provide a focus for educational activities in the medical record. These forms can provide visibility for patient education; they can cue desirable provider–patient interactions.

Figure 13-20 (p. 306) provides an example of a patient teaching documentation form that has been developed for a specific teaching protocol; it lists the subjects to be taught, the method used, and outcome. On the opposite side of the patient teaching documentation form, an abbreviated teaching guide is provided for the patient educator's reference. It lists the title, purpose, and directions for using the Teaching Guide/Documentation Form.

This form serves many purposes. It prompts the patient educator as to what should be taught, lists methods and teaching aids, and forces the patient educator to assess teaching outcome by providing questions to stimulate patient feedback. Many times, well-developed teaching programs do not meet their goals because health care providers are so busy providing care and teaching that they do not assess whether the patient actually learned the information.

Documentation is an important form of communication and feedback among health care providers. A form can indicate to various members of the health care team what has been taught and learned in previous interactions with patients or in group interventions.

Figure 13-19. Chemotherapy Instructor In-Service Guide

Objectives	Content	Time Frame	Faculty	Outcome Criteria
Day 1: Review Chemotherapy Class Content Outline	Chemotherapy is	20 mins.	Stewart	Participants familiar with chemotherapy class content outline
Prioritize the outcome criteria related to standards of care.	Discuss the standards of care as related to the Chemotherapy Class Content Outline			Participants prioritize the outcome criteria.
Coffee break	Questions and answers	10 mins.		
Day 2: (Adult Learning Theory) Describe 5 characteristics of the Adult Learner	The Adult Learner 1. Is problem oriented 2. Builds upon past experience 3. Wants autonomy and control in a learning experience 4. Prefers to take an active role in the learning process 5. Needs reinforcement, but resents drill/repetition	10 mins.	Webber	Lecture and dialogue Overhead
Participant will begin to integrate theory with practice.	Break out into groups of four: Work together as a team. Plan a short teaching session utilizing principles of Adult Learning and content from one segment of the chemotherapy class content outline. Demonstrate a mock teaching session in front of class. You may team teach if you wish, or just have one instructor with a group of learners.	40 mins.	Co-facilitator circulates through the room	Group practice Group practices presentations.
(Health Belief Model) Describe the basis for Health Belief Model	Health Belief Model 1. Person believes he is at risk for certain health related problems. 2. Person perceives this risk as a serious threat. 3. Person believes that intervention is worth the effort in order to avoid the threat. 4. Person responds to a cue for action.	10 mins.	Hernandez	Lecture: Overheads
Relate a similar cycle from one's own professional experience.	Dysfunctional Health Belief Model. Discuss the broken appointment cycle.			
Explore different ways of changing a negative health belief cycle into a positive one.	Participants break up into groups to brainstorm and problem-solve about different health belief cycles.	20 mins.		Exercise

Figure 13-19. (Continued)

Objectives	Content	Time Frame	Faculty	Outcome Criteria
(Principles of Self-Efficacy) Define self-efficacy using an operational construct and a constitutive construct.	*Self-efficacy* is the belief in one's ability to change behavior in order to effect or enhance one's well-being. Constitutive definition: (1) self-esteem, (2) past experiences, (3) role models, (4) reinforcement Operational definition: Belief in one's self results in changes in behavior. Give one example of Dodd's Research Study.	10 min. 50 min.	Webber	Lecture Overhead
Participants will be able to use self-efficacy model after participating in the compass exercise. Coffee Break	Instruct participants in use of the compass sheet.	10 min.		Group exercise Handouts
(Presentation Skills) Describe the characteristics of a dynamic speaker	Vocal clarity Vocal variety Organization Good eye contact Appropriate body language Avoidance of annoying mannerisms	12 min.	Sayles	Presentation by Texas Medical Center Toastmasters
Participants will be able to give a 2-5 minute icebreaker speech. Participants will be able to give a short written evaluation of each other.	Participants break up into small groups of three or four. Each participant gives a short talk to the group about him/herself. All participants fill out an evaluation and discuss each other's strengths.	18 min.		
Applies to STD programs only—curriculum strands listed on the first page of the overview form. Total minutes _____ divided by 50 _____ (Deduct coffee and lunch breaks from total time)				

Reprinted, with permission, from the U.T.M.D. Anderson Cancer Center, Houston.

Communication must also link outpatient and inpatient educational interventions. By knowing what patient education has taken place, providers in different settings can better reinforce learning and ensure continuity of teaching approaches.

☐ Evaluating the Quality and Effectiveness of Patient Education Programs

After discussing what evaluation is and why it is needed, the next sections explain the factors involved in several types of evaluation. Decisions about evaluation that need to

Louise A. Villejo, M.P.H., C.H.E.S.

Figure 13-20. Patient–Family Teaching Guide and Documentation Form for Self-Care after Gynecological Surgery

U.H.#		**Patient–Family Teaching**
Name:		**Self-care After Gyn Surgery**
D.O.B.:		The University of Texas Medical Branch at Galveston
Address:		

Initial and Date Each Entry *Denotes Nurses Note Entry — Teaching Subjects	Method				Outcome			Information Handouts
	Explanation	Audio/Visual Used/Given	Demonstration	Reinforcement	Acknowledges Understanding	Satisfactory Return/ Demonstration	Follow-up Needed	**Facts about** ( ) *Your Care After Surgery*
I. Surgical Procedure and Effects								*Questions Women Ask* ( ) *Rocking Chair Exercises*
II. ADLs Post-op								( ) *Premarin*
III. Dietary Changes								( ) *Tylenol #3*
IV. Managing Pain/Discomfort								( ) *Iron* ( ) *Surfak*
V. Vaginal Discharge								( ) *MOM*
VI. Potential Problems (decision making)								( ) *Bactrim* ( ) *Macrodantin*
VII. Health Promotion Behaviors								( ) *Pyridium*
								( ) ( )
								Pamphlets
								( ) *Breast Self-exam*
								( ) *Smart Advice for*
								Women Over 40
								( ) *Have a Mammogram* ( ) *What Is A PAP?*
								( ) ( )
								Class(es) Attended

Comments _____

_____

_____

_____

_____

Name of Translator: _____

Nurse's Initials Signature	Nurse's Initials Signature	Nurse's Initials Signature

Form 5635-Rev

Figure 13-20. (Continued)

Teaching Guide

Title: Self-care Following Gyn Surgery

Purpose: 1. To provide the patient with enabling information/skills necessary for self-care following a surgical procedure.
2. To assist the patient/family in learning the decision-making and self-management skills necessary to maintain the medical regimen.

Directions for use of Teaching Guide/Documentation Form:
1. Provide copies of appropriate printed materials to the patient for reference before teaching sessions begin.
2. Check (or write) name of FACT sheet or pamphlet in "Information Handouts" column.
3. As teaching proceeds, ask the questions listed below.
4. Evaluate patient's response based on criteria listed and document on front of form.
5. If patient cannot provide appropriate verbal feedback or demonstration, document plan for follow-up intervention(s) in "Comments" column or in nursing narrative notes.

Question	Outcome Criteria	Comments
I. What kind of surgery did you have? What effect will this have on your body?	I. **Patient will describe body part removed or repaired and effect to be expected on her body.** eg., uterus—can no longer have children or will not have monthly period.	
II. How should you manage your daily routine for the first few weeks after surgery?	II. **Patient can state 5 of the following:** • get more rest, avoid getting overtired • understand that energy levels may vary • do not lift more than 5 pounds at any time for the next 4 weeks (e.g., no grocery bags, laundry baskets, children) • keep body clean—shower or tub daily • resume the following only after discussion with doctor: —douching —driving —regular housework or work schedule —sex	
III. What changes should you make to your regular eating habits?	III. **Patient can state that she should** • eat small portions, take more frequent meals. • drink 8 glasses of water or liquids a day. • eat extra fruits/vegetables to keep bowels regular.	
IV. Tell me at least two ways that you can manage pain or discomfort.	IV. **Patient can state that she should** • take pain medication specifically as ordered • use breathing and relaxation exercises • use visualization techniques • use distraction (TV, a special activity)	
V. Tell me three things you know about your vaginal discharge.	V. **Patient can state that** • it may last 3–6 weeks. • its color may change from red to dark brownish red. • she should use pads, **not** tampons.	
VI. I'm going to name nine problems you *might* have after your surgery. For each one, tell whether you would • *call your doctor or clinic* or • *go to the nearest emergency room*	VI. **Patient can decide for each possible problem:** 1. Unexpected heavy bleeding (ER) 2. Constipation (Call MD) 3. Pain or burning when urinating (Call MD) 4. Sharp pain not relieved by medicine (ER) 5. Redness, swelling or pain around the wound size (Call MD) 6. Chest pain, difficulty breathing (ER) 7. Pain, swelling (redness) of leg or legs (ER) 8. High fever over 100°F. (ER) 9. Discharge from vagina with foul smell or itching (Call MD)	
VII. Tell me three things you can do over the next year to help prevent "female" health problems.	VII. **Patient will (if applicable)** 1. describe trick she will use to remind herself to do BSE regularly. 2. state when her next PAP test is due. 3. state when her next mammogram is due.	

SDHE/992

be made include determining the timing for evaluation, defining the parameters of the evaluation, and determining who should conduct the evaluation.

What Evaluation Is

Evaluation consists of establishing criteria and collecting information that enable a person to judge the appropriateness, effectiveness, and efficiency of a patient education program. There are numerous types and levels of evaluation, depending on the questions to be answered, the methodology used to answer them, and the goal of the evaluation.

Understanding Why Evaluation Is Needed

The most obvious and common reason for performing evaluation is to determine whether program objectives were achieved. If they were written correctly, they should provide the standard against which the program's results can be compared. Other powerful and persuasive reasons to incorporate evaluation into program development efforts are that administrators, boards of directors, staff, funding sources, and many others want to know what was accomplished by educational programs and the resources they consumed. Evaluation can serve many purposes, including:

- Demonstrating the impact of a program on the patient or target population
- Demonstrating the quality and efficiency of a program
- Determining staff and participant satisfaction with the program
- Suggesting ways to improve the program
- Justifying the program's budget or attracting additional resources
- Fulfilling grant, contract, or other requirements
- Contributing to performance assessment of staff involved in patient education
- Providing feedback for patients
- Providing feedback for health care providers and volunteers (those who make referrals and those who educate patients)
- Building administrative, staff, or community support for patient education or the hospital
- Contributing new knowledge to the field of patient education
- Enhancing job satisfaction/professional development

Evaluation of these outcomes would be very helpful in enhancing a patient education program and building support for its activities. Of the major elements of the program development cycle, however, evaluation is probably the least attended to and, to some, the least understood. It is mentioned here to emphasize that evaluation activities suited to a program's particular needs should be planned from the start. Unfortunately, evaluation is often developed as an afterthought. The long process of program planning and implementation leaves everyone hoping that the program is going well and meeting its objectives. Another problem is that PEMs usually wear many hats and are often overcommitted. They usually do not have the time, staff, funds, or expertise to conduct evaluative research. They barely have enough time to implement the program. Thus it is helpful for the PEM to decide whether he or she needs to conduct a scientifically rigorous research project or implement a simple monitoring activity to meet evaluation needs.

Practical prioritizing and decision making are in order here. Why is evaluation needed? The PEM might consider the potential purpose in the preceding list and assess what is most important to do in the limited time available. What are the resources available? Is there a School of Public Health or other related institution of higher learning in the area? Professors may be able to assist in developing an evaluation plan, and students may be able to help implement it.

Process and Impact Evaluation

Evaluation terminology can be confusing, but the levels of process and outcome have fairly common meanings. Process objectives may suggest evaluation questions such as:

- Was the patient education plan implemented consistently?
- Was it implemented correctly?
- What proportion of the target population was reached?
- How much of which resources (for example, staff time, dollars, materials) did it utilize?
- Were there any implementation problems?
- Were participating patients and families satisfied?
- Were participating staff and volunteers satisfied?

In contrast, the impact and outcome objectives may reflect such evaluation questions as:

- Did the hoped-for changes occur? These usually are changes in knowledge, attitudes and beliefs, skills, and/or behaviors that can usually be seen in the short term after patient education is provided. These changes are not always included in objectives because factors other than patient education can be so influential and because long-term follow-up would be needed to detect them.
- Was the program cost-effective?
- Were changes maintained over time?
- Did any unanticipated changes occur as a result of the program?

Determining the Timing for Evaluation

Although it is usually listed as the last of the major program development steps, evaluation considerations should emerge at the time objectives are written and should strongly influence all subsequent steps. For example, when someone wants to compare skill proficiency before patient education has been provided, it is important that the assessment of preprogram proficiency be done in such a way that it can be repeated afterward. If staff want to observe and record a patient's ability to perform a skill, record-keeping procedures must be built into the patient education plan and staff training. To be most useful, evaluation should be an ongoing process rather than a "snapshot" of program status at one point in time.

As programs evolve from planning through pilot testing, through revision and widespread implementation, evaluation shifts from being formative to summative. *Formative evaluation* is primarily process-oriented and focuses on monitoring a program in its early developmental stage so that any problems are identified and corrected as they occur. As experience with the program grows and formative data indicate successful implementation, emphasis may be placed on *summative evaluation*, in which program outcome is of primary interest. Formative evaluations will become less frequent and less intense, but will never be phased out completely. Evaluation should be integrated into a program for as long as that program is implemented.

The timing of data collection for evaluative purposes varies from program to program. Options for data collection include:

- Prior to provision of patient education. Unless a randomly assigned control group is available for comparison, it is usually necessary to determine the target population's level of knowledge, practices, and so on before the program. Identifying these levels will help determine the gap between their preprogram status and the level of achievement specified in the objectives.
- During provision of patient education. Monitoring the process is best done as education occurs. Some of the ways to record this process were discussed in the earlier

section on documentation. It is sometimes possible to collect monitoring information retrospectively, but completeness and accuracy are more likely in close proximity to the teaching itself.

- At the end of a patient education intervention, or shortly thereafter. Immediate changes in knowledge, attitudes, and behaviors can usually be detected at this point.
- At one or more follow-up points, which may be weeks, months, or years after patient education has been provided. This may be important for many different reasons:
  - Determining whether learning was transferred from one setting to another (for example, home to hospital, hospital to home)
  - Detecting any delay in effect (for example, the adoption of a behavior several weeks after discharge, when a patient might be feeling better and be taking more responsibility for self-management behaviors)
  - Identifying decay in effect (for example, initial increases in knowledge are lost as time passes)
  - Tracking patterns of service utilization, which tend to spread out over time

To determine timing, it is important to look at the objectives and questions that form the framework for the evaluation and think about when the best time will be to collect data. Published literature and the input of knowledgeable colleagues should be used to make this decision.

Defining the Parameters of an Evaluation

Within the many reasons to evaluate and the numerous process and impact considerations that can be included in an evaluation, a program evaluation should be focused so that the program ultimately makes use of the data collected and collects only what it will be able to use. A natural starting point is the objectives, which, if properly written, can serve as a framework for determining the questions to be answered and the approaches utilized to answer them. Following are some of the decisions that must be made to guide the development, conduct, and application of a program evaluation:

- What is needed and needs to be known about the program in order to make decisions about it?
- Who are the audiences for evaluation of the results, and what questions will they want to have answered? Not everyone will be primarily interested in program impact; some will be more concerned about the amount of time the program took, the amount of visibility it achieved, or whether participants were satisfied.
- What source(s) of data must be tapped to answer these questions, and what is the best data collection method, given the resources available? Whenever possible, it is preferable to locate existing sources of information rather than to collect original data. When needed data do not exist, direct measures (for example, test results, trained observations) should be developed rather than utilizing patient self-reports, whether in person, by phone, or on written questionnaires. The goal is to gather the best-quality data possible, balanced against feasibility and cost.
- What will the standards be for making judgments about the program? Evaluation results are not meaningful if they are simply reported statistically. Interpretation is important but should be based on a predetermined standard for comparison. How will it be known whether a program was a success? What kind of response determines satisfaction?

Determining Who Should Conduct the Evaluation

Determining who should conduct the evaluation depends on resources (for example, availability of skilled personnel and time) and political considerations (for example, Who is interested in the results? Who has credibility?). It is usually more practical, cost-efficient, and desirable to have in-house staff evaluate programs; if the PEM feels that he or she lacks evaluation expertise, other hospital staff may be able to help. There may be individuals in the local area—university faculty or students, for example—who could become involved in the program as a special project. If resources are available and a rigorous approach is desired, an outside evaluator might be hired, especially if there is concern that the results might be skewed if generated by the same people with an investment in the success of their programs. A mixed model—using hospital staff plus a consultant to provide counsel and technical assistance for aspects of the evaluation that may require expertise not accessible in their settings—works well for many patient educators. The result should be information that guides the PEM in making decisions about a program (for example, whether to continue, change, or expand it) and guides other decision makers who affect the program (for example, those who decide whether to provide institutional, staff, or financial support).

☐ Conclusion

Designing a patient education program for a specific target population must be sufficiently fluid to reach from hospital to home, but also provide the information and skills necessary to develop a confident, autonomous patient and family unit that is comfortable functioning outside a health care setting. Keys to the success of a population-based patient education program include involvement in all phases of the program by the target population and hospitalwide support from upper-level administration to management to staff. Also vital to success are the patience, perseverance, skills, and resources to move through the program planning process, as outlined in this chapter. The outcome of this process will be empowered patients and families who are able to function confidently both within and outside the health care environment.

References

1. What is the educational model of health care? International Patient Education Resource Sheet. Rockville, MD: International Patient Education Council, 1990, catalog number: RS9005.

2. Lerman, B., and Kobernick, M. S. Return visits to the emergency department. *Journal of Emergency Medicine* 5(5):3359–62, Sept.–Oct. 1987.

3. Feher, M. D., Grout, P., Kennedy, A., Elkeles, R. S., and Touquet, R. Hypoglycemia in an inner-city accident and emergency department: a 12-month survey. *Archives of Emergency Medicine* 6(3):183–88, Sept. 1989.

4. Powers, R. D. Emergency department patient literacy and the readability of patient-directed materials. *Annals of Emergency Medicine* 17(2):124–26, Feb. 1988.

5. Bone, L. R., Mamon, J., Levine, D. M., Walrath, J. M., Nanda, J., Gurley, H. T., Noji, E. K., and Ward, E. Emergency department detection and follow-up of high blood pressure: use and effectiveness of community health workers. *American Journal of Emergency Medicine* 7(1):16–20, Jan. 1989.

6. Kernich, C., and Robb, G. Development of a stroke family support and education program. *Journal of Neuroscience Nursing* 20(3):193–97, June 1988.

7. Lewis, F. The impact of cancer on the family: a critical analysis of the research literature. *Patient Education and Counseling* 8(3):269–89, Sept. 1986.

8. Fleming, S. Supporting the family's role in patient recovery, rehabilitation. *Promoting Health* 8(1):1–12, Jan.–Feb. 1987.

9. Green, L., and Kreuter, M. *Health Promotion Planning: An Education and Environmental Approach.* Mountain View, CA: Mayfield Publishing Company, 1991.

10. Green, L., and others. Selection of educational strategies. *Health Education Planning: A Diagnostic Approach*. Mountain View, CA: Mayfield Publishing Company, 1980, pp. 86–115.

11. Fredette, S. A model for improving cancer patient education. *Cancer Nursing* 13(4):207–15, 1990.

Bibliography

This chapter has provided an overview of the principles, steps, and considerations involved in the design of patient education programs for specific populations. For further information, readers are referred to the bibliography at the end of the book, especially to the section on Target Population Patient Education Programs, and the section that lists Books. The following references will be useful to those who are specifically interested in program evaluation.

Evaluating the Quality and Effectiveness of Patient Education Programs

Aday, L. *Designing and Conducting Health Surveys*. San Francisco: Jossey-Bass, 1989.

Campbell, D., and Stanley, J. *Experimental and Quasi-Experimental Designs for Research*. Chicago: Rand McNally, 1966.

Cook, T., and Campbell, D. *Quasi-Experimentation Design and Analysis Issues for Field Settings*. Boston: Houghton Mifflin, 1979.

Eddy, M., and Coslow, B. Preparation for ambulatory surgery: a patient education program. *Journal of Post Anesthesia Nursing* 6(1):5–12, Feb. 1991.

Flay, B., and Best, J. Design problems in evaluating health behavior programs. *Evaluation and the Health Professions* 5:43–69, Mar. 1982.

Green, L., and Lewis, F. *Measurement and Evaluation in Health Education and Health Promotion*. Palo Alto, CA: Mayfield Publishing Company, 1986.

Lorig, D., and González, V. The integration of the theory with practice: a 12-year case study. *Health Education Quarterly* 19(3):355–68, Fall 1992.

Morris, L., Fitz-Gibbon, C., and Herman, J. Program Evaluation Kit. Nine volumes. Newbury Park, CA: Sage Publications, 1987.

Mullen, P., and Iverson, D. Qualitative methods for evaluative research in health education programs. *Journal of Health Education* 13(3):11–18, May–June 1982.

Rossi, P., and Freeman, H. *Evaluation: A Systematic Approach*. 2nd edition. Beverly Hills, CA: Sage Publications, 1982.

Ruzicki, D. Evaluation: it's what you do with what you've got that counts. *Promoting Health* 6(5):6–8, Sept.–Oct. 1985.

Windsor, R., Baranowski, D., and others. *Evaluation of Health Promotion and Education Programs*. Palo Alto, CA: Mayfield Publishing Company, 1984.

Chapter 14

Using the Research Base to Improve Program Design

Patricia Dolan Mullen, Dr.P.H.

☐ Objectives

The reader will be able to:

- Discuss research that evaluates the effectiveness of patient education and counseling programs
- Use research results to plan more effective programs
- Evaluate research reviews

☐ How Research Affects Patient Education

Recognition of the important role that patients play in managing their own chronic illnesses and acute conditions has prompted numerous studies evaluating patient education programs. It has become increasingly important to clarify and summarize what is known about patient education. Third-party payers and administrators need to know whether patient education works and, if so, how much it will cost. When clinicians refer their patients for patient education programs, they need to know whether the education will increase the patients' chances of recovery or help them regain their independence. Patient education practitioners need to know what works best, and for which patients.

In the past, dispersion of study reports in journals and theses of the various behavioral and health sciences has made this literature difficult to track. Differing methods of measurement and reporting have further complicated the task of summarizing the research. Fortunately, numerous recent reviews of patient education studies have made use of more reliable and appropriate techniques for assessing study findings.[1-3]

This chapter reviews research in patient education. It summarizes what is known from patient education research that will help practitioners prove that patient education programs accomplish their goals and improve programs already in place. And it covers some of the research into the overall effects of patient education as well as patient education efforts aimed at specific patient groups.

The reviews that served as the data base for this chapter can best be viewed as just a few of the pieces of a puzzle. The pieces that are missing include more diverse diagnoses, research on highly prevalent conditions, research with other populations deserving high priority, comparison of patient education techniques and approaches, investigation of state-of-the-art educational interventions, and stronger data on which to estimate both short- and long-term effects.

☐ The Research Data Base

The data base consisted of 16 reviews published since 1981 of various studies that measured the impact of education and counseling in health care settings on behavior and/or other clinically significant variables for patients with chronic or acute conditions. These reviews were found through consultation with experts in patient education and from a search of computerized data bases. Eleven of the reviews were of studies conducted for either specific (asthma, arthritis, coronary heart disease, diabetes, and hypertension) or mixed chronic conditions. Four reviews focused on studies of education and counseling for individuals with acute conditions, painful procedures, surgery, and pregnancy; and one review was for a broad set of chronic conditions, addictive behaviors, and weight management. Table 14-1 (p. 316–321) lists the criteria used to select the studies that were reviewed, the method used to analyze study findings, the behavioral and/or clinical outcomes measured, the number of studies reviewed, and the overall findings of the review.

Techniques Used

Most of the reviews used quantitative techniques known as meta-analysis to represent the findings of individual studies and to combine those findings. Such techniques also have been used recently in the medical literature to summarize the results of clinical trials, and they can be very helpful in measuring diverse outcomes with a common yardstick.[4] In a meta-analysis, the test of each dependent variable yields an estimate of effect size. (The prototypical formula is the difference between the posttest mean of the experimental and control groups divided by the pooled standard deviation of the two groups.) An effect size can be interpreted as the change, in standard deviation units, attributable to the experimental intervention.

The advantage of effect sizes is apparent when it is recalled that *statistical significance* is a function of number of subjects and effect. Thus, a 10-point difference in the percentage of patients in the control and experimental groups whose blood pressure is under control may not be statistically "significant" if the number of subjects is small. On the other hand, with a very large number of subjects, a small and clinically insignificant difference in blood pressure control might well be statistically significant. This can become a problem when the reviewer relies on significance tests and simply counts how many studies had "significant results." If the studies have few subjects, for example, as in the case of many of the studies of arthritis patient education reviewed,[5] the reviewer using significance tests to gauge the study results might wrongly conclude that the intervention programs did not have an effect. The opposite problem could occur in interpreting the results of very large studies. Thus, relying on significance tests is not recommended.

As an alternative to significance tests, effect sizes pose a problem of interpretation for those not accustomed to thinking in standard deviation units. One way that an effect size can be interpreted is illustrated by the following example. In the review by Brown[6] of controlled studies of patient education for persons with diabetes, the average effect size in standard deviation units was 0.41 improvement for glycosylated hemoglobin. Assuming that the control population has a near-normal distribution for most health parameters, a 0.41 average improvement for diabetic control indicates that the average patient who receives education will demonstrate a physiologic response to therapy better than 66 percent of control patients. (This translation is accomplished by looking up 0.41 in a standard or cumulative normal distribution table found in most statistics books.)

Another way to look at the 0.41 standard deviation improvement is to impose this number on real data. For example, Mazzuca used such a procedure with data from a diabetes research and training center.[7] In his group's data, the mean fasting blood glucose was 233 mg/dl, with the standard deviation of 101 mg/dl. Using the 0.41 standard deviation improvement, it can be anticipated that these patients would lower their mean fasting blood glucose to 192 mg/dl (that is, 233 − [0.41 × 101]). Mazzuca noted that this value of 192 mg/dl exceeds the limits of normal for diagnosed diabetics, but pointed out that under routine care only about 18 percent of patients reach the criterion value of 140 mg/dl or lower. With an education program this percentage of patients under control would nearly double.

☐ Average Effects of Patient Education and Counseling

Overall, the reviews concluded that education and counseling can significantly affect the activities and health status of people with chronic and acute conditions. Although some outcomes were based on self-report, for example, self-reported adherence to a dietary regimen or self-reported distress, other effects were more objective, such as blood pressure, glucose control, and hospitalization. On average, the effects were positive and clinically significant. However, a few reviewers questioned the findings, or acknowledged their limitations, and made recommendations for future research.

Goodall and Halford, for example, pointed out that when a physiologic outcome is measured, for example, glycemic control for studies of people with diabetes, and self-management is not measured, it is not clear that the cause of any improvement observed is the self-management per se.[8] (See Lorig and others[9] and chapter 15, which notes the lack of analysis of the relationship between behavior [compliance] and health outcome.)

It is possible that cases showing small effects on physiologic measures are the result of inappropriate regimens or intervening factors that reduce the effectiveness of self-management. However, a review of 19 programs developed to teach self-management skills to children with asthma and their parents concluded that improvements can be attributed to self-management. When self-management skills were practiced, the children, together with their parents, made several positive contributions to preventing and controlling asthma attacks and reducing financial and social costs associated with the disorder.[10]

Some reviewers noted limitations on the sensitivity of measures for populations with chronic illnesses, for example, pain scales for people with arthritis.[11] This may limit the effect that can be demonstrated. The strong average effects reported most often were from studies with short-term follow-up, making it difficult to estimate how much of the short-term success will be maintained over long-term regimens for chronic conditions.[12,13]

In the reviews of studies on the effect of patient education on acute conditions, the evidence is very strong for a consistent and clinically significant effect. The strongest application is in the preparation of adults for surgery. Devine and Cook's review of this area not only showed a significant effect, but it also was particularly careful in evaluating the effects of factors that might unduly influence the study results. Thus the conclusions drawn from their review are highly credible.[14]

An important feature of the surgery preparation literature is the emphasis on measures with cost-saving potential, including shorter length of stay and fewer complications. Devine and Cook are cautious regarding conclusions about length of stay, because of the dramatic economic pressures that have been brought to bear on this indicator in recent years. Nevertheless, any erosion of the effect on length of stay is offset by the reduction in complications, a highly relevant outcome from both patient and hospital perspectives.

Table 14-1. Reviews of Primary Studies on the Impact of Patient Education and Counseling on Behavior and Clinical Outcomes

Diagnosis	Study Selection Criteria	Analysis Method	Outcomes	Number of Studies	Findings[a]	Citation
I. Chronic Conditions						
Arthritis	Studies, 1981–86, with a control group and reporting usable data measuring pain, depression, and/or disability; n = 10	Meta-analysis: average effect sizes in standard deviation units, 95% confidence intervals	Pain	11	+0.21* (CI=.08,.33)	Mullen, Laville, Biddle, and Lorig, 1987
			Depression	11	+0.28* (CI=.15,.42)	
			Disability	13	+0.09 (CI=−.03,.21)	
Arthritis	Studies, 1970–87, with a control group measuring knowledge, behavior, psychological status, and/or health status	Percent of studies with statistically significant changes	Exercise, relaxation, joint protection, other behaviors	28	77%	Lorig, Konkol, and González, 1987
			Depression, mood, coping, other psychosocial behaviors	32	61%	
			Pain, disability, depression, other health status	?	61%	
Asthma	Studies, 1972–87, measuring the effect of education and self-management programs on children's asthma	Narrative discussion	Pulmonary function	19 Total		Wigel and others, 1990
			Medication taking, other self-management behaviors			Creer and others, 1990
			Use of health services			
			School attendance, activities			

Condition	Description	Measure	Outcome	N	Effect size	Source
Coronary heart disease	Studies, 1971–88, with a control group measuring the effect of patient education on behavior and health status	Meta-analysis: average effect sizes in standard deviation units, 95% confidence intervals	Exercise	12	+0.18* (CI=.07,.29)	Mullen, Mains, and Velez, in press
			Diet	9	+0.19* (CI=.05,.34)	
			Smoking	9	+0.07 (CI=−.08,.22)	
			Medication	3	−0.09 (CI=−.39,.22)	
			Morbidity	9	+0.05 (CI=−.04,.13)	
			Return to work	6	+0.08 (CI=−.11,.27)	
			Death	7	+0.24* (CI=.14,.33)	
			Blood pressure	5	+0.51* (CI=.24,.77)	
Diabetes mellitus	Studies, 1976–86, with a control group measuring knowledge, psychological status, compliance, and/or metabolic control; − 5 subjects/group	Meta-analysis: average effect sizes in standard deviation units, 95% confidence intervals	Physical	71	+0.60 (CI=−.05,1.25)	Padgett, Mumford, Hynes, and Carter, 1988
			• Didactic	5	+0.36* (CI=.16,.56)	
			• Enhanced education	17	+0.62* (CI=.23,1.01)	
			• Diet instruction	12	+0.31* (CI=.12,.50)	
			• Exercise instruction	5	+0.50 (CI=−.19,1.19)	
			• Self-monitoring instruction	10	+0.60* (CI=−.19,1.19)	
			• Social learning/ behavior modification	7	+0.60* (CI=.29,.91)	
			• Counseling	5	+0.39* (CI=.15,.63)	
			• Relaxation training	0	+0.28 (CI=.30,.90)	

Table 14-1. (Continued)

Diagnosis	Study Selection Criteria	Analysis Method	Outcomes	Number of Studies	Findings[a]	Citation
Diabetes mellitus	Studies, 1954–88, with a control group measuring knowledge, psychological status, self-care behavior, and/or metabolic control	Meta-analysis: average effect sizes in standard deviation units, 95% confidence intervals	Weight control	28	+0.17* (CI=-.08,.27)	Brown, 1990
			Dietary compliance	15	+0.57* (CI=-.44,.70)	
			Glycosylated Hg	27	+0.41* (CI=.31,.52)	
			Blood sugar	28	+0.34* (CI=.25,.43)	
			Urine sugar	5	+0.39* (CI=-.15,.63)	
			Insulin dose	10	+0.16* (CI=.03,.28)	
			Cholesterol	9	+0.24* (CI=.09,.38)	
			Blood pressure	3	+0.34* (CI=.14,.55)	
			Medical care	6	+0.35* (CI=.21,.50)	
			Psychological	14	+0.27* (CI=.12,.42)	
Diabetes	Studies, 1983–87, with a control group measuring a glycemic control	Percent studies with statistically significant change	Glucose control			Goodall and Halford, 1991
			• Information giving ±peer support groups	5	0%	
			• Skills training + feedback + didactic	4	100%	
			• Behavioral for weight loss	4	100%	

Condition	Description	Method	N	Outcome	Effect	Citation
Hypertension	Published studies, 1977–83, funded by the National Heart, Lung, and Blood Institute, with control groups measuring the effect of patient education on adherence and blood pressure control	Narrative review	7	Adherence, blood pressure control	Interventions with active patient themes, contingency contracting, and home visits were more effective than fear arousal or didactic. Mix of strategies was the most successful.	Garrity and Garrity, 1985
Chronic disease, general	Studies, 1961–80, with a control group and reporting usable data measuring the effect of patient education on adherence, therapeutic progress, and/or long-range health outcomes	Meta-analysis: median effect sizes in the standard deviation units	18 Total 13 Total 5 Total	Adherence • Didactic • Behavioral Therapeutic progress • Didactic • Behavioral Long-range health outcomes • Didactic • Behavioral	+0.26 +0.64* +0.18 +0.74* +0.19 +0.31*	Mazzuca, 1982
Chronic disease with medication regimes	Published studies, 1961–84, with controlled designs measuring the effect of patient education on knowledge and adherence to a regimen that included drugs	Meta-analysis: average effect sizes in standard deviation units, 95% confidence intervals	55	Adherence, health status	+0.37* (CI=.31,.43) Largest effects were for interventions with highest ratings on principles of education, regardless of communication channel	Mullen, Green, and Persinger, 1985
Chronic disease, general	Studies, 1961–81, with controlled designs measuring the effect of patient teaching on knowledge, adherence, physical well-being, psychological well-being, and self-care	Meta-analysis: average effect sizes in standard deviation units	2 ? 4	Psychological well-being Self-care Physical well-being	+0.59* +0.55* +0.43*	McCain and Lynn, 1990

Table 14-1. (Continued)

Diagnosis	Study Selection Criteria	Analysis Method	Outcomes	Number of Studies	Findings[a]	Citation
II. Acute Conditions						
Painful procedures	Studies, 1962–86, with a control group measuring the effects of pain management techniques on children's behavioral, self-report, and/or physiologic response	Meta-analysis: Fisher's combined test and effect size estimated as r	Behavioral, including verbal and nonverbal body reactions	21	+0.82[b]*	Broome, Lillis, and Smith, 1989
			Self-reported distress	9	+0.68*	
			Physiologic distress, for example, galvanic skin response	11	+0.60*	
Pregnancy	Studies, 1960–81, with a control group measuring the effect of childbirth education on the parent–infant relationship	Meta-analysis: average effect sizes in standard deviation units	Behavioral • Women • Men	27 Total	+0.44* +0.54* +0.31*	Jones, 1986
Surgery	Studies, 1963–83, with a control group measuring the effect of preoperative instruction on physiologic and/or psychophysiologic variables in adults	Meta-analysis: average effect size in standard deviation units, variance	Physiologic outcomes Psychologic outcomes Psychophysiologic outcomes	64 Total	+0.47* (CI=−.59,1.53)[c] +0.27 (CI=−.87, 1.41) +0.28* (CI=−.53,1.09)	Hathaway, 1986
III. Mixed Chronic Conditions, Addictive Behaviors, Weight						
Surgery	Studies, 1961–83, with a control group measuring effect of psychoeducation on adults hospitalized for elective surgery, measuring recovery, pain, and/or psychological well-being	Meta-analysis: average effect size in standard deviation units, 95% confidence intervals	Recovery Pain, including amount of analgesic, pain scales	73 51	+0.50* (CI=.41,.59) +0.39* (CI=.30,.48)	Devine and Cook, 1986

Mixed chronic conditions, addictive behaviors, weight	Studies, 1968-71, measuring the effects of contingency contracting on behavior	Narrative discussion	Psychological well-being	36	+0.40* (CI=.22,.58)
			Length of stay, medical complications (published 1979–83)	6	+0.54* (CI=−.54,1.64)[d]
			Weight change	5	The studies demonstrate at least short-term positive effects
			Smoking cessation	2	
			Alcohol use	1	
			Drug use	3	
			Renal disease regimen	2	
			Blood pressure control	1	

Janz, Becker, and Hartman, 1983

a = + (plus) indicates improvement in the experimental group on the outcome.
b = Confidence Interval calculated by author, based on reported corrected variance.
c = Confidence Interval calculated by author, based on reported standard deviation.
d = Average effect size estimated by author, based on Fisher's combined test and effect expressed as r.
* = $p \leq 0.05$, statistically significant difference.

Fewer studies have been done on preparation of children undergoing painful procedures. However, this appears to be an area with good potential for effectiveness in improving behavior and reducing distress.

For three of the four reviews of educational programs for acute conditions, short-term outcomes are appropriate, moderate, and positive. Overall, the numerous studies that have been conducted to reduce pain and other negative postsurgical outcomes have shown consistently positive results. However, in such cases, the main problems with estimating how well the interventions to reduce pain would work in another population are whether usual staff care givers could execute the intervention as well as specially trained staff under the close scrutiny of an experiment.

The results of the reviews discussed above did not discriminate state-of-the-art patient education and counseling from programs that would not stand up to scrutiny by knowledgeable practitioners such as Neufeld.[15] Reviewers often criticized the types of patient education programs that were tested and called for both stronger interventions and those that more closely followed patient education theory. For example, Janz and her colleagues looked at studies of contingency contracting.[16] Despite weaknesses in some of the studies, the consistency with which the reviewers found moderate and positive effects makes a conservative case for the effectiveness of patient education. Practitioners planning patient education programs should consult authoritative sources regarding specific educational techniques.

☐ Relative Effectiveness of Specific Types of Patient Education

Some reviewers who attempted to compare different types of education programs were unsuccessful in finding sufficient numbers of studies of similar programs that could be grouped for analysis.[17] Even though those who did explored different aspects of the interventions, their reviews are helpful in suggesting directions for effective programming.[18-23]

Principles of education—namely *individualization of education, explicit feedback on learning* or *clinical progress*, and *reinforcement* (other than feedback)—are associated with the larger effects on behavior and clinical progress.[24-26] Other educational principles also measured and found to have an effect were *enabling a patient to take action or removing barriers to action; relevance of the education to the needs, interests, and abilities of the learner;* and *use of multiple communication channels for conveying information.* These principles have a long history in patient education, and they are predictors of intervention effect, despite the type of communication medium used, whether interpersonal or audiovisual media.[27,28] Patient package inserts (inserts included with medication) were the only channel of information found to have no effect on patient behavior or clinical progress regarding medication regimens for individuals with chronic conditions.[29]

One other review designed to investigate the relative effectiveness of various communication media found that few of the studies actually provided for a valid test of the communication medium.[30] Another finding consistent with the principles of education is that programs relying exclusively on information approaches designed to increase knowledge consistently showed lesser effects than those with behavioral and skill-training approaches.[31-33] An exception was from a review of interventions for cardiac patients where behavioral emphasis was not significantly associated with outcome.[34] This may have been the result of including in the didactic group relatively intensive interventions that were neither behavioral nor instructional. These interventions focused, instead, on feelings and used group therapy.

Mazzuca found a clear advantage for behavioral intervention programs over didactic programs for people with diabetes.[35] He concluded that a patient education program "conceived and designed to help patients cope with their unique self-management plan is much more likely to improve the course of chronic disease than is a standard presentation of medical facts and treatment rules which all hypertensives, or all diabetics, or all asthmatics should know."[36]

Behavioral approaches do not necessarily develop real self-management. Instead, they may emphasize adherence to a set treatment or recovery regimen. Thus newer types of self-management studies emphasize decision-making skills and self-confidence in management ability. As expressed by one group of reviewers, the most successful arthritis self-management programs seemed to be those that used "an interactive, experimental approach with emphasis on developing a daily routine of self-management activities."[37] This was termed the *active patient theme* by Garrity and Garrity in their review of hypertension education programs, and they viewed it as a promising theme for improving adherence and blood pressure control.[38] However, they acknowledge that it is not fully clear what makes this intervention approach work. It may be that the shift of responsibility to the patient or some other element, such as increased interest or support on the part of the health care provider, improved teaching of the skills, or patients' anticipation of rewards.

The relative advantage observed for behavioral approaches does not imply that there is no place for relevant health information. Indeed, didactic methods appear to be supportive of self-management activities when they are used in combination with behavioral techniques.

The reviewers who looked at studies of contingency contracting found that most of them were conducted with motivated volunteers rather than random samples of some defined population.[39] The intervention evidently was not acceptable to substantial numbers of potential subjects. The reviewers reported that many patients declined participation in the studies included in their review. This seems to limit the broad-scale application of contingency contracting, but might suggest its usefulness as an optional component of a patient education program.

In summary, for those reviews where sufficient numbers of studies evaluating specific types of patient education programs could be found, there is support for several conclusions. Adherence to principles of education as previously described results in larger effects. A cognitive approach by itself is not effective, and it is best to combine cognitive with behavioral techniques. Behavioral techniques such as feedback and reinforcement are among the principles of education. No single channel of communication is inherently superior to other channels.

☐ Considerations in Evaluating Reviews

Based on guidelines and evaluation criteria described by several authors, the reader of a research review should ask the following questions:[40-44]

1. What was the purpose of the review? Or put another way, what question(s) did the reviewer try to answer? The question or hypothesis should be stated clearly. Although it can sometimes be useful to focus on the average effect of a broad group of patient education and counseling programs, it is generally more helpful to also ask the question, Which approaches work better and with whom?

2. Were the criteria for including/excluding studies stated? This is as important as knowing which patients were studied in a clinical trial. The reviewer should also give a rationale for the criteria so that the reader can evaluate the wisdom and consequences of the choices.[45,46]

3. How were the relevant studies located? Did the reviewer conduct a systematic search that is fully described in the report? Did he or she look systematically and search beyond computerized data bases, for example, ask experts in the field and look at the bibliographies of articles already retrieved?

4. Did the reviewer code or otherwise make note of study characteristics that might influence the results? Important characteristics include study design, sample, and measures.[47,48] Analysis of specific aspects of a given patient education intervention

is especially important when the reviewer has used a broad definition of patient education and counseling for including studies.[49] Ideally, an intervention is examined along several dimensions, for example, contact frequency and duration; communication channel(s), including one-on-one and group education, media, and so forth; use of specific educational techniques such as social support and self-monitoring; educational orientation, didactic or cognitive and behavioral; and adherence to principles of education.[50,51]

5. Did the reviewer represent each relevant study finding with a common metric, for example, standard deviation units, and avoid reliance on tests of significance? Although reviewers who use techniques of meta-analysis sometimes use inappropriate techniques or replace thinking with numeric hocus-pocus, much is to be gained from their proper and thoughtful application.

6. Did the reviewer look at conceptually different effects (dependent variables) separately? It is not a good idea to combine highly different effects, such as, for example, measures of knowledge and attitude change and behavioral change.

7. Did the reviewer examine the distribution of findings, paying close attention to the lessons that could be learned from those that were extremely positive or negative? Average effects should not be reported unless they come from a similar range. Much can be learned from looking at dissimilar findings, although a reviewer should guard against the tendency to look only at positive findings.

8. Does the review attempt to interpret the findings and pursue the whys in depth? It is not sufficient to rely solely on numeric data as if they speak for themselves.

☐ Conclusion

This data base of 16 reviews of several hundred primary studies evaluating patient education and counseling across numerous diseases and acute conditions demonstrates that patient education yields positive behavioral and health status changes. More effective programs appear to follow basic principles of education (relevance, reinforcement, feedback, facilitation, and multiple channels), emphasize self-management, and teach behavioral skills.

References

1. Cook, T. D., and Leviton, L. C. Reviewing the literature: a comparison of traditional methods with meta-analysis. *Journal of Personality* 48(4):449-72, 1980.

2. Glass, G. V., McGaw, B., and Smith, M. L. *Meta-Analysis in Social Research.* Beverly Hills, CA: Sage Publications, 1981.

3. Light, R. J., and Pillemer, D. B. *Summing Up: The Science of Reviewing Research.* Cambridge, MA: Harvard University Press, 1984.

4. Hedges, L. V., and Olkin, I. *Statistical Methods for Meta-Analysis.* Orlando, FL: Academic Press, 1985.

5. Mullen, P. D., Laville, E. A., Biddle, A. K., and Lorig, K. Efficacy of psychoeducational interventions on pain, depression, and disability in people with arthritis: a meta-analysis. *Rheumatology* 14(S15):33–39, 1987.

6. Brown, S. A. Studies of educational interventions and outcomes in diabetic adults: a meta-analysis revisited. *Patient Education and Counseling* 16:189–215, 1990.

7. Mazzuca, S. A. Does patient education in chronic disease have therapeutic value? *Chronic Disease* 35:521–29, 1982.

8. Goodall, T. A., and Halford, W. K. Self-management of diabetes mellitus: a critical review. *Health Psychology* 10(1):1–8, 1991.

9. Lorig, K., Konkol, L., and González, V. Arthritis patient education: a review of the literature. *Patient Education and Counseling* 10:207–52, 1987.

10. Wigal, J. K., Creer, T. L., Kotses, H., and Lewis, P. A critique of 19 self-management programs for childhood asthma: part II. Development and evaluation of the programs. *Pediatric Asthma, Allergy, and Immunology* 4(1):17–39, 1990.

11. Lorig and others.

12. Goodall and Halford.

13. Mullen and others, 1987.

14. Devine, E. C., and Cook, T. D. Clinical and cost-saving effects of psychoeducational interventions with surgical patients: a meta-analysis. *Research in Nursing and Health* 9:89–105, 1986.

15. Neufeld, V. R. Patient education: a critique. In: D. L. Sackett and R. D. Haynes, editors. *Compliance with Therapeutic Regimens.* Baltimore: The Johns Hopkins University Press, 1976, pp. 83–92.

16. Janz, N. K., Becker, M. H., and Hartman, P. E. Contingency contracting to enhance patient compliance: a review. *Patient Education and Counseling* 5(4):165–78, 1983.

17. Goodall and Halford.

18. Garrity, T. F., and Garrity, A. R. The nature and efficacy of intervention studies in the national high blood pressure education research program. *Hypertension* 3(1):S91–S95, 1985.

19. Lorig and others.

20. Mazzuca.

21. Mullen, P. D., Green, L. W., and Persinger, G. Clinical trials of patient education for chronic conditions: a comparative meta-analysis of intervention types. *Preventive Medicine* 14:753–81, 1985.

22. Mullen, P. D., Mains, D. A., and Velez, R. A meta-analysis of controlled trials of cardiac patient education. *Patient Education and Counseling* 19:143–62, 1992.

23. Padgett, D., Mumford, E., Hynes, M., and Carter, R. Meta-analysis of the effects of educational and psychosocial interventions on management of diabetes mellitus. *Journal of Clinical Epidemiology* 41(10):1007–30, 1988.

24. Mullen, P. D., and Green, L. W. Educating patients about drugs. *Promoting Health* 6:6–8, 1985.

25. Mullen and others, 1985.

26. Mullen and others, 1992.

27. Mullen, P. D., and Green, L. W. From theory and research to principles of education and counseling for prevention. In: R. B. Goldbloom and R. S. Lawrence, editors. *Preventing Disease: Beyond the Rhetoric.* New York City: Springer/Verlag, 1990, pp. 474–79.

28. Padgett and others.

29. Mullen and others, 1985.

30. Broome, M. E., Lillis, P. P., and Smith, M. C. Pain interventions with children: a meta-analysis of research. *Nursing Research* 38(3):154–58, May–June 1989.

31. Garrity and Garrity.

32. Goodall and Halford.

33. Mazzuca.

34. Mullen and others, 1992.

35. Mazzuca.

36. Mazzuca, p. 528.

37. Lorig and others.

38. Garrity and Garrity.

39. Janz and others.

40. Cooper, H. M. The integrative research review: a systematic approach. In: L. Bickman and D. Rog, editors. *Applied Social Research Methods Series.* Vol. 2. Beverly Hills, CA: Sage Publications, 1984.

41. Glass and others.

42. Goldschmidt, P. *Information Synthesis: A Practical Guide.* (Health Services Research and Development Document RES #29-07-110.) Washington, DC: Department of Veterans Affairs, 1984.

43. Light and Pillemer.

44. Mullen, P. D., and Ramirez, G. Information synthesis and meta-analysis. *Advances in Health Education and Promotion* 2:201–39, 1987.

45. Bryant, F. B., and Wortman, F. B. Methodological issues in the meta-analysis of quasi-experiments. *New Directions in Program Evaluation* 24:25–42, 1984.

46. Tabak, E. R., Mullen, P. D., Simons-Morton, D., Green, L. W., Mains, D. A., Eilat-Greenberg, S., and Glenday, M. The definition and yield of inclusion criteria for a meta-analysis of patient education studies in clinical services. *Evaluation and the Health Professions* 14(4):388–411, Dec. 1991.

47. Creer, T. L., Wigal, J. K., Kotses, H., and Lewis, P. A critique of 19 self-management programs for childhood asthma: part II. Comments regarding the scientific merit of the programs. *Pediatric Asthma, Allergy, and Immunology* 4(1):41–55, 1990.

48. Sackett, D. L., and Haynes, R. B. *Compliance with Therapeutic Regimens.* Baltimore: The Johns Hopkins University Press, 1976, pp. 193–260.

49. Glass and others.

50. Mullen and Green, 1990.

51. Neufeld.

Chapter 15

Using Self-Efficacy Theory in Patient Education

Kate Lorig, Dr.P.H., R.N., and Virginia M. González, M.P.H.

☐ Objectives

The reader will be able to:

- Define self-efficacy theory and differentiate it from similar theories
- Identify the importance of using self-efficacy theory in patient education
- Briefly describe some of the research on the use of self-efficacy in patient education
- Outline four specific patient education strategies for enhancing self-efficacy
- Discuss methods for implementing self-efficacy in practice

☐ Uses of Theory and Self-Efficacy Theory in Patient Education

This chapter describes the general role of theory in patient education program planning and illustrates that role through a discussion of self-efficacy theory. It defines the self-efficacy theory and discusses how research has shown this theory to be useful in predicting health behavior and behavioral change. The chapter then identifies strategies for enhancing the self-efficacy of patients and describes how self-efficacy theory may be implemented in patient education programs.

☐ The Role of Theory in Patient Education

The ultimate objectives of patient education are to improve health and to limit the effects of disease. To achieve these objectives in the most efficient and effective way, patient education managers (PEMs) must *plan* the approaches to be taken. One approach to planning proceeds from common sense or the experiences of people involved in the process. That is, the PEM may rely on the experience of a single patient educator or may include

Parts of this chapter were published previously in V. González and others. Four psychological theories and their application to patient education and clinical practice. *Arthritis Care and Research* 3(3):132–43, 1990.

other health care professionals, administrators, patients, and the general public in planning. Unfortunately, the experience guiding such a planning process is often based on an individual's personal beliefs or reflects the consensus of a group, and the resulting plan is thus limited by the knowledge and experience of the individuals involved. Depending on the quality of information on which program planning is based, the program may or may not be effective—and even if it is effective, it may not be efficient.

This is not to say that personal experience or the experiences of others should be ignored. However, consideration of *theory* can take PEMs one step beyond personal beliefs or group consensus and provide a framework within which to *integrate* or *focus* these experiences.

Theory is a set of relatively abstract and general statements that collectively purport to explain some aspect of the empirical world.[1] In other words, theory is an explanation of how or why things happen. In *Health Behavior and Health Education: Theory, Research, and Practice,* Glanz and her colleagues discuss three important criteria that a theory should meet if it is to be useful to health education practice:[2]

1. It must have been tested on health-related behavior.
2. There must be evidence of its utility in predicting or changing health behavior.
3. It must be useful to health education practitioners.

Because a theory has usually been tested in several situations, it is often a more accurate guide to program planning than are personal beliefs or group consensus. Nonetheless, theories remain tools that, like any others, must be applied more or less precisely as the situation dictates. If properly applied, theory can increase the probability of both effective and efficient patient education.

To illustrate the application of theory to patient education practice, the balance of this chapter examines self-efficacy theory. Self-efficacy theory in patient education has a strong research base, has been proven useful in changing health behaviors and health status, and, equally important, has specific strategies through which it can be integrated into patient education practice.

☐ Self-Efficacy Theory in Patient Education

Perceived self-efficacy refers to people's beliefs in their capabilities to mobilize the motivation skills, cognitive resources, and courses of action needed to meet given situational demands.[3,4] *Self-efficacy* is most simply described as an individual's confidence in his or her ability to do something. It is concerned not with actual skills, but rather with the *judgments and perceptions* of what the individual can do with the skills he or she possesses.

Self-efficacy theory states that:

- The strength of the individual's beliefs in his or her ability to achieve a specific behavior, thought, cognitive state, or emotion is a good predictor for the actual achievement of that behavior or state.
- Personal belief or self-efficacy can be enhanced through skills mastery, modeling, reinterpretation of physiological symptoms, and persuasion.
- Enhanced self-efficacy leads to improved behaviors, thoughts, cognitive states, or emotions.

Self-efficacy is behavior-specific, relating the use of specific types of performance and/or cognitive strategies to specific situations. In this way, self-efficacy differs from two related constructs: learned helplessness and locus of control.[5,6]

Learned helplessness theory asserts that a sense of helplessness occurs when people feel their actions have no effect; that is, they believe they have no control over their lives in general.

Locus of control theory refers to people's generalized perceptions of the sources of control over their lives. For example, some individuals feel that their health is controlled internally, that is, by their own behavior or actions; whereas others feel that their health is mainly determined externally, that is, by physicians, chance, or a higher power.

Both these constructs, learned helplessness and locus of control, imply that a person's feelings or perceptions can be generalized, affecting more than one aspect of his or her life across different situations. These theories differ from self-efficacy, where beliefs or expectations pertain only to the individual's ability to carry out *a specific behavior in a specific situation*. For example, a person may have very high self-efficacy for leading a small group discussion but very low self-efficacy for giving a speech before 300 people.

Self-efficacy theory deals with the individual's *perception or belief* that he or she can accomplish some future behavior. In this way it is predictive: The individual's efficacy for a given behavior becomes a predictor of actual future performance. Thus, if a circus owner had to hire a new unicycle rider quickly, self-efficacy theory would direct the owner to ask job applicants how certain they were that, given some brief instruction, they could ride a unicycle. The circus owner would do best to hire the applicant with the highest self-efficacy, because that applicant is predicted to be more likely to quickly master the art of unicycle riding.

This same principle can be applied to patients. For example, patients could be asked how certain they are, on a scale of 1 to 10, that they will exercise as directed to improve their health, with 1 being totally uncertain and 10 being very certain. Their stated level of certainty is a good predictor of actual future exercise.

In summary, self-efficacy is the individual's belief in his or her ability to perform a specific action or achieve a specific cognitive state, such as mental relaxation. There is no such thing as an "efficacious person." Rather, self-efficacy is always specific to precise behaviors. The following section examines some of the research that has demonstrated the usefulness of self-efficacy theory in working with patients.

☐ Research on Self-Efficacy in Patient Education

The self-efficacy theory has been the basis for a number of studies directly related to patient education. In one study, self-efficacy was studied as a predictor of the ability to manage pain during childbirth.[7] Women who had participated in childbirth preparation classes judged their self-efficacy for managing their labor without the use of pain medications. These judgments were made immediately after their training and during the early stages of labor. As self-efficacy theory would predict, women with higher self-efficacy for managing a medication-free labor did so more often than did women with lower self-efficacy. The amount of the medication used was negatively correlated with self-efficacy (that is, the higher the efficacy, the less medication used). Surprisingly, there were no associations between the amount of pain control training or the amount of pain control practice with the amount of medication use. In other words, neither the skills taught in the childbirth classes nor the practice of these skills were related to medication usage during labor. Instead, the correlation was strongest for those persons with higher self-efficacy for managing medication-free labor.

Another experiment studied the effects of self-efficacy on the ability of patients to control future episodes of tension headaches.[8] Patients were randomly taught one of two forms of relaxation. One technique was believed to help control tension headaches, and the other was believed not to help tension headaches.

Next, all subjects were asked to practice the technique they had been taught while being monitored by a biofeedback machine. The machine gave them random feedback unrelated to their actual state of relaxation. Subjects receiving feedback that indicated they were successfully relaxing increased their efficacy for controlling headaches, whereas subjects who were told they needed to practice relaxation more in order to become effective did not raise their efficacy.

Subjects were then followed for several months. Those having high self-efficacy for controlling tension headaches had fewer headaches than those with lower self-efficacy. Headache control was not related to the type of relaxation practiced nor to the actual success of subjects in reaching a relaxed state.

This finding suggests that (1) self-efficacy can be manipulated by feedback and (2) self-efficacy may act as a mediator of headache pain, independent of actual relaxation techniques. This latter finding is especially important because it suggests that self-efficacy predicts not only future behaviors but also future health status, in this case, how often patients will have tension headaches.

In a third study, the interaction of achievement and self-efficacy was studied in cardiac rehabilitation patients.[9] Their self-efficacy for exercise was measured before treadmill testing. Those patients with higher self-efficacy for their abilities to exercise achieved higher-peak heart rates during the treadmill test than those with lower self-efficacy for exercise.

In addition, when patients were told that they had achieved higher-peak heart rates after exercise, they had higher self-efficacy for future exercise. Finally, posttreadmill judgments of self-efficacy predicted the level and amount of future exercise, whereas treadmill peak heart rates alone did not.

This experiment demonstrates that self-efficacy predicts future behavior and levels of performance for that behavior. This finding also suggests that patient education interventions using self-efficacy theory may also be self-reinforcing; that is, success leads to enhanced efficacy, which, in turn, leads to future success.

A large program developed at Stanford in the late 1970s also helped prove the value of self-efficacy in patient education.[10] During this period, the Stanford Arthritis Center was funded by the National Institutes of Health to develop an arthritis patient education program. A needs assessment was conducted to determine what to include in the program. More than 100 persons with arthritis completed questionnaires, and 20 health care professionals with experience in treating people with arthritis were interviewed. As a result, the Arthritis Self-Management Program (ASMP) was designed.

The ASMP is a twelve-hour program given two hours a week for six weeks. Patients are taught by two trained lay leaders, usually people with arthritis. The program is held in community sites such as churches, senior centers, hospitals, or libraries. Each course is attended by approximately 15 individuals, including both people with arthritis and their significant others.

The program is taught according to a detailed protocol.[11] Program content includes an overview of osteoarthritis and rheumatoid arthritis, pain management, use of medications, design of individualized exercise programs, problem solving, patient–physician communication, and nutrition. All sessions are highly interactive and emphasize a problem-solving approach.

Because the ASMP was funded as a research project, the program has been carefully evaluated since its earliest days. From the beginning, upon applying for the course patients were randomized to either take the course immediately or serve as controls by waiting four months before taking the course. All applicants filled out self-administered questionnaires at the beginning and again four months later. These data were used to evaluate the effectiveness of the course.

In the early days, ASMP staff believed that by teaching such skills as exercise and pain management techniques, patients would in turn use these skills to reap such benefits as reduced pain and disability as well as fewer arthritis-related visits to their physicians.

Data from the first 500 people who took the course showed that the practice of specific behaviors, including pain management and exercise, had increased, whereas pain and depression had decreased.[12] In addition, there was a trend toward fewer physician visits associated with arthritis. However, using statistical tests of correlation, *no* clear association was found between the increased practice of behaviors and the decrease in pain and depression. In other words, the people who did the things they were taught were not necessarily the people who reduced their pain or depression. This was puzzling.

Because the improvements in health status were not related to behavioral changes, a qualitative study was conducted to search for a different explanation as to how the ASMP might have affected the health status of patients.[13] Twenty-five ASMP participants who had decreased their pain and 25 participants who either had no change in their amount of pain or had experienced increased pain were interviewed. However, neither participants nor interviewers knew how subjects for the study were chosen. All 50 subjects were asked how the ASMP had affected their levels of pain and to explain why their pain had either increased or decreased. People who had lessened their pain talked about having more control over their symptoms. Those people who had not decreased their pain as a result of the program talked about how nothing could be done for arthritis so there was no point in trying. Overall, this study discovered that people who had benefited from the ASMP seemed to be people who had gained a sense of *control* over their symptoms.

Based on this qualitative study, it was hypothesized that the ASMP had enhanced the participants' *self-efficacy for managing their symptoms.* Before this hypothesis could be tested, however, it was necessary to develop an arthritis-specific self-efficacy scale to measure the self-efficacy of patients both before and after the program.[14] Once the scale was developed, researchers measured self-efficacy before the ASMP and again four months later. The findings indicated that even though there had been no systematic efforts to change self-efficacy in patients, participants in the ASMP enhanced their self-efficacy; the controls, those randomized to wait four months for the course, had not. More important, increased self-efficacy, unlike increased practice of self-management behaviors, was associated with improved health status. This finding was similar to those in the childbirth and tension headache studies discussed earlier. Thus, there was further evidence that self-efficacy may be at least one mechanism by which patient education affects health status.

To further explore this finding, the Arthritis Self-Management Program was revised. Like the original program, this enhanced version was taught two hours a week for six weeks by trained lay instructors. Although the content was much the same as in the original program, endurance exercise—walking, bicycling, or swimming—was further emphasized, and a wider variety of cognitive pain management techniques was included. However, the biggest change was the systematic inclusion of self-efficacy-enhancing techniques throughout the course. These included contracting between patient and educator for behavioral change in every session, as well as exchanging feedback about the previous week's contract. Modeling was emphasized by having ASMP patient group members discuss problems and provide solutions, rather than having the leaders give all the answers. In addition, when discussing symptoms such as pain or fatigue, participants were taught that there are many causes for most symptoms and that they could do many things to manage their symptoms.

When the new ASMP was given to a new group of patients, it was found to be more effective than the original course. Pain and depression were even further reduced, as were arthritis-related outpatient visits to physicians.[15]

In a final study of the ASMP program, research staff surveyed approximately 400 participants four years after they had taken the original program. This number represented 80 percent of the original sample. They found that the gains patients had made at four months had continued and had been enhanced over the four years. Pain had been reduced by approximately 20 percent, and arthritis-related visits to physicians had been reduced by more than 40 percent. This occurred despite an expected increase in disability due to the arthritis.[16]

These findings are similar to those of the self-efficacy study with peak treadmill heart rates and future exercise. It appears that self-efficacy creates a self-reinforcing cycle in which people with enhanced efficacy are more willing to try new behaviors that, in turn, further enhance efficacy. From the ASMP studies, this self-reinforcement appears to last for at least four years.

There are at least two reasons, then, for using self-efficacy as a theoretical basis for patient education programs:

- Efficacy enhancement leads to improved health behaviors and health status.
- Self-efficacy may help to make patient education self-reinforcing.

The following section addresses strategies for enhancing self-efficacy in patient education.

☐ Strategies for Enhancing Patient Self-Efficacy

Having identified the potential usefulness of self-efficacy theory to patient education, it is important to examine the four key strategies to enhance patient self-efficacy: (1) skills mastery, (2) modeling, (3) reinterpreting physiological signs and symptoms, and (4) persuasion. These strategies should help PEMs successfully integrate the theory into actual practice.

Skills Mastery

Probably the best way to enhance self-efficacy is through *skills mastery*. Skills mastery is generally achieved by breaking goals into small, manageable tasks and then ascertaining that each small task is successfully completed. The key to skills mastery is the word *mastery*. It is very important that people be successful at or *master* whatever they are trying to do if they are to become more efficacious with regard to that behavior. To help patients increase their skill levels, each step or task in skills mastery is skill-specific and short term. The objective is to gradually increase the skill levels of patients to perform a task.

Some of the original work in skills mastery was done with agoraphobics, who gradually learned the skills to open up their personal and physical boundaries. They first walked through the door, then took a few steps, then walked to the sidewalk, and so on.

Whether planning patient education programs for specific groups or working with patients one on one, it is best to have people start with what they are sure they can master at the time. For example, the person with arthritis who can walk half a block is encouraged to do so four times a week and then to add to the distance walked, gradually increasing the distance by no more than 10 percent each week.

One of the best ways to foster skills mastery is to have patients set goals for themselves in a particular area or for a specific behavior. These may be written in the form of a self-contract in which the patient states what he or she agrees to do, or in a contract between educator and patient in which they state what they will do together. These goals provide direction and incentive for action or change.[17]

To increase effectiveness, the goal setting or contracting should be patient driven. The patient, not the educator, decides what behavior is to be mastered; this serves as a greater incentive for the individual to work toward the goal. The patient-driven contract *enhances* self-efficacy, and this differentiates it from the professionally driven contracts that are often used to enhance compliance. For example, the patient may need to lose weight and have a desire to do so. The patient educator and the patient can then list all the behaviors that lead to weight loss (daily exercise, not eating between meals, eating only at mealtime, avoiding fried foods, and so on). Then the patient chooses the specific strategies he or she wishes to use, and these are included in the contract.

The goal or contract should also be clear and specific, describing the behavior as well as the amount of effort needed to accomplish it successfully. This specificity helps the individual regulate his or her performance (for example, how often or how much of the activity to do) so that the goal is both realistic and attainable.[18,19] (For example, "I will walk four blocks five days next week before dinner.") Writing out the specific behavior in the form of a contract may also help remind the individual to practice the behavior or skill until mastered.

Equally important are opportunities for the patient to receive feedback about his or her performance and to make mid-course corrections in the contract, increasing the likelihood of mastery. For example, every session of a patient education program should begin with feedback from the previous visit or session in which the patient reports on progress toward the goal. Every session might end with a goal-setting or contracting activity in which the patient writes a contract for a specific goal. As much as 30 percent of patient education time may be necessary to provide feedback and develop contracts with patients.

If education is given on a one-to-one basis, the feedback mechanism can be formalized and documented. This can be done by noting the patient's contract in the chart and asking about it during each visit. Even more effective is a follow-up telephone call in a week to 10 days to see how work on the contract is proceeding. Effective feedback and follow-up are keys to using self-mastery to enhance patient self-efficacy.

Modeling

Another excellent way to enhance self-efficacy and change patient behavior is to provide a *model*. Allow the person attempting to change behavior to see someone else with the same problem who has been successful in achieving this change. This is the principle used by several voluntary organizations and self-help groups, including Alcoholics Anonymous. With modeling, people who have the same disease or problem are actively involved in working with other patients, be it teaching courses or providing peer counseling. This is one of the reasons why support groups of persons with common problems are so popular.

In choosing models, the patient educator should look for someone who is as much like the patient as possible. Matching age, sex, ethnic origin, and socioeconomic parameters is important.

Unfortunately, educators sometimes select the wrong types of models. For example, they sometimes select "super achievers," those people who have had problems and have overcome them in some spectacular manner. An example is the cancer patient who has had an amputation and walks across the country. Although this type of person is certainly inspirational, he or she is not always the best model for many cancer patients. These "super" achievements are not realistic goals for most people with cancer. A better model would be someone who is struggling to manage cancer and is coping "pretty well" on a day-to-day basis. This is the type of person with whom most patients can readily relate.

Several ways of using models in patient education have been tried. For example, lay instructors with the same health problem could be used. This is the model used by the Arthritis Foundation's Arthritis Self-Help Course and by the American Cancer Society's Reach to Recovery program. Given a structured curriculum, good training, and adequate professional backup, lay people experiencing the same problems as their classmates can make excellent health education instructors. Or people with related illnesses or problems can also be invited to patient education classes to talk with patients and share their own experiences.

Another way of using models is to encourage class members to help resolve problems others are having, rather than having only the instructor suggest solutions. Every time a problem is stated, the instructor should ask group members if anyone has ever had a similar problem or has any ideas about how to solve the problem. The leader can still be the expert of last resort.

This teaching strategy has several advantages. First, it teaches class members that they really are experts and have useful knowledge to share. It also teaches them that they do not always have to rely on professionals for expert help. Finally, this approach generates many innovative solutions to problems that might not always occur to professional instructors.

Patient education managers considering the use of media as part of a patient education program or in clinical practice should choose the models carefully, based on the types of clients needing the program. This includes videotapes, audiotapes, books, and pamphlets. For example, if a patient educator is teaching elderly people how to get up from the floor after falling, the pictures used should be of an older person rather than a young one. This point is not always obvious. In fact, until recently, media producers did not consider the "appropriateness" of models; rather, models were chosen for their photogenic or charismatic qualities and their experience or natural talent in front of the camera. However, for patient education it is truly important to consider the audience. When appropriate models are used, modeling can be a successful strategy for enhancing patient self-efficacy.

Reinterpretation of Physiological Signs and Symptoms

The job of patient educators is to determine what and why people believe and behave as they do and, when possible, help them change or reinterpret these beliefs regarding their illness or injury. By doing so, patient educators can help patients reinterpret their physiological signs and symptoms, change their behaviors, and increase their self-efficacy.

When judging capabilities, people rely on information from their physiological states;[20] therefore, what people believe about their problems or how they interpret symptoms can affect their self-efficacy to manage illness. For example, people with emphysema, when encouraged to exercise to improve fitness, might incorrectly interpret the increased breathing associated with exercise as a sign of worsening symptoms. Thus, as far as they are concerned, their disease prevents them from exercising. To be able to achieve the benefits of exercise, then, these people might be taught to *reinterpret* their beliefs about exercise and accompanying symptoms. For example, it might be pointed out that increased breathing occurs in everyone as exercise increases, and this is the body's normal way of getting more of the oxygen it needs.

In another example, many people with chronic disease are fatigued. They interpret this to be a symptom of the disease and thus believe that the fatigue should be treated with rest. In fact, fatigue can also result from poor nutrition, physical deconditioning, or depression. In many cases the treatment is not rest but rather improved nutrition, exercise, and/or counseling. Rest, in fact, may exacerbate the fatigue.

Determining someone's beliefs about a disease is not difficult. All the educator needs to do is ask. Among the questions that are helpful in soliciting beliefs are:

1. If you "start exercising," "take a particular medication," and so forth, what are you afraid might happen?
2. When you think of "dieting," "diabetes," and so forth, what do you think of?
3. What barriers prevent you from beginning to "lose weight" or "exercise"?

Once the belief has been identified, the patient educator can set about helping the person to reinterpret it.

When using this method, it is important not to give mixed messages. For example, for years health care professionals have told patients with osteoarthritis that it is a "wear-and-tear" disease, resulting from some behaviors. Is it, then, any wonder that these same patients are confused when told to exercise? In fact, activity helps the osteoarthritic joint remain supple and is not counterproductive.

The message must be simple, clear, and direct. Keeping the language regarding diseases and symptoms simple and explicit serves everyone's best interests. Almost any symptom can be explained as having multiple causes. When this is understood and believed by patients, they can then begin to see how symptoms may be managed by using many different approaches. Such reinterpretations allow people to view their disease and symptoms differently. This, in turn, affects their judgments about their abilities and self-efficacy to manage the disease.

Persuasion

The last way to enhance self-efficacy, and probably the method most familiar to patient educators, is to use persuasion. It is often used to get people to believe they have the capability to attain goals.[21] Verbal persuasion can help people believe it is possible for them to develop the skills needed to meet a given situation.[22]

One way patient educators and PEMs can use persuasion without arousing fear is to urge patients to do slightly more than they are now doing by setting *goals*. However, goals that are set with the patient should be short term and realistic. More important, they should be manageable and not beyond what the patients believe they can accomplish at that point in time. Thus, instead of saying, "You could lose 20 pounds if you tried," it would be better to say, "By making small changes in your diet or by increasing your exercise, you can lose 1 to 2 pounds this week." In this way, the task becomes more manageable and the goal more realistic.

Another way to use persuasion to enhance self-efficacy is through the use of small patient groups in which each member helps "persuade" other members to change behavior. Patients working together to solve problems and set goals not only model and provide support for each other but they also provide the power to influence or persuade each individual.

Furthermore, experience suggests that the individual who is resistant or has difficulty doing certain activities, such as starting to exercise, modifying a diet, or setting goals, can often be influenced by the group. After seeing his or her peers, the individual is often more willing to participate in the activity and, from this participation, is able to begin to master skills. In this way, verbal persuasion as a form of gentle encouragement or positive feedback can help increase self-efficacy.

☐ Methods for Implementing Self-Efficacy Theory in Practice

Thus far, this chapter has defined self-efficacy theory, provided examples of its use in different patient education programs, and provided information on how to incorporate efficacy-enhancing strategies into patient education programs. However, experience shows that the biggest problem in implementing efficacy-enhancing strategies is *time*. Because self-efficacy strategies emphasize process rather than content, it is impossible to include all the program content and efficacy-enhancing strategies without expanding teaching time. There are two choices to deal with this problem: (1) keep all the content and do not try to enhance efficacy, or (2) eliminate a considerable amount of the content in favor of including efficacy-enhancing strategies.

From the research and case studies presented in this chapter, there is good evidence that enhancing self-efficacy is at least as important as content knowledge when it comes to improving health status. Therefore, the preferred strategy is to cut some program content and add efficacy-enhancing strategies. As much as 50 percent of the available educational time could be used to enhance self-efficacy, 30 percent for providing feedback and developing contracts and another 10 to 20 percent for other efficacy-enhancing strategies.

This means making hard decisions about what specific content needs to be cut. Although these decisions must necessarily be based on specific situations, there are some general practical guidelines:

- *Keep the teaching of anatomy and physiology to a minimum.* People can read such information on their own time if they really want to know. For example, in a 12-hour arthritis class designed by the Stanford Patient Education Research Center, only 15 minutes are spent on joint anatomy and the types of arthritis.[23] In Stanford's 14-hour chronic disease self-management course, no anatomy or physiology is taught.[24]

- *Content should be something that patients can act on or use to make decisions.* Thus, instead of teaching everything there is to know about all medications, the arthritis self-management instructors at Stanford teach patients how to recognize side effects, to remember to take medications, and to contact their physician if, for any reason, they cannot or will not take a particular medication.
- *Don't get sidetracked by questions.* It is very important to answer patients' questions. However, some patients will ask all kinds of questions, especially if new behaviors are being taught. This is not so much because they want to know, but because it is a way of avoiding having to do something. Patients' questions can sometimes be deflected by suggesting that they be asked during the break or after class, especially if they are not of general interest. Also, by supplying good written materials, educators can suggest that patients read the information first and then come back if they still have questions. This advice is not to say that patients' questions and interactions are not important; rather, their questions must be *channeled* so as not to detract from the educational process.
- *Post an agenda with times assigned to each major topic.* When patients can see the time allotted for each topic, they are much less likely to get sidetracked. The posted agenda also allows the patient educator to point out when it is time to move on.

In summary, in order to implement self-efficacy, some program content may have to be shortened or curtailed. However, the role of self-efficacy in patient education has been well supported, and use of this approach should enhance education efforts overall.

☐ Conclusion

Self-efficacy theory deserves careful consideration in the planning and implementation of patient education programs. Self-efficacy is the individual's belief that he or she can perform some behavior or use some cognitive strategy to meet the demands of a given situation. Research with a variety of patient types has proven the worth and practical application of self-efficacy theory in patient education. Patient self-efficacy can be enhanced through skills mastery, modeling, reinterpreting physiological signs and symptoms, and persuasion.

In developing patient education programs, there will always be a trade-off between content (*what* one teaches) and process (*how* one teaches). By carefully incorporating self-efficacy theory into the program planning process, a balance can be made between imparting program content and enhancing self-efficacy. In applying this theory to patient education, emphasis should be on the teaching process rather than on including more content.

References

1. Chafetz, J. *A Primer on the Construction of Theories in Sociology.* Itasca, IL: Peacock, 1978, p. 2.

2. Glanz, K., Lewis, F. M., and Rimer, B. K. *Health Behavior and Health Education: Theory, Research, and Practice.* San Francisco: Jossey-Bass, 1990, pp. 17–32.

3. Bandura, A. Self-efficacy: toward a unifying theory of behavior change. *Psychological Review* 84(2):191–215, Mar. 1977.

4. Bandura, A. *Social Foundations of Thought and Action.* Englewood Cliffs, NJ: Prentice-Hall, 1986.

5. Seligman, M. *Helplessness: On Depression, Development, and Death.* San Francisco: W. H. Freeman, 1975.

6. Wallston, B. S., Wallston, K. A., Kaplan, G. D., and Maides, S. A. Development and validation of the health locus of control (HLC) scale. *Journal of Consulting and Clinical Psychology* 44(4):580–85, Aug. 1976.

7. Manning, M. M., and Wright, T. L. Self-efficacy expectancies, outcome expectancies, and the persistence of pain control in childbirth. *Journal of Personality and Social Psychology* 45(2):421–31, Aug. 1983.

8. Holroyd, K. A., Penzien, D. B., Hursey, K. G., Tobin, D. L., Rogers, L., Holm, J. E., Marcille, P. J., Hall, J. R., and Chila, A. G. Change mechanisms in EMG biofeedback training: cognitive changes underlying improvements in tension headache. *Journal of Consulting and Clinical Psychology* 52(6):1039–53, Dec. 1984.

9. Ewart, C. K., Taylor, C. B., Reese, L. B., and DeBusk, R. F. Effects of early post-myocardial infarction exercise testing on self-perception and subsequent physical activity. *American Journal of Cardiology* 51(7):1076–80, Apr. 1983.

10. Lorig, K., Cox, T., Cuevas, Y., Kraines, R. G., and Britton, M. C. Converging and diverging beliefs about arthritis: caucasian patients, Spanish-speaking patients and physicians. *Journal of Rheumatology* 11(1):76–79, Jan. 1984.

11. Lorig, K. *Arthritis Self-Help Leader's Manual.* Atlanta: National Arthritis Foundation, 1990.

12. Lorig, K., Seleznick, M., Lubeck, D., Ung, E., Chastain, R., and Holman, H. R. The beneficial outcomes of the arthritis self-management course are inadequately explained by behavior change. *Arthritis and Rheumatism* 32(1):91–95, Jan. 1989.

13. Lenker, S. L., Lorig, K., and Gallagher, D. Reasons for the lack of association between changes in health behavior and improved health status: an explanatory study. *Patient Education and Counseling* 6(2):69–72, Spring 1984.

14. Lorig, K., Chastain, R. L., Ung, E., Shoor, S., and Holman, H. Development and evaluation of a scale to measure perceived self-efficacy in people with arthritis. *Arthritis and Rheumatism* 32(1):37–44, Jan. 1989.

15. Lorig, K., and González, V. The integration of theory with practice: a twelve-year case study. *Health Education Quarterly* 19(3):355–68, Fall 1992.

16. Lorig and González, 1992.

17. Bandura, 1977.

18. Bandura, 1986.

19. Locke, E. A., Shaw, K. N., Saari, L. M., and Latham, G. P. Goal-setting and task performance: 1969–1980. *Psychological Bulletin* 90(1):125–52, July 1981.

20. Bandura, A. Self-efficacy mechanism in human agency. *American Psychologist* 37(2):122–47, Feb. 1982.

21. Bandura, 1982.

22. Lazarus, R. S., and Folkman, S. *Stress Appraisal and Coping.* New York City: Springer, 1984.

23. Lorig.

24. Lorig, K., González, V., and Laurent, D. *Chronic Disease Self-Management Leader's Manual.* Stanford, CA: (publisher not available), 1992.

Chapter 16

Using Technology to Enhance Patient Education Effectiveness

Patricia Agre, M.S., Ed.D., R.N.

☐ Objectives

The reader will be able to:

- List four technologies used in patient education
- List some of the potential benefits of closed-circuit television (CCTV)
- Discuss research studies on the use of video in patient education
- List the steps to be taken in planning for CCTV and the equipment needed to run the system
- Discuss the importance of evaluating the CCTV system
- Compare computer-assisted instruction (CAI), videodisc, and interactive video

☐ Technology Used in Patient Education

Technology, in the form of electronic media, adds important dimensions to patient education. Because it can save staff time and add interest, depth, and breadth to teaching programs, it is increasingly being integrated into the process of educating patients. Technology enables individual teachers to bring the outside world into the learning setting, take advantage of talent and expertise in many areas, and engage many senses. Some forms of electronic media demand interaction in much the same way that an individual teacher might; but with these, the learner advances at a time and pace that he or she chooses.

This chapter describes four electronic and computer technologies helpful to patient educators. The strengths of these mediums are discussed, as well as their applications and uses. The most common technology, *closed-circuit television* (CCTV), is covered in some detail; topics include the potential of CCTV, the theory behind it, practical implementation issues, and the argument for system evaluation. CCTV enables patient educators to program their own or commercially developed videotapes. The research data on CCTV are meager, but the literature has many examples of studies showing that patients gain knowledge and skills and change behaviors after exposure to educational videotapes.

Therefore the argument in favor of the use of CCTV to reach and teach patients is based on the success of individual video programs. The second technology, *computer-assisted instruction* (CAI), has been around for years. Common in staff education, it is less so in patient education. In either case, CAI is a first-line interactive technology with research data supporting its ability to educate.[1] An example of CAI would be a program offering a menu of topics containing questions and responses for each selection. The third technology is *videodisc.* It works on the same principle as compact audio disks (CDs) in that viewers can go instantly to a specific video selection. Videodisc is much less expensive to develop than interactive video. The fourth technology, *interactive video,* is a new and rising star in educational media and integrates video, text, art, and graphics. Its appeal lies in the breadth of media it contains and the choices it gives users in the depth of information they desire.

☐ Closed-Circuit Television

Simply described, CCTV allows selected television channels to be electronically designated as "in-house" or "closed-circuit." This means that the programs transmitted are seen only on the television sets wired to receive them. These channels are on video frequencies not used by broadcast networks such as ABC, NBC, or CBS. (Later sections of this chapter explain more about how a CCTV system works.)

The capability to direct programs to select patient groups is an obvious boon to patient educators who want to use electronic media to teach patients and also ensure that programs are aimed at patient needs. As illustrated in the following section, CCTV's potential for teaching patients is enormous.

It is important to note that, although the potential uses of CCTV are broad, the following discussion deals exclusively with patient education programming. However, other health care staff investigating CCTV should be aware that some systems can be used to document vital signs, order meals, and provide movies or other entertainment. These other uses may be limited by the specific CCTV system. Some CCTV systems can be initially used only for narrowly defined purposes, but can be easily upgraded at a later time; others are upgradable only at great expense.

The Uses of CCTV in Patient Education

Practically speaking, any teacher, whether a nurse, physician, social worker, or other professional, has only a limited number of teaching aids available. However, learning theory says that the greater the number of sensory channels used by learners in the learning process, the greater is the actual amount of learning.[2] Although the patient educator has his or her voice, style, presence, and possibly some visual aids, a CCTV program can include music, graphics, color, motion, and the voices, opinions, and experiences of other experts, patients, and families. These elements, used in conjunction with one-on-one educational methods, can increase patient learning. CCTV can stand alone or be part of a comprehensive instructional program. It can include programs designed with varied learning styles in mind and can be aimed at many levels of interest and ability.

The potential of CCTV to teach, divert, or relax patients and families is enormous. It can be used to deliver the fundamental or basic facts needed by specific patient groups, transmit panel discussions or interviews, convey interesting stories about individual patients, describe innovative technologies or treatments, provide health messages, and test learner knowledge.

CCTV, especially when used in concert with other methodologies, can also address some of the barriers affecting the adult's ability to learn. As people age, short-term memory declines and it becomes difficult to organize complex material and discriminate between what is relevant and irrelevant.[3] New information often conflicts with previous learning.[4]

Programs can be structured to provide repetition, progress gradually from simple to more complicated concepts, explain the same facts in many ways, eliminate irrelevant material, and provide pause time for taking notes.

CCTV can be used to reach groups of patients who challenge traditional methods of education. For example, if a large percentage of hospital patients do not speak English, a second channel can be designated as the Spanish or other foreign language channel. The economic feasibility of this depends on the hospital's market area.

Depending on the variety of patient types, CCTV channels can be designated for specific patient categories. For example, one channel can be designated as the maternal/child health channel, with only programs relating to this population, whereas other channels might be designated to cover only relaxation, surgery, or oncology. Or one channel can include programs for all audiences, with individual programs scheduled at specific times.

In some hospitals CCTV provides the information patients need to make an informed decision about a procedure or other aspects of their care. Results of research beginning to appear in the literature suggest that patients learn important facts from television programs or video as well as they do from one-on-one encounters with physicians.[5-7] Using CCTV for informed consent saves staff time and ensures that all patients have the opportunity to make a decision based on adequate and consistent information. Before actually getting the signed consent form, physicians could then spend their time on specific explanations that are individualized for each patient.

CCTV is an ideal mode for helping patients relax. Many hospitals program videotapes with soothing music and scenery, alternating or combined with instruction on relaxation techniques on a channel devoted solely to relaxation.

CCTV sometimes reinforces the information given in one-on-one encounters. Programs can be repeated in a daily schedule, allowing for multiple viewings. Programs may have complementary written materials and include self-quizzes so that patients can test themselves on what they have or have not learned.

Because the content in any CCTV patient education program is unchanging, evaluation of what specific information a patient has learned is made considerably easier. The professional, who has seen the program and knows what information the patient should have learned, can easily determine in either casual conversation or more formally in a quiz whether the patient has understood the material and learned the important facts. In addition, by directing a patient to watch a program and take a quiz, the professional has a head start on filling in learning gaps.

To summarize, CCTV can eliminate some of the time currently needed for one-on-one teaching; appeal to the visual and audio learner; provide consistent, comprehensive information; incorporate adult-learning theory; help in relaxing patients; expedite the informed-consent process; and facilitate the evaluation of learning.

Related Research on the Effectiveness of Video

Although there are cogent reasons why CCTV can help educate patients, do data exist to support the idea? Research that has been done on using video in patient education has implications for the use of CCTV.

Most published research compares particular video programs with other methods of teaching and learning. Research to date has not evaluated learning from programs viewed on CCTV. However, a growing body of research says that patients do learn from video programs, and most CCTV channels are programmed with videotape. Nielsen and Sheppard summarized findings for more than 100 articles published on the use of television as a patient education tool.[8] In the majority of articles in which the study design included randomization and control groups, videotape helped patients gain knowledge, learn skills, and change behavior. Three examples follow of studies demonstrating knowledge gain, one of knowledge gain and skills acquisition, and one of knowledge gain and behavior change.

Knowledge gain was demonstrated by Alkhateeb, Lukeroth, and Riggs in a venereal disease clinic population.[9] Three educational techniques to improve patient knowledge, attitudes, and behavior were compared: a one-on-one interview, a programmed learning guide, and an audiovisual program. All three interventions significantly increased knowledge, and patients generally responded well to the experimental technique they experienced.

Videotape was also found useful in educating glaucoma patients and offering healthy controls about glaucoma at two outpatient centers, one in England and one in California.[10] Each group was pretested for its knowledge of glaucoma and then shown the video on glaucoma. All groups substantially improved their knowledge of glaucoma immediately after viewing the videotape. In addition, because video explanations save staff time, the study investigators suggested that video in an outpatient setting may be a simple and economical method of patient education.

The methods used in a study to determine the most effective means of providing contraceptive information to clinic patients included pamphlets, one-on-one dialogue, and a precursor of video, a slide and tape presentation. The audiovisual (slide and tape) approach was found to be the most effective method of providing contraceptive information.[11] The authors of this study also suggest that an audiovisual approach is a cost-effective method of successful patient education.

Another study focused on parenting skills. This study compared four instructional methods using a control group. Seventy-seven mothers of young children were taught the "time-out procedure" as a method of teaching the child to either do or not do something. The four instructional methods used included a lecture, videotaped modeling, a written presentation, and videotaped modeling combined with role-playing.[12]

Although knowledge gain was demonstrated equally in all groups when assessed by questionnaire, the groups varied considerably when they were asked to apply the knowledge. In this case, modeling, as presented in the videotape, was significantly better than written presentations and approached significance compared to the lecture group. Videotaped modeling coupled with role-playing was superior to all three other groups, probably because it allowed immediate translation of learned information into behavioral practice.[13]

McColloch and others assessed knowledge gain and compliance with a diabetic diet among 40 adults with long-standing, poorly controlled diabetes.[14] Patients were randomly assigned to three teaching methods: conventional diet sheet instruction, lunchtime demonstrations, and videotape education. The greatest improvement in both knowledge and compliance was seen in the group assigned to videotape education.

Research on the Current Reality of CCTV

The number of hospitals using CCTV in patient education is growing, yet some general issues concerning its use still need further study. Are patients watching? Are they learning? Has CCTV freed professional staff from repetitive teaching and allowed them to individualize effectively? Esdale and Harris published one of the few articles on an actual hospital experience with CCTV.[15] Although their planning process was built on solid theory and much time and effort went into it, results of two surveys showed that few patients watched. Furthermore, their report is supported by anecdotal evidence.

An acknowledged gap in existing patient education programs and the observation that patients watched television led the patient education coordinator and head librarian in a 558-bed acute care facility to work with various hospital departments, committees, and task forces to establish a CCTV program. Six to 10 days after the CCTV system was implemented, 60 patients were surveyed about their use of it. Half of the 60 patients were aware of the channel and had a brochure about it, but only 7 percent had the channel turned on, only 16 percent had watched it at all, and none had returned the evaluation sheet. A second survey, conducted 10 months later, was limited to ascertaining only whether the channel was tuned in. Of 120 rooms visited, only 2 patients were watching the channel.[16]

This sobering report, rather than discouraging patient educators from using CCTV, should provide the impetus to plan CCTV programs better and integrate them into patient education efforts. In setting up a new system or improving an existing one, the authors suggest:[17]

- Formalizing accountability for the various components of the CCTV system
- Forecasting the time needed to plan, operate, market, and evaluate such a system
- Securing more active involvement of nursing staff to build a base of interest for the system
- Undertaking a more thorough assessment of the target population's capabilities and needs

Steps in Implementing a CCTV System

The following sections discuss the basic steps that should be followed when planning and implementing a CCTV system in a hospital-based patient education program. Although some steps after initial planning may occur concurrently, they are presented here in a roughly chronological order.

Conduct Initial Planning

Lawrence Green's *PRECEDE/PROCEED* model should be reviewed for an in-depth discussion on how best to begin planning a CCTV system.[18] It can help determine who would benefit, what illnesses they have, and what interventions appear to be most effective. Although the model also covers examining the resources available to support the CCTV channel and evaluation issues, only the planning issues are discussed here. Briefly, the model starts with quality-of-life issues, and asks about general population hopes or concerns.[19] For example, in a cancer hospital, patients might hope for cure or freedom from pain. Then it surveys the target population's specific needs that relate or contribute to the health goals identified under quality of life. Using the cancer hospital again, this phase would look at what kind of information or services would contribute to cure or a pain-free state.

Next, it asks about behavioral and environmental risk factors, in this case, related to health goals (cure or pain-free state), that the CCTV programs hope to address. Using this information, those factors that might affect the success of the CCTV channel as an educational tool are identified. First are the predisposing factors (knowledge, attitudes, perceptions that hinder or facilitate change). Patients might need information about treatment possibilities for cancer, or they might need more facts to persuade them that taking pain medication does not lead to addiction. Next, it looks at enabling factors (skills or barriers that help or hinder change). Is it lack of insurance that prevents patients from getting a treatment for cancer, or is it a belief that pain medication leads to addiction that prevents them from taking medication and getting relief? Finally, the model examines reinforcing factors (rewards or feedback encouraging or discouraging continuation of behavior change). Here it might look at how patient-to-patient volunteers affect health goals or how professional staff or family support contributes to compliance with cancer treatment regimens. This information is used to determine the system goals and objectives[20] that are covered later in this chapter.

Surveys, focus groups, or other methods can be used to discover the attitudes of staff and the target audience (patients) toward CCTV as an educational tool. Staff should be queried on the following points:

- Would they use CCTV in their teaching?
- What kinds of programs would they recommend?

- What kinds of supporting materials should be available to inform them about programs or to help them make a program part of an overall teaching plan?

Patients should be asked the following questions:

- Would they watch CCTV?
- What kinds of programs would interest them?
- What format (such as a panel discussion or true story) would they prefer?
- Which language would they prefer?
- Would they want programs to include pauses or quizzes or have supplementary written summaries?

Based on this information, decisions can be made about how and when to use a CCTV channel.

Another early step, one that might precede, coincide with, or follow the surveys of patients and staff, is to determine what kinds of CCTV technology options exist. Each year, more new and exciting technology is available, and all possibilities should be considered before final decisions are made on the kind of system to install. In most hospitals the decision is made by a high-level administrator, not a patient educator.

Prepare Program Goals and Objectives

A very important part of developing a CCTV system is writing clear overall goals and specific patient education objectives for it. The goals and objectives should fit with the hospital's overall strategic plan, as mentioned in chapter 2, and they should draw from the initial research information obtained from patients and staff.

Goals for the system may be stated broadly, but the objectives should have measurable outcomes. One goal might be that medical and nursing staff use CCTV as an integral part of their teaching. An objective, though, should state who will do what and by when. Some examples of objectives include the following:

- By _____ (date), 50 percent of the medical staff or 100 percent of the nursing staff will recommend specific programs to patients.
- All conscious and alert patients will watch one or more programs during their hospital stay.
- Eighty percent of patients will express satisfaction with CCTV as a teaching methodology.
- After watching a program, 80 percent of patients will be able to relate one fact that they learned.

Objectives should also be program-specific. For example:

- For preoperative education, 80 percent of patients will be able to describe important parts of the preoperative routine after watching a CCTV program.
- For maternal/child health, after watching a CCTV program on care of the umbilicus, 80 percent of new mothers will be able to describe signs and symptoms of infection.

Without clear objectives, it is difficult to judge the worth of the CCTV system. With measurable objectives, however, the system and individual programs can be evaluated and improved. (Evaluating whether goals and objectives were achieved is discussed under Evaluate the System later in this chapter.)

Determine Staff Responsibility for the System

Another important aspect of developing a CCTV system is establishing who will be in charge of making the system work. Often the person in charge of the CCTV system is the patient education manager (PEM), but in some institutions the director of the audio-visual department has this responsibility. It is generally a one-person effort.

Select Equipment and Evaluate Necessary Support

Once goals and objectives have been established and responsibility for the system has been assigned, the next phases of developing the CCTV system are more technical. The type of system determines the equipment needed; and the company selected to install, operate, and service it will recommend the necessary components. However, knowing what equipment already exists in the hospital and what it can handle will help in making decisions.

Understand the Types of CCTV Equipment and How They Work

Figure 16-1 provides a schematic on the basic components of a CCTV system and how they work. The following brief discussion elaborates on the schematic.

In the simplest possible terms, a radio band has a limited number of separate and distinct frequencies. Think of listening to the radio while driving across country. At some point, one radio station fades, another competes, and the reception is fuzzy and irritating. As the miles pass, the former station fades entirely and the new one becomes crystal clear. These stations are on the same frequencies in bordering communities. Each frequency is assigned a call number and a location on the band. This arrangement is similar to that of CCTV. For television, the radio frequency has overtones that constitute the video signal.

To pick up these radio/video signals, an antenna is needed. Most hospitals have a master antenna (MATV), but it may not be adequate to transmit closed-circuit signals. The consultant or company retained to advise on systems should evaluate the capability of the MATV before equipment is purchased. It may be necessary to buy a new MATV. The master antenna receives a signal (RF, or radio frequency) and feeds it to the modulator, which decodes it and directs it to a specific channel that can be picked up on the facility's television sets.

Most hospitals have television sets, and if these can accommodate a CCTV channel, it can be used for patient education purposes. The newer 54-or-more-channel systems are far better able to accommodate CCTV than the older 12-channel systems. Originating in a videocassette player in some central location, CCTV sends its radio/video signals to the modulator. The modulator then takes those signals and redistributes them to an assigned unused broadcast channel.

In addition to a master antenna, a modulator, and television sets, the basic equipment necessary to run a CCTV channel includes a programmer, at least one videocassette player, and cables to attach the system to the MATV. Programmers switch a videocassette player on and off at a predetermined time(s) each day.

A character generator, which can be included in the programmer but is usually a separate piece of equipment, creates text for announcing messages such as special programs, hours of operation, or other information the hospital would like to give viewers. These messages can be stored and programmed to play at specific times, either following specific programs or between programs. A character generator can also be used to provide specific emergency information or instructions.

The videocassette player plays the tape on which the program is recorded. There are three kinds of videocassette players: ¾ inch, super VHS (½ inch), and regular VHS (also ½ inch). The ¾-inch videocassette players are considerably more expensive and play only one hour of programming at a time, but generate a superior-quality image. Super VHS plays two hours of programming at a time and generates a better image than standard VHS players, but is not as expensive as ¾-inch players. Standard VHS players, the least expensive and most widely used of the three types, usually generate an acceptable image and, like the super VHS, can play two hours of programming.

Gather Information for Equipment Decisions

In gathering information for equipment decisions, it is necessary to evaluate the capacity of the MATV and existing television sets to handle CCTV and to decide what kind of programmer and videocassette players to purchase. The resource list at the end of this chapter suggests several directories that may be helpful. Many hospitals have an audiovisual department with knowledgeable staff who can advise and assist, if not in actual purchasing recommendations, at least in where to go for help in making decisions. In addition, many communities have independent audiovisual consultants who can evaluate existing equipment and make specific recommendations based on the hospital's needs. Because

Figure 16-1. How the CCTV System Works

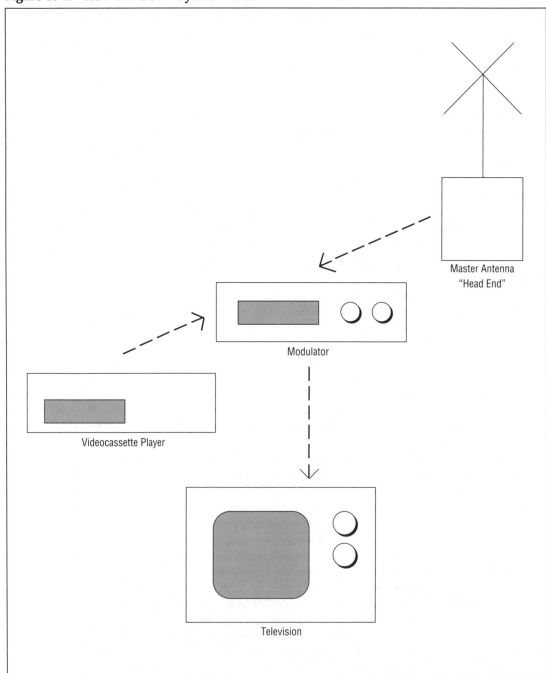

patient educators in larger hospitals and medical centers may have had to answer some of the same questions, they may be able to share their solutions and provide the names of other knowledgeable resource people. Equipment suppliers, especially those dealing with more than one manufacturer, can often recommend components for the system and can compare the advantages or strengths of each brand or model. Whatever the recommendations, one general rule of thumb is to purchase equipment *designed for industrial or frequent use.* Equipment for the home user, although less expensive, is not meant to hold up to the kind of day-in, day-out, long-term usage a hospital's CCTV will require.

Audiovisual magazines have articles on systems and specific equipment and also advertisements from manufacturers and dealers. A magazine's editorial staff or byline writers might well respond to queries. Regardless of how equipment decisions are made, the overall quality and reliability of the system depend on them.

Plan for Maintenance and Servicing of Equipment

A final but extremely important decision is determining who will be responsible for maintaining and servicing the system. The following must be considered (and budgeted for) in the planning stage before the system is purchased and installed:

- Should a service contract be negotiated at the onset?
- Can the equipment be serviced by the hospital's electrical engineering department?
- Can it be returned to the supplier for repair?
- Who will come in to troubleshoot if a problem cannot be easily diagnosed or fixed?
- Is the audiovisual department willing or able to take on the responsibility?

Even the best mechanical device can and probably will need repair. A system that consistently breaks down breeds resentment on the part of staff who want to use it or recommend it and among patients who have been told it is available. Every effort should be made to ensure that technical difficulties interfering with programming are short-lived.

Select or Produce Tapes

Once the goals and specific objectives for each target audience are known and the specific equipment is selected, decisions about whether to select commercially produced tapes or produce new ones can be made. Selection criteria might be based on the patient education objectives or more practically (but less ideally) on a comparison of available tapes, with the best one chosen.

Selecting from among commercially produced tapes can be tedious. Most medical libraries have source books for commercially produced tapes, but there is currently no reliable rating service. (See the resources listed at the end of this chapter for source books and directories.)

Tapes can be ordered for preview, sometimes for free, sometimes for a fee. Patient educators should establish their own system for previewing tapes and obtaining approval. The chief of service in the particular specialty for which the tape is intended should be given the opportunity to preview the tape or to designate someone else to view it. Nursing and other care-giver staff from each relevant discipline should also preview it. Then the tape can be reviewed by the hospitalwide committee that oversees operation of patient education services or the patient education television system. Ideally, appropriate patients would also preview the tapes. However, because of the time required, arranging for patient viewing may be difficult.

If no acceptable tape can be found for a specific group of patients, there are two possibilities. The project can be put on hold until an appropriate commercially produced tape becomes available, or a new tape can be produced, in-house or with the assistance of a professional video service.

Producing a videotape can range in cost from inexpensive to very expensive. To save money, scripts can be written by staff and produced with standard home video equipment.

The quality of "home-grown" videos may be limited, but they may have good teaching potential, depending on the interest and needs of the target audience. At the other end of the cost spectrum, video companies can usually provide scriptwriters, technical expertise, and location or studio production services. To help produce programs, the creative patient educator will write grants or seek funding from voluntary organizations or other private sources.

One advantage of producing tapes in-house is the opportunity it provides for evaluating and improving the production process along the way. It is easier to change a script that does not meet patient or staff needs after a trial run. Focus groups are a good way to gauge response to the script. Focus groups generally consist of 10 to 12 people with similar backgrounds (for example, all new mothers or all preop patients) and a group leader. The focus group can be videotaped or audiotaped so that comments can be transcribed and analyzed. Appropriate patient groups may be given the script to read before the appointed time and asked to participate in the group discussion.

A note of caution: When using the focus group process, it is important that the focus group discussion leader be neutral in encouraging comments from participants. Any slight or apparent approval or disapproval by the leader can color, direct, influence, or sway the group, who will want to avoid displeasing the leader.

Another advantage of producing videotapes in-house is the control over content, format, and choice of talent (actors or actresses). For example, hospitals may provide care (for example, catheter care) in a very specific way and want only that methodology represented. Or they may have many minority patients whom they would want to "reach" with minority talent. Or they may have a large percentage of patients who, based on their level of education, might respond more readily to a particular teaching format. For example, well-educated patients might best be reached through a panel discussion offering sophisticated decision-making techniques. On the other hand, patients with low-literacy skills might learn best by having a single host simply explain a procedure, using colorful graphics or actual patient demonstrations.

Fill Time between Programs

Most videos produced commercially or in-house do not last a full 15, 20, or 30 minutes. The remaining minutes until the next time slot can be filled in a variety of ways that can help to increase the value and usefulness of the system. For example, a program lasting 11.5 minutes gives the programmer 3.5, 8.5, or 13.5 minutes for "messages" or "shorts." These messages can be static, that is, they can remain on screen the entire time, or they can roll or flash, as in movie credits. Messages might include the times and locations of patient support groups or classes, the titles and times of programs aimed at the same target audience as the just-finished program, a schedule of events in the recreation room, the various hospital services and how to access them, gift or coffee shop hours, or parking information.

Examples of shorts might include brief "visits" to hospital locations (that is, nuclear medicine, physical therapy, occupational therapy), explanations of "Who We Are" programs (that is, social work, chaplaincy, primary nursing, respiratory therapy) and "How We Work" programs (that is, the dietary department, billing and financial services, or housekeeping). The president of the hospital could explain hospital philosophy; appeals could be made for donations to various charitable programs or community health services such as Medic Alert®, Planned Parenthood, Basic Cardiac Life Support (BCLS), or Lamaze classes could be described. Short-answer or multiple-choice quizzes can be designed to entertain while giving the patient information. For example, "An intern is . . . " would be followed by four choices. Either the correct answer would then appear or the patient would be told that answers would be shown at a specified time. Here, the CCTV coordinator can be creative and add some light educational entertainment.

There are several ways to create messages or shorts. The easiest is with a character generator. A character generator can be programmed to *roll*, that is, have the messages slowly move from the top of the screen to the bottom. A message created with a character generator can be videotape-recorded and edited onto the videotape immediately after the program. Alternatives include using typewriter- or computer-generated messages, which are videotaped as stills and then edited onto the videotape after the program.

Determine Programming

Once tapes have been selected and material is available to fill gaps between programs, the PEM (or committee) must tackle the difficult task of *programming,* or scheduling, when tapes are to be shown to patients. Programming patient education videos is a science, an art, and in many hospitals a political skill. Even in hospitals specializing in only one type of patient, the number of services performed and the different stages of treatment that patients require make programming a challenge.

Whether one person (such as the PEM) or a committee is charged with responsibility for programming, the responsibility is to *all services and all patients.* This means that it is important to determine the scheduling needs of all hospital services. The key is to be flexible and work with service providers to determine the best available time for each service.

The staff and patient survey used for initial planning is the best place to begin the process of sorting out what programs to show when. Another source of information is informally asking staff about the best time to show programs. For example, if staff relate that patients on a specific service are frequently off the unit in the morning for testing or procedures, programs for those patients should be scheduled in the afternoon or evening.

Programming can begin at any time—on the quarter hour, every 20 minutes, or every half hour. Unfortunately, there may be competition for prime viewing hours; the same two or three hours may be chosen for all services. Or there may be no consensus, even within a single hospital service, as to the best time to schedule programs. In these situations the programmer may want to work with larger blocks of patient categories. For example, preop teaching can be scheduled in the evening, perhaps as a lead-in to a class or as reinforcement to individualized teaching by the nurse, or early in the morning for same-day surgery patients. Programs for new mothers might work best just before or after class sessions or before babies are delivered to rooms, or perhaps during visiting hours so that fathers can also watch. A program on chemotherapy or radiation therapy might reach its largest audience in the early morning or evening.

With cable or network programming, each show tries to hold or attract the audience for the next show. However, for patients watching CCTV, successful programming may mean not showing important programs back-to-back, but spreading them over the course of a day. This allows patients to process and digest information from each program.

Sometimes video programs come in parts. If so, the best approach might be to schedule part one at 2 p.m., part two at 2:30 p.m., and part three at 3 p.m. In this way, patients will not have to remember totally different times, can stay tuned throughout all three parts if desired, or can tune in on succeeding days for each new part.

Programming can be provided on different days for specific patient groups. For example, Monday, Wednesday, and Friday may feature programs for the surgical, perinatal, and pediatric patients, while Tuesdays and Thursdays may be devoted to oncology and general medicine. General health messages could be shown every day.

Most patient education programs, especially those aimed at major patient populations, should be repeated at least once a day to provide a chance for review. A fixed or permanent schedule should never be determined until it is clear that the best compromises have been reached. (There is, however, a fine line between having many trial runs and losing staff enthusiasm. Each time program times are changed, even if staff request the change, they have to remember the new time before they can tell patients.) Successful programming depends on staff input.

Promote the CCTV System

As shown by anecdotal experience and confirmed by the Esdale and Harris article[21] discussed earlier in this chapter, patients may not watch patient education CCTV for a variety of reasons. The key is to promote the channel to ensure staff commitment to its use in patient education.

Staff who provide direct patient care must be the major targets when promoting CCTV. Ideally, staff members will get to the point that they do not remember what it was like not to use CCTV as a patient education tool. When staff recognize the time-saving potential of using CCTV to help fulfill a portion of their patient education responsibilities, they will begin to ask patients to watch specific programs and rely on them as vital tools in their education efforts. (For example, a program on catheter care became so integral to patient teaching among nurses at Memorial Sloan–Kettering Cancer Center in New York that they were furious when the CCTV system went down for a time and they had to rely on a portable VCR.)

There are a number of ways to ensure staff commitment to using CCTV as a patient education tool. For example, as each new tape is added to the programming system, staff in that specialty area must be informed, given an opportunity to view the tape, and provided with suggestions on how to use it in their teaching. Also, the coordinator of the CCTV program should consider writing teaching plans that include the video program for major areas of teaching (that is, colostomy care, recovery from myocardial infarction, care of the newborn, diabetic teaching). Supplementary written materials and/or brief quizzes should be used whenever possible. A video program directory or TV "guide" summarizing each program, giving the schedule, and outlining the key points covered should be available on each unit.

Physicians should be notified of all general-health CCTV programs in addition to those that pertain to their specialties, and asked to include these programs in their instructions and recommendations to patients. Prescription pads with the physician's name and the name and time of the program could be preprinted to make the recommendation carry more weight.

A single, initial effort to inform staff is rarely enough. Until nurses and others get used to using a program in their teaching and see how it saves them time and helps their patients learn, they will often forget to recommend it. Each PEM has his or her own techniques for winning staff support, but whatever they are, *they must be ongoing*.

Once hospital staff are committed, patients must also be informed of the existence of the patient education CCTV channel and the program schedule. Hospitals have done this in a variety of ways. Many hospitals produce a formal TV guide and distribute it either with an admission packet or at the time the room is readied for a new patient. Others have a volunteer describe the channel during an initial patient visit. Often the schedule is posted permanently in the patient's room—on the TV itself, in a drawer, on the back of the room door, or on a wall. The channel itself can serve as a reminder of programming. Patients flipping channels might take note of messages describing various programs. However, the best way to get patients to accept the idea of CCTV is for them to be encouraged to use it by staff members who believe in its value.

Evaluate the System

To constantly improve the CCTV system, its offerings, and its value to staff and patients, evaluations should be done on two fronts: the entire system and individual programs. The first question regarding the system might be, Is it reliable? Many CCTV channels suffer equipment breakdowns, making staff wary of recommending programs to patients. After several experiences of having a patient say, "I tried to watch it, but it wasn't on," nurses and other staff may lose faith in the system. All-out promotion of the system should not begin until the PEM is sure it is working consistently well.

If the system itself is working well, the next step is to evaluate how well it is being used. Based on goals and objectives for the channel and specific programs, patients can and should be surveyed to see if they watch, learn, and enjoy the programs. They can be quizzed individually on paper or verbally by nursing staff to see whether they have understood the key points covered in a program. They can be asked for critical reviews or suggestions to improve on or add to specific programs.

Staff members should also be surveyed to see if they can name three or more programs and the times they are on; they can be asked if they have recommended programs to patients or if they routinely use the channel in their patient teaching. Staff members can be asked if the channel is generally helping them in their teaching activities and for suggestions on how it could be improved.

All suggestions for improvement, whether from patients or staff, must be addressed. If the channel seems to be well received and is being used but specific programs are weak, a careful needs assessment should be done and the programs replaced with ones that meet the learning objectives. If the channel is not well received, if patients are not aware of it and encouraged to watch it, or if staff are not using it in their teaching, a more thorough assessment should be done.

The success of patient education CCTV is determined by how often it is used, how well it meets staff and patient needs, and how successfully it teaches. With all the work that goes into planning and program development, it is unfortunate that so many channels appear not to have a following. This is the major reason that evaluation of both the system and specific programs should be built into the process at the beginning.

☐ Computer-Assisted Instruction

Another technology used in patient education is computer-assisted instruction (CAI), also known as computer-assisted learning (CAL). Many hospitals use CAI in outpatient areas or for specific patient populations (for example, diabetics or patients with post-myocardial infarction). It is entirely computer-based and may include graphics, illustrations, sound, or animation. CAI technology is *interactive* in that it offers choices and directions for further instruction. It generally requires the patient–learner to proceed in a given direction to reach a successful conclusion.

The simplest CAI programs ask the participant to push a button for a list of topics. Once the selection is made, it is followed by a list of questions with a variety of possible answers. After an answer is chosen by the participant, a response appears with an accolade such as "You're absolutely right" or "Too bad, try again," or it simply shows the correct answer. More elaborate CAI programs guide learners through some base information, then ask them to use the information to respond or react to situations that require assimilating this information.

Overall, CAI can be very "user friendly." It does not require any computer experience because the directions for what keys to press appear clearly on the computer screen. This is an important feature for all patients who are not computer-literate.

However, one study of nurses' responses to a computer-assisted learning program for patients on continuous ambulatory peritoneal dialysis found that nurses were apprehensive about using the "machine," worried that it might replace them as the teacher, and felt they might look foolish to patients if they did not fully understand how to operate the program. They also voiced concerns about how older patients might respond to the program. This study was conducted in England, however, and had only 14 subjects. It is possible that attitudes toward patient teaching responsibilities and computer experience might be very different from those in the United States.[22]

One very exciting CAI program is the VIVA! (Voice Interactive Visual and Aural) Spinal Injury Series produced by Health Enhancement and Learning Programs of Dallas, Texas. This series includes nine programs, most with several component parts, that cover the extensive information a spinal injury patient needs regarding rehabilitation. As described by Jo Ann Wells, a patient educator at the Dallas Rehabilitation Institute, the system can work for even ventilator-dependent quadriplegics.[23]

VIVA begins with a menu offering logically sequenced information categories. Ten to 25 minutes of information, conveyed visually with graphics and text and orally with voice-overs, is followed by three questions. Each question is followed with the prompt "Are you ready to answer, or do you want the information repeated?" If the patient elects to answer and does so correctly, the program proceeds to the next step. A wrong answer results in a 30- to 60-second review, followed by a repeat question.

In Ms. Wells's experience, patients respond enthusiastically to the program and seem to retain and use the information they learn. She relates that it is particularly rewarding to see spinal injury patients progress from using the program in the voice-activated mode to being able to use the keyboard. She also appreciates seeing how the program motivates patients to learn.[24]

The advantage of CAI over CCTV or video is that it is interactive. Also, compared to interactive video, it is less expensive to develop. It meets many learning needs and may prove a durable format for educating patients.

☐ Videodisc

Another tool that can be used in patient education is videodisc technology. Laser-operated videodiscs hooked up to a computer use a laser beam to read video stored on a disc. Users can access any piece of information on the disc in any order.

Although not necessarily interactive in the truest sense of the word, videodisc does allow the viewer to skip around in sequencing, avoid subjects of no interest, and review material easily. Unlike CAI, videodisc technology uses motion. As more and more children who grew up with television become adult patient learners, technology that uses motion—such as videodiscs—may evolve as important visual learning sources.

With videodiscs, a menu of choices allows the learner to go directly to his or her specific area of interest. For example, suppose a patient wanted to know only the risks of a particular surgery. To get this information from a patient education program on that surgery offered on CCTV, he or she would have to watch until the information was given, perhaps not until halfway or later through the program. To get it on a CAI program, the patient would most likely (though not always) have to proceed through each step in the program until that information was covered. However, with a videodisc, the patient could go immediately to it without having to wade through extraneous information. This immediate access to specific and relevant information may be particularly satisfying for adult patients.

Olevitch and Hagan used a videodisc as a tool in rehabilitating patients diagnosed with schizophrenia or schizo-affective disorder. The videodisc, called *How to Get Out and Stay Out: The Story of Cathy*, described how Cathy, a fictional psychiatric patient, was discharged from the hospital and had some minor problems. The responses of two groups who watched the videodisc were compared. The experimental group had repeated opportunities to make different behavior decisions for Cathy and based on these, see how her story ended. For example, Cathy could either take her medication or not, engage in stress management techniques or not. The control group saw selected sequences and were then asked some questions about their reaction to the videodisc and their predictions for Cathy. All participants enjoyed the videodisc. The experimental group significantly increased their scores on the Wellness-Maintenance Questionnaire.[25]

Currently more health education/patient education videodiscs are available than interactive programs, though the selection is not extensive. Videodisc technology may not be within the reach of many patient educators. Although the initial purchase of the hardware is expensive, even the videodiscs themselves are generally priced around $1,000.[26] Videodiscs can also be pressed using the educator's own in-house video source, thus allowing a fully customized program.

☐ Interactive Video

Interactive video is the newest and most sophisticated technology used in patient education. It offers patients a selection of video, text, art, and graphics; the chance to explore information superficially or in-depth; and the ability to proceed in their own preferred direction. Weyer described the many levels of user choice offered in interactive video in *As We May Learn*[27] (see table 16-1).

The hardware and programs are still expensive (about $1,000 per program, plus hardware) and the selection of programs for patients is limited. But as with other new technologies, the costs are bound to come down and the number of available programs is likely to increase.

Interactive video generally offers learners a choice of options at almost every stop. One excellent patient education program was developed by the United States Pharmacopeial Convention and the American Diabetes Association. This touch-screen program, called *About Your Diabetes,* offers users menu choices covering what diabetes is, diet, exercise, traveling, long-term problems, education, foot care, treatment, and general information.

The program begins by asking the patient a series of questions about his or her own disease and situation. For example, it asks what type of diabetes the patient has, what kind of insulin he or she uses, and the dosage. The prompts on the screen use pictures and symbols, making it appropriate for all literacy levels.

After establishing the baseline patient-specific information, the presentation is then customized to relate to that patient. A section on treatment offers options on injections/self-administration, insulin, oral antidiabetics, precautions, and side effects. The specifics of the information given are based on the kind of insulin the patient takes. Questions are interspersed throughout the program to test the patient's comprehension of covered material. An on-screen report generated at the end of the program identifies areas of low comprehension so that the health care professional can provide reinforcement or additional instruction.

Interactive video programs are especially good at entertaining while they teach. Children's and general interest museums have developed a wide variety of innovative interactive programs combining video, narration, text, graphics, and still photographs.

The range in the depth of information and participative value makes interactive video ideal for patient education. Patients can learn what they want, when they want, and how they want. The interactive video program meets needs at all levels of interest and learning ability.

☐ Conclusion

The four technologies discussed in this chapter—CCTV, CAI, videodisc, and interactive video—all hold promise for meeting patient education goals and objectives. CCTV can

Table 16-1. Levels of User Choices

Learner's Goal	System's Interpretation
Tell me.	Give me the facts, no embellishments.
Inform me.	Give me facts plus optional background and other points of view.
Amuse me.	Find me interesting connections or perspectives.
Challenge me.	Make me find or create creative connections.
Guide me.	Let me browse, but give me over-the-shoulder advice.
Teach me.	Give me more step-by-step guidance, fewer irrelevant links.

Reprinted, with permission, from S. A. Weyer. As we may learn. In: S. Ambon and K. Hooper, editors. *Interactive Multimedia: Visions of Multimedia for Developers, Educators, & Information Providers.* Redmond, WA: Microsoft Press, 1989, p. 92.

reach hundreds or even thousands of people at once, but compared to CAI and interactive video, it is a passive medium. CAI allows instant feedback as patients learn, while videodisc allows learners to proceed directly to their areas of interest. Interactive video programs, however, may prove to be the most rewarding in terms of patient knowledge gain, interest, and satisfaction. They may also expedite the necessary behavior changes or skill acquisitions required of different types of patients.

None of these technologies replaces dialogue between the nurse or physician and the patient. Patient educators need to determine which method can best supplement that dialogue, under what conditions, and for which patients. Comparative evaluations of patient learning, staff time expended, and patient and staff satisfaction using various methodologies will be important in improving the potential of technology used in patient education.

References

1. Jolicoeur, K., and Berger, D. E. Do we really know what makes educational software effective? A call for empirical research on effectiveness. *Educational Technology*, Dec. 1986, pp. 7–11.

2. deS. Brunner, E., Wilder, D. S., Kirchner, C., and Newberry, J. S., Jr. *An Overview of Adult Education Research.* Chicago: Adult Education Association of the U.S.A., 1959.

3. Knox, A. B. Quoted by: Darkenwald, G. G., and Merriam, S. B. *Adult Education: Foundations of Practice.* New York City: Harper and Row, 1982, pp. 108–9.

4. Knox.

5. Chamorro, T., and Apelbaum, J. Informed consent: nursing issues and ethical dilemmas. *Oncology Nursing Forum* 15(6):803–8, 1988.

6. Faden, R. R. Disclosure and informed consent: does it matter how we tell it? *Health Education Monographs* 5(3):198–214, 1977.

7. Barbour, G. L., and Blumenkrantz, M. J. Videotape aids informed consent decision. *JAMA* 240(25):2741–42, 1978.

8. Nielsen, E., and Sheppard, M. S. Television as a patient education tool: a review of its effectiveness. *Patient Education and Counseling* 11(1):3–16, Feb. 1988.

9. Alkhateeb, W., Lukeroth, C. J., and Riggs, M. A comparison of three educational techniques used in a venereal disease clinic. *Public Health Reports* 90(2):159–64, 1975.

10. Rosenthal, A. R., Zimmerman, J. F., and Tanner, J. Educating the glaucoma patient. *British Journal of Ophthalmology* 67:814–17, 1983.

11. Marshall, W. R., Rothenberger, M. A., and Bunnell, S. L. The efficacy of personalized audiovisual patient education materials. *The Journal of Family Practice* 19(5):659–63, 1984.

12. Nay, W. R. A systematic comparison of instructional techniques for parents. *Behavior Therapy* 6:14–21, 1975.

13. Nay.

14. McColloch, D. K., Mitchell, R. D., Ambler, J., and Tattersall, R. B. Influence of imaginative teaching of diet on compliance of metabolic control in insulin dependent diabetes. *Patient Education and Counseling* 287:1858–61, 1983.

15. Esdale, A., and Harris, H. L. Evaluation of a closed-circuit television patient education program: structure, process and outcome. *Patient Education and Counseling* 7:193–215, 1984.

16. Esdale and Harris.

17. Esdale and Harris.

18. Green, L. W., and Kreuter, M. W. *Health Promotion Planning: An Educational and Environmental Approach.* Mountain View, CA: Mayfield Publishing Co., 1991, p. 27.

19. Green and Kreuter.

20. Green and Kreuter.

21. Esdale and Harris.

22. Firby, P. A., Luker, K. A., and Coress, A. L. Nurses' opinions of the introduction of computer-assisted learning for use in patient education. *Journal of Advanced Nursing* 16:987-95, 1991.

23. Telephone interview, Jo Ann Wells, Dallas Rehabilitation Institute, Dallas, TX, 1991.

24. Telephone interview, Jo Ann Wells.

25. Olevitch, B. A., and Hagan, R. J. An interactive videodisc as a tool in the rehabilitation of the chronically mentally ill: a preliminary investigation. In: *Computers in Human Behavior,* vol. 7, 1991, pp. 57-73. (No further information available.)

26. Mageau, T. Laser-disc technology. *Electronic Learning,* Mar. 1990, pp. 23-28.

27. Weyer, S. A. As we may learn. In: S. Ambon and K. Hooper, editors. *Interactive Multimedia: Visions of Multimedia for Developers, Educators, & Information Providers.* Redmond, WA: Microsoft Press, 1989, p. 92.

Resources

AV Market Place 1991. *The Complete Business Directory of: Audio, Audio Visual, Computer Systems, Film, Video, Programming.* New York City: R. R. Bowker, A Division of Reed Publishing Inc., 1991

Educational Film and Video Locator of the Consortium of College and University Media Centers and R. R. Bowker, 1990-1991. 4th ed. Vols. 1 and 2. New York City: R. R. Bowker, 1991.

Frank, C. D., ed. *Patient Education Sourcebook,* Vol. II. St. Louis: Health Sciences Communication Association, 1990.

1991 Interactive Healthcare Directory—CD-ROM. Alexandria, VA: Stewart Publishing, Inc.

1991 Interactive Healthcare Directory—Computer-Assisted Instruction. Alexandria, VA: Stewart Publishing, Inc.

1991 Interactive Healthcare Directory—Videodisc. Alexandria, VA: Stewart Publishing, Inc.

Weiner, D. J., editor. *The Video Source Book.* 12th ed. Vols. 1 and 2. Detroit: Gale Research Inc., 1991.

Chapter 17

Promoting Effective Use of Print Materials in Patient Education

Annette Rykwalder Mercurio, M.P.H., C.H.E.S.

☐ Objectives

The reader will be able to:

- Describe how to determine the need for print materials
- Apply a set of criteria for critiquing print materials
- Outline steps in development of effective patient education materials
- Refer to writing guidelines for developing low-literacy materials
- Define elements of culturally sensitive materials
- Determine whether to initiate development of an institutional policy for print materials
- Examine the need to strengthen the materials distribution system within the hospital
- Distinguish the role of materials consultant from that of materials producer
- Cite ways to advocate for improvements in the quality of patient education materials
- Locate existing patient education materials

☐ The Materials Maze

Print materials have great potential to enhance the effectiveness, efficiency, and quality of patient education efforts. For example, pamphlets, brochures, instruction sheets, posters, and flip charts are all tools that can help stretch limited teaching time. Because print materials can convey basic, repetitive information, they free the patient educator to concentrate on individualized follow-up instruction. Additionally, because print tools can reinforce teaching and serve as an at-home reference for patients, patients are better able to manage their own health. Further, print materials can promote consistency of teaching throughout a patient care area.

However, realizing the full potential of print materials requires considerable skill in negotiating the materials maze. What is the materials maze? For many patient education managers (PEMs), this maze is similar to a dense forest thicketed with trees (materials). The constant proliferation of patient education materials is causing this forest to grow in size and complexity. Some PEMs become lost in this forest because they see an abundance of trees, but lack the necessary guideposts to tell them which trees are worth their attention.

For other PEMs, the problem in negotiating the materials maze is that they are unaware of all the trees that surround them. They invest time and energy in planting their own trees without realizing that there is already a mature forest within reach.

Regardless of how PEMs perceive the materials maze, they tend to race through it. They often embark on their journey without receiving maps from colleagues in education, instructional technology, library science, and other disciplines. Eager to reach their goal, they omit the stages of assessment and planning. They run through the maze with great determination and expend considerable energy, time, resources, and sanity. They begin to wonder why they entered the maze in the first place. Finally, they pant across the finish line and their prize is produced. They are not sure what that prize is worth or what they can do with it, but it is a product!

Although traveling through the materials maze can be overwhelming, progress has been made in charting pathways through it. This chapter presents keys to the effective use of print materials. Those keys will enable PEMs to successfully negotiate the materials maze and reap the full potential of print materials.

☐ Defining the Need for Materials

Patient education managers are often so eager to respond to requests for materials that they bypass steps essential to effective use of those materials. The first of these essential steps is to define the need for print materials. The following section poses three questions that PEMs can use to determine whether print materials are needed.

What Is the Educational Need?

How often do PEMs assume that print materials are necessary when told that patients are ill-informed? Before investing in materials selection or development, PEMs should ensure that print tools are part of the solution to a defined need.

For example, suppose a nurse from the newborn intensive care unit (NICU) approaches the PEM with a materials development request. The nurse explains that NICU staff are finding that parents of infants on the unit are constantly asking questions that have been previously answered in a brief, oral orientation to the NICU. NICU staff are convinced that an orientation booklet would reduce the amount of time they devote to repeating basic information.

Is an orientation booklet the solution to the problem identified by this staff? First, the problem must be explored and more clearly defined. For example, by interviewing parents of former NICU infants, the PEM may ascertain that their anxiety blocks comprehension of detailed information and is most acute during an infant's first two days on the unit. Discussions with nurses who transport infants to the hospital might reveal that they usually have three to five minutes to talk with parents before the infant is transported. The transport nurses feel that tips on how to more effectively counsel parents during that brief period would enable them to lower parental anxiety.

As a result of the needs assessment, the PEM may decide to organize a discussion among NICU and transport staff on methods for reducing parental anxiety. The PEM could use all the information from the needs assessment to determine whether development of an orientation booklet would in fact be a valuable intervention.

Questions such as the following need to be considered:

- Whose needs are being served?
- What is known about that population?

- What is the educational need?
- How has that educational need been identified?
- What is being done now to address that need?

The scope of a given project, its priority, and the available resources help determine how formally those questions must be addressed. When developing a one-page sheet of medication instructions, for example, those questions could be adequately addressed in less than an hour. On the other hand, a more extensive materials development project (such as a series of pamphlets for one of the hospital's priority service areas) may require a more formal needs assessment involving interviews with patients.

Developing a profile of patients and needs also helps shift the focus from patient education as a product to the broader view of patient education as a process. Materials are then perceived as tools for accomplishing an overall educational plan rather than as the total patient education effort. Maintaining a focus on that expansive view of patient education and engendering that perspective among other health care professionals is perhaps the most important key to the effective use of print materials.

Can That Need Best Be Addressed through Print Materials?

Once the educational need has been defined and assessed to the extent possible, how that need can best be addressed must be considered. Reaching a decision about the "best" approach involves weighing factors such as educational effectiveness and extent of resources. Some of the questions that are helpful in determining whether print materials can best address the defined need are:

- What action does the patient need to take?
- What is currently being done to help patients take that action?
- Would a teaching tool support staff by increasing the effectiveness and/or efficiency of their efforts?
- Would a print, video, or audio tool be most effective in helping patients take that action?
- What funds are available to purchase or develop materials?

Considering these questions can be a fairly simple, rapid process. However, proceeding through them is another step that helps ensure print materials really will enhance efforts to address a need.

Is New Material Really Necessary?

Before developing new materials, it is essential to identify and obtain existing materials, and then critique them to determine if they are appropriate. If appropriate materials are available, the PEM can determine whether to purchase them or develop new ones by assessing funding resources and relative costs.

Locating Existing Materials

Tapping into existing resources promotes more effective use of print materials. After determining that print materials will help meet an identified need, the PEM should identify and obtain existing materials that may address that need. (Consulting the guides to print materials in the appendix to this chapter is a useful place to begin.) PEMs may then wish to request samples of materials from voluntary associations, government agencies, and commercial producers. In addition to those sources, colleagues in other health care organizations can be contacted to determine whether they have materials to suggest or share.

For example, consider a search for materials dealing with pediatric cancer. An excellent starting point is the Cancer Patient Education subfile of the Combined Health

Information Database (CHID). CHID is a computerized bibliographic data base developed and managed by several federal agencies; the National Cancer Institute developed and manages the Cancer Patient Education subfile. A search of CHID's Cancer Patient Education subfile reveals descriptions of materials and programs on pediatric cancer as well as contact information on PEMs with expertise in pediatric cancer. (Information on how to access CHID is available in the appendix to this chapter.)

What might the search process look like if the PEM wants to collect materials on smoking cessation, a topic for which a plethora of materials is available? Again, the search might begin with the pertinent CHID subfiles. Material could also be obtained directly from local offices of the American Heart Association, the American Lung Association, and the American Cancer Society. (The guides referenced in the appendix to this chapter list smoking cessation materials available from government agencies and commercial producers.)

Critiquing Materials

Following collection of existing materials, the next step is to assess their appropriateness for the target population. Figure 17-1 presents a form for reviewing print material. It requires critique from four perspectives: clinical, educational, technical, and affective. In order to critique materials on all four dimensions, reviewers should include clinicians with content expertise, individuals with educational expertise, and laypeople. Although this form does not yield a numerical score for materials reviewed, it is possible to establish criteria for reviewer acceptance. For example, 10 factors could be selected on the form that appear to be most critical and materials would be deemed appropriate only if at least 80 percent of the reviewers circled "agree" for those 10 factors.

Readers may also wish to consult Gibson and others[1] for an example of a print materials review form that employs a numerical rating scale. Patient education colleagues may also be able to provide fine examples of tools for critiquing print materials.

Deciding Whether to Purchase or Develop Materials

Costs and funding resources enter heavily into the decision to purchase or develop materials. How does the purchase cost compare with the cost of materials development and production? Are there political benefits to developing materials in-house (for instance, gaining increased support for patient education by collaborating with medical staff on a materials development project)? Who will assume the expense? Can multiple areas share the expense of purchase or development? Can cost be recovered through patient charges?

Regardless of whether the decision is to develop or purchase materials, the PEM should be able to answer the following questions before using the materials:

- How will the materials be integrated into the teaching plan?
- Who will give patients the materials, and when?
- How can those providers be helped to learn about this tool and how to use it?
- How will staff access this material?
- How will supplies of this material be replenished?

At the very least, reviewing existing materials offers ideas that improve the quality of any new materials produced. Being able to document that no appropriate tool exists may also help secure funds for materials development.

☐ Developing Effective Print Materials

The references in the appendix to this chapter list several excellent guides to development of health communications.[2-4] Consulting those sources will enhance the quality of materials that are developed. The following section offers general guidance for developing

Figure 17-1. Form for Reviewing Print Patient Education Materials

Date: _____ Title: _____

Format:
Single-page handout _____ Pamphlet _____ Booklet _____ Other _____

Source: _____ Cost: _____

Evaluated by: _____

Intended audience: (please circle response(s))

| High education | Moderate education | Low education | Pediatric | General | Other _____ |

Desired use/purpose for this material (include identified educational need):

Overall, how would you rate this material for use with identified audience?

| Very useful | Somewhat useful | Not useful |

For the following factors, please circle the appropriate response.

Clinical Assessment:

Information is current.
   Agree   Neutral   Disagree   N/A

Information is accurate.
   Agree   Neutral   Disagree   N/A

Information is sufficient for purpose.
   Agree   Neutral   Disagree   N/A

Educational Assessment:

Organization of information is appropriate (logical, easy to follow, builds on prior content).
   Agree   Neutral   Disagree   N/A

Learning objectives are identified *and* appropriate.
   Agree   Neutral   Disagree   N/A

Language level is appropriate for intended audience.
   Agree   Neutral   Disagree   N/A

Technical terms are identified.
   Agree   Neutral   Disagree   N/A

Amount of information delivered is appropriate.
   Agree   Neutral   Disagree   N/A

Maintains interest and attention.
   Agree   Neutral   Disagree   N/A

Visuals/graphics are used to illustrate concepts.
   Agree   Neutral   Disagree   N/A

Summary/review of important points is included.
   Agree   Neutral   Disagree   N/A

Self-assessment or practice is solicited.
   Agree   Neutral   Disagree   N/A

(Continued on next page)

Figure 17-1. (Continued)

Technical Assessment:

Text is clearly legible.

      Agree   Neutral   Disagree   N/A

White space minimizes concentration of text.

      Agree   Neutral   Disagree   N/A

Paragraphs are short and simple.

      Agree   Neutral   Disagree   N/A

Informational headings are used.

      Agree   Neutral   Disagree   N/A

Main points stand out clearly.

      Agree   Neutral   Disagree   N/A

Illustrations are simple and easy to understand.

      Agree   Neutral   Disagree   N/A

Illustrations clearly promote the textual information.

      Agree   Neutral   Disagree   N/A

Affective Assessment:

Overall appearance is appealing.

      Agree   Neutral   Disagree   N/A

Overall message is clear and evident.

      Agree   Neutral   Disagree   N/A

Tone is personalized and positive.

      Agree   Neutral   Disagree   N/A

Stereotyping is avoided.

      Agree   Neutral   Disagree   N/A

Commercial product promotion is not noticeable.

      Agree   Neutral   Disagree   N/A

Would this material be useful to patients independently, or should its use be guided by a nurse or other health care professional?

      Independent use   Guided use

Does the program contain information or visuals that might be offensive to a certain population?

      Yes   No

If so, please explain _____

_____

Does the program contain information that is inappropriate to the needs of patients at our hospital?

      Yes   No

If so, please explain _____

_____

Is there important relevant information that is not covered in this material and should be?

      Yes   No

If so, please identify _____

_____

Developed at the Department of Patient and Community Health Education, University of Virginia Health Sciences Center, 1991.

Used, with permission, from the University of Virginia Health Sciences Center, Charlottesville.

print materials for patients.[5] First, eight steps in developing materials are described. The challenge of developing materials for low-literacy populations is then broadly addressed. The section concludes with an overview of considerations in developing culturally sensitive materials.

Eight Steps in Materials Development

The following steps are generic guidelines for development of print materials. They begin with developing a portrait of the target audience and conclude with using evaluation results to improve the materials development process.

Step 1. Focus on the Audience and What It Needs to Know and Do

Gathering information on the target audience and formulating clear objectives for the material are the initial steps in developing effective print materials. The profile of the target population and the objectives then drive development of the content outline.

Identify with the Target Audience

All information on the target population should be reviewed. What does this group look like in terms of age, educational level, urban versus rural residence, average background in the content area, and so on? This information creates the portrait of the target audience.

Focus should then be directed to the "typical" patient to whom the material is targeted. What might be some of his or her questions, concerns, and fears? These should be addressed in the material being developed.

Define Objectives for the Material in Behavioral Terms

With the target population clearly in mind, objectives for the material should be formulated. Specifically, what should the patient be able to know and do after reading the material? (Examples of objectives are provided in Step 7.)

Focus on Objectives While Developing the Content Outline

The behavioral objectives are used to define the content of the material. Only information that is necessary to help the patient accomplish the learning objectives should be included. One of the greatest mistakes made in developing health communications is to bury vital information among unnecessary details. A pamphlet on taking medications does not need to include discourses on the history of pharmacology and primers on organic chemistry. Confining the outline to the essential "what" and "how" information helps streamline content from the beginning.

Step 2. Write a Draft

The content outline is used as the basis for writing a draft of the material. Following are specific guidelines for writing patient education materials.

Write as Though Talking with the Patient

The writing should be in a conversational tone. The text should begin with an introductory paragraph that helps establish a positive and personal relationship. The patient should be informed of the purpose of the information and exactly what he or she should be able to know or do after reading this information.

Keep Writing Simple and Direct

It is important to try to say exactly what is meant, using as few and as simple words as possible. Sentences should be short but not choppy. Paragraphs should be limited to four or five sentences and one key concept. If technical terms will be helpful to patients in managing their condition, they should be used but couched in simple language.

Some patients and family members wish to study more detailed and technical information. To encourage their participation in care, it is useful to identify supplemental materials and make them or a bibliography available.

Simple, direct language should not sound condescending, even to the most highly educated patients. Rather, such good writing should enable patients to readily understand what they need to know and do.

Use Active Voice

Sentences should be active rather than passive; for example, "Take this medication with breakfast" rather than "This medication should be taken with breakfast."

Make Text Interactive and Build in Review

A number of simple devices should be used to help the reader assume an active role in learning from the material. In addition to conveying a personal tone, using *you* and *your* helps engage the reader's attention. Information seems more personally relevant when addressed to "you" rather than to "the patient."

Building in application and review of information is essential if materials are going to be effective learning tools. A summary of key points should be included at the end of the text. Incorporating sections that require readers to apply information helps them translate content into practice. Figure 17-2 illustrates sections from a booklet on pulmonary diet that enables readers to apply content to their daily lives.

Step 3. Edit and Rewrite

Once the draft of the text is written, it needs to be edited for clarity and relevance of information. It is also advisable to have the draft reviewed and to incorporate any pertinent suggestions.

Eliminate Unnecessary Information and Simplify Wording

After completing the first draft, the text should be edited with a determination to keep it as simple as possible. The content should be critically examined to ensure that it is confined to information that the reader must have to carry out his or her behavioral objectives. These are the steps to follow:

- Read the text out loud.
- Weed out unnecessary information.
- Turn passive sentences into active ones.
- Simplify wordy sentences.
- Substitute simple, common words for less familiar ones.
- Reorganize information to achieve greater clarity.

Have a friend or Colleague Review the Draft

It is useful to ask a friend or colleague to review the draft and offer feedback. Feedback from someone who is unfamiliar with the content area is especially valuable. The draft should then be revised to incorporate useful suggestions.

Step 4. Design the Visual Appearance

Once the text of the draft has been informally reviewed, the visual dimension of the health message should be developed. Visuals include a range of components such as illustrations, color, typeface size and style, spacing of text on the page, and so on. Visuals can emphasize key points, help motivate patients to use instructions, and reduce the amount of reading in the text.[6] The following brief discussion highlights several simple methods that can be used to strengthen print materials with visuals.

Figure 17-2. Making Text Interactive: Examples from a Pulmonary Diet Book

For your review . . .

List some examples of foods from each group that you might eat.

Fruits and vegetables   Dairy

_____   _____

_____   _____

_____   _____

_____   _____

Grains and cereals   Meat and proteins

_____   _____

_____   _____

_____   _____

_____   _____

Place a check by the following changes you could make to improve your eating and breathing habits.

_____ Get regular exercise.
_____ Avoid or reduce anxiety.
_____ Drink plenty of liquids.
_____ Plan your medication times.
_____ Rest before and after your meals.
_____ Keep your mouth and teeth clean.
_____ Avoid eating very hot or very cold foods.
_____ Keep a good posture while eating.
_____ Eat foods that are easy to chew and swallow.
_____ Develop a positive take-charge attitude.

Reprinted, with permission, from I. Hagerty and A. L. Mason, *Your Pulmonary Diet,* published by the University of Virginia, Charlottesville, 1989, pp. 11–12.

Use White Space

White space is the space on the page that does not contain print. Using white space helps to visually highlight specific information and creates a less intimidating appearance. Ways to increase white space include:

* Using wide margins and borders
* Using bullets (lists like this with a dot or other notation preceding each main point)
* Skipping spaces between paragraphs, sections, and so on

Highlight Important Information

Headings, bold type, and bullets in front of phrases are effective ways to highlight information. Using all capital letters to emphasize points should be avoided because a combination of uppercase and lowercase letters is easier to read.

Choose Simple, Clear Illustrations

Simple line drawings are the best illustrations. They should relate directly to the text and include labels where appropriate.

Step 5. Conduct a Simple Field Test

Unlike automotive executives, who test their products rather than proceed from the design board directly to the production line, PEMs frequently distribute their products to customers without field-testing, or pretesting, the products with representatives from the target population to ensure that the products actually work.

Field-testing a draft of the proposed product can help:

- Assess comprehension
- Assess attention and recall
- Identify strong and weak points of material
- Determine personal relevance
- Gauge sensitive or controversial elements[7]

Often field-testing is omitted because it appears to be a complex, time-consuming undertaking. However, it does not need to be. In fact, feedback obtained from 10 to 15 patients is sufficient in most cases. Open-ended questions can be used in individual patient interviews or discussions with groups of patients. It may be feasible to obtain feedback from both providers and patients and involve unit staff in conducting field tests. (A more extensive discussion of field-testing may be found in the guides referenced in the appendix to this chapter.[8-10])

The field test of the draft may well reveal problems with both text and illustrations, and the results from the field test can help strengthen those weak points. If major revisions are made, it may be helpful to also field-test the revised material.

Step 6. Coordinate Production

Once material has been field-tested and revised, the production phase of materials development can proceed. Production includes word processing, graphic design, layout, and illustration as well as photocopying or printing steps. Because "the baby is finally born" at the end of this phase, this step can be the most rewarding one in materials development. However, materials production can also be time-consuming, frustrating, and costly if the PEM is not familiar with keys to negotiating this phase.

One of those keys is knowing what resources are available for production—funds, computer support, graphic design services, printing services, and so on. Resource assessment should occur early on in the development process and not at the point when the material is ready for production.

Determining whether the material will be photocopied or printed is a key decision. Answering the following questions will assist in making that decision:

- Is printing needed to meet the objectives of this material (for example, color or photographs are necessary, material will be a marketing tool, and so on)?
- What quantity of material will be needed over the next year or so?
- Is it less expensive to print or photocopy that quantity?
- Is it likely that funds will be available to reprint this material, or would a continuing supply be better assured if copies could be reproduced as needed?
- Will this material need to be revised frequently or in the near future?

Regardless of whether the material is to be printed or photocopied, desktop publishing capability produces a high-quality product at relatively low cost. Skillfully combining word processing with graphics software provides a product that is ready for the printer or the copy machine. Camera-ready artwork (clip art) and simple line drawings can be used when only word-processing capability is available. The cost of graphic design services and printing is usually lower if text can be supplied on diskette; the graphic designer or printer should be consulted beforehand regarding hardware and software requirements.

Photocopying has become a more attractive option since desktop publishing revolutionized the production of patient education materials. Materials can look quite professional if high-quality copying services are used. Ease of revision is another advantage of photocopying materials rather than printing them. Using colored paper or card stock for covers can add interest to photocopied materials.

However, sometimes the need for color or photographs dictates that the material be printed. Although photocopying is generally less expensive, in the long run printing can be the more economical option if large quantities of materials are required.

The following factors contribute to the cost of printing:

- Dimensions of the material
- Use of photographs
- Number of pages
- Binding, folding
- Number of ink colors
- Number of copies
- Paper weight
- Paper color
- Completion time frame

Effective communication with the printer is key to obtaining the product on time and for the expected cost. If in-house printing services are not required, at least three written estimates and work samples should be obtained from outside printers. Once a printer is selected, the PEM and the printer should meet to discuss the job in detail. Printers can offer expert assistance in choosing paper, ink, and so on, and in working with the PEM to meet his or her budget.

After the meeting, the PEM should send the printer written specifications and request a confirmation of the cost and the delivery date. Printers provide proofs that enable errors to be corrected; at least one person other than the PEM should carefully review the proofs. Proof review should not be regarded as an opportunity for further editing; unnecessary changes at the proof stage will add both delay and cost to the finished product.

When the finished product is in hand, all those involved in its development should receive proper appreciation and recognition. For example, an article in the hospital newsletter featuring staff and patients using the material can provide recognition as well as promote visibility of patient education.

Step 7. Evaluate

Once materials are finally produced, expending more time and energy to evaluate them is not an appealing thought. It is not surprising that most PEMs consider a materials development project completed when the finished product is at last in hand. By that point, a tremendous amount of time and energy has been invested in development of that material and the PEM is already immersed in other projects. Although evaluation of materials can be a major research project, it can also be practical, simple, and inexpensive.

Why is it worthwhile to invest effort in evaluation? Evaluation can help:

- Determine how staff and patients are using the material
- Assess whether the material is helping patients learn what it was intended to help them learn
- Improve other materials projects by applying lessons learned
- Provide feedback to those who contributed to materials development
- Demonstrate accountability for funds used to develop materials

One of the first steps is to decide what type or types of evaluation to conduct. A *process evaluation* helps examine such factors as how materials are being used, and how and why certain elements associated with their use are or are not working. A process evaluation can suggest changes that could be made in procedures, staff training, or materials management in order to enhance use of the material.

For example, the PEM may decide to examine how staff are using a new pamphlet. In this case, the process measure could be the number of pamphlets distributed to patients over a two-week period or the percentage of patient charts documenting that nurses reviewed the pamphlet's content with patients.

Another process approach would be to interview staff to find out how they are using the materials. If the materials are intended to be used in combination with one-on-one teaching, are staff using them that way? If not, what do staff perceive to be the barriers to that usage? Are the materials easily accessible? What problems are staff experiencing in obtaining and using the materials?

An *outcome evaluation* helps determine whether the objectives for the material are being met. This form of evaluation helps document short-term results such as changes in knowledge, attitudes, or behavior. For example, a pamphlet on diabetes pills may be conducted using a pretest and a posttest. Areas in which knowledge change could be assessed might include how to take pills, their side effects, and when to call a physician.

Most PEMs usually want to know whether reading the material makes any difference. To find out, they must have some understanding of what difference the material was intended to make. What specific knowledge, attitudes, and/or behavior was the material designed to effect? If effort was devoted to specifying measurable objectives during the planning phase of materials development, it is possible to assess whether those objectives were achieved.

For instance, following are two objectives:

1. This pamphlet will help patients with arthritis learn how to take aspirin.
2. After reading this pamphlet, patients will be able to state:
   - How much aspirin they should take each day
   - How often they should take it
   - Two problems to watch for in taking aspirin
   - Two steps they can take to alleviate each problem

It is impossible to measure whether the desired learning outcome in the first objective has been achieved. However, the second objective specifies measurable outcomes that can be assessed through an evaluation.

Short length of stay, lack of resources for follow-up, and inability to pinpoint material as the cause of change are some of the factors that frustrate PEM efforts to assess behavioral change. Patients' self-reports of the likelihood of their making a behavioral change is a strong predictor of actual change. This is a fairly simple measure to employ and appears to be one that is underutilized by patient education managers.

As an example, suppose the PEM wishes to evaluate a smoking cessation booklet. Before patients read the booklet, he or she could ask: "On a scale from 1 to 10, where 1 is 'extremely likely' and 10 is 'no likelihood,' how likely do you think it is that you will be able to quit smoking within the next month?" The question could then be repeated after the patient has read the booklet and the difference determined between the two responses.

In summary, PEMs can promote effective use of print materials by employing simple and practical evaluation methods. Those interested in further discussion of evaluation of health communications may wish to consult *Making Health Communication Programs Work*.[11]

Step 8. Use the Evaluation Results
The last step in materials development is to reap the benefits of the investment in evaluation. The evaluation results can be used to:

- Promote more effective use of the material by addressing problems that were identified
- Improve other materials projects by using the information that was gained about elements that worked or did not work
- Demonstrate accountability for the organization's investment in the patient education project by reporting results to decision makers
- Recognize the efforts of those participating in the materials project
- Encourage others to incorporate evaluation into their patient education efforts
- Foster awareness of the benefits of using patient education tools as part of an educational plan
- Help advance the professional development and efforts of others involved in patient education by sharing the evaluation design and results with them

A more in-depth discussion on the use of evaluation findings is contained in *Making Health Communication Programs Work*.[12]

Considerations in Developing Materials for Special Populations

The eight steps just described are basic to development of materials for all populations. Developing materials for special populations requires additional effort to understand the unique needs of those populations and how to effectively address them. PEMs are challenged to strengthen their response to the growing problem of low literacy and to view readability formulas as useful but limited tools. PEMs must also enhance their skills in developing materials that are culturally appropriate.

Addressing the Needs of Low-Literacy Populations

An estimated 23 million American adults lack the reading, writing, and numerical skills needed to function effectively in everyday life.[13] In other words, one out of five American adults is functionally illiterate. These adults cannot read a restaurant menu, address an envelope, or understand directional signs. Contrary to popular belief, illiteracy is found among all socioeconomic groups and races, and this has implications for patient education materials.

What is the relationship between literacy and health? In examining that question, the staff of the Literacy and Health Project in Canada found that illiteracy appears to significantly affect health in both direct and indirect ways.[14] The direct effects of illiteracy on health include incorrect use of medications, not following medical directions, and safety risks. The indirect effects of illiteracy on health are overwhelming:

Illiteracy leads to poor lifestyle practices, stress, unhealthy living and working conditions, and results in lack of access to health information and to inappropriate use of medical and health services. It also frequently results in unemployment and in poverty.[15]

The Centers for Disease Control (CDC) have published an annotated bibliography designed to help health care professionals meet the needs of low-literacy populations.[16] Items in the publication *Literacy and Health in the United States: Selected Annotations* are also listed in the Combined Health Information Database (CHID).

Learning to communicate effectively with patients who have low-literacy skills is one small step that PEMs can take toward resolution of this global problem. Influenced by the pioneering work of Leonard and Cecilia Doak and Jane Root, the writing guidelines in the preceding section apply to development of low-literacy materials. The references[17,18] at the end of this chapter offer a more in-depth treatment of principles and strategies for teaching patients with low-literacy skills.

Exercising Caution in Using Readability Formulas

Enhanced awareness among PEMs of the low-literacy problem has stimulated intense interest in readability formulas. By focusing on sentence length and vocabulary difficulty, these formulas enable the PEM to estimate the reading level of material. To achieve the best fit between materials and patient needs, it is important to treat reading level as one of many elements that affect ability to learn from materials.

In selecting and developing print materials, the following limitations of readability formulas should be kept in mind:[19,20]

- Readability formulas do not consider many of the factors that are critical to clear writing. For example, a text with short, choppy sentences may earn a low reading score and yet be very difficult to read. The fact that an item is written at a low reading level does not mean that it is clear and well written.
- Readability formulas do not address visual elements, which are key determinants of reading ease and appeal.
- The precision of readability formulas is misleading; the scores they yield are approximations.
- By nature, readability formulas do not consider patient characteristics. Level of knowledge, prior experience, cultural background, motivation, and interest are key determinants of how much patients learn from reading materials.

In summary, reading level should be treated as one of many elements to be considered when assessing the appropriateness of print materials for low-literacy populations. The materials review form in figure 17-1 can be used to achieve the best fit between patients and materials.

Developing Culturally Sensitive Materials

What are culturally sensitive patient education materials? They are materials that reflect intimate familiarity with, and respect for, the language, values, and customs of the target culture. As Hall[21] states:

To create culturally appropriate nutrition and health education materials for America's growing ethnic minority population, more than translation services are needed. Materials need to be adapted or even redesigned, using concepts, methods, activities and meal plans that are relevant to the culture.[22]

Simply translating materials from English into another language rarely, if ever, yields culturally sensitive materials. As Hall notes, "Literal translations fail to modify the content to make it relevant to the members of the target culture."[23] To illustrate her point, Hall uses the example of a Spanish-language booklet on diabetes that defines one bread exchange as equal to one-half bagel; a more relevant example would have used the daily staple of tortillas.[24] References at the end of this chapter[25,26] should be consulted to further skills in development of culturally sensitive materials.

The Office of Minority Health Resource Center in the Department of Health and Human Services responds to inquiries on minority health-related topics by distributing materials and providing referrals. Among the excellent resources available from the Office of Minority Health are listings of health materials for African-Americans and Spanish-language materials. Contact information is listed in the appendix to this chapter.

☐ Developing Hospitalwide Approaches to Promoting Effective Use of Materials

One way to encourage more effective use of patient education materials throughout a hospital is to implement a policy for producing and approving them. Another key approach is to develop a system that ensures that staff have ready access to the materials.

Developing a Hospitalwide Policy and Approval Mechanism

Instituting a hospitalwide policy for development and approval of patient education materials can be an important vehicle for promoting the effective use of print tools. What are the benefits of a patient education materials policy?

A materials policy can promote consistently high-quality educational tools. It can incorporate the development guidelines discussed earlier in this chapter. Incorporating a requirement for review during the conceptual or draft stage of materials development can provide formative evaluation and improve the effectiveness of the final product. By encouraging use of development guidelines and by using the review process, the policy can advance the perception of materials as tools within a planned patient education effort.

A hospitalwide materials policy can also aid efforts to promote patient education and the hospital. By specifying standards for production, the policy can help ensure that the materials present a uniformly excellent image for both the program and the institution. It may be advantageous to require that all patient education materials follow a standardized format or at least incorporate the patient education or institutional logo. Such standardization helps internal and external customers readily identify materials as patient education products developed within the hospital.

A hospitalwide policy for materials development and approval can also promote coordination and cooperation among service areas. By requiring that all materials under development be channeled through one department or committee, the policy can prevent duplication of effort and increase awareness of resources.

How does the PEM go about instituting a policy on development and approval of patient education materials? One of the first steps is to investigate the feasibility of instituting such a policy. In some cases, such as in a highly decentralized organization where individual units have great autonomy, a first step may be to offer guidelines for materials development rather than pursue a policy mandate.

As with any patient education effort, determining who needs to be involved and how to win their support is critical to the success of this policy endeavor. What individuals or committees need to be involved in development and approval of policies? What needs to be done to ensure that the policy receives the support required to translate it from paper to practice? Who should and can be involved in the review of materials?

After investigating those fundamental questions, a materials policy can be drafted. The statement should specify:

- The rationale for the policy
- What materials are subject to review
- The stage at which materials should be reviewed
- Guidelines for development
- How to submit materials for review
- Approximate time required for review

To aid in formulating a policy statement, the PEM may wish to review samples of materials policies from other hospitals. Those who will be affected by the policy should have input into its development, with respect to both content and means to translate it into practice.

Developing Materials Distribution Systems

No matter how much work has been invested in selecting and developing materials, they will not be used to their full potential if an effective distribution system is not in place. The basic goal of a materials distribution system is to provide staff with ready access to the teaching materials. Some of the key factors that determine what type of system will most effectively accomplish that goal within a given organization are: complexity of the organization, extent to which patient education is centralized, flow of communication within the organization, availability of computer support, and staff and financial resources that can be dedicated to establishing and managing a system. No one system works best in all hospitals. (See chapter 19 for a discussion of the potential roles of consumer health information centers in materials distribution systems.)

Materials distribution systems fall along a continuum from decentralized to centralized approaches. Although a system can be developed that leans toward one end of the continuum, incorporating decentralized and centralized elements into a single system may enable the PEM to draw on the strengths of both.

A decentralized approach is typically one in which individual patient care units, floors, or departments maintain primary responsibility for funding, ordering, organizing, and storing materials. A totally decentralized approach to materials distribution would represent an inefficient use of institutional resources. In addition, it would be difficult to ensure the quality of materials provided to patients under a completely decentralized approach. However, a decentralized approach does enable each patient care area to exercise a high degree of autonomy and flexibility in developing and controlling a materials system that meets its unique needs.

Under a centralized approach, responsibility for purchasing and copying materials, maintaining an inventory, providing listings of available materials, and distributing materials to patient care areas is retained by one or a few areas. For example, the patient education department, hospital library, and storeroom may collaborate in managing a centralized materials distribution system.

A centralized approach can produce cost savings. Consolidating materials management may free unit staff to perform other care functions and result in greater system efficiencies. Additionally, costs of materials may be reduced as a result of ordering materials in greater quantity.

Establishing and managing a highly centralized materials distribution system obviously requires staff time, space, and operating resources. To obtain those resources, it is useful to conduct a needs assessment in order to document materials management problems and estimate costs being incurred by individual patient care areas in ordering materials, photocopying them, and so on. If the decision is made to proceed with development of a centralized system, resources could be extended by drawing on volunteers to assist with functions such as receiving and filling orders from patient care areas.

One of the disadvantages of a highly centralized approach is that staff may feel less ownership in the system. Involving representatives from all areas in development of the system can help staff assert a stronger role in ensuring that the distribution system works for their service area. Building decentralized elements into the system can also help staff experience a greater sense of ownership. For example, two service areas with similar materials needs may be able to jointly manage materials ordering and storage. This approach may provide staff with more rapid access to materials and entail less expense than the centralized system alone would.

Providing staff with a directory of available teaching aids is key to ensuring the effectiveness of both centralized and decentralized approaches. The directory promotes staff awareness of available teaching materials and can help reduce potential duplication of effort in developing materials. When the materials system is more decentralized, the directory can reduce inefficiencies by promoting collaboration among areas with similar materials needs.

Compiling, distributing, and updating a directory of teaching aids requires the collaboration of a hospitalwide team. Representatives from patient care areas should be involved in identifying teaching materials that are presently being used, and the expertise of health librarians should be drawn on to help develop materials categories. Once the directory is produced, representatives from patient care areas should again be employed to help introduce staff to the directory, distribute copies, and report updated information.

Computer-Supported Systems

An increasing number of organizations are integrating patient education resources into their computer information systems. One of the first steps that many of these organizations have taken is to develop an on-line catalog of patient education resources. In more sophisticated systems, materials can be ordered on-line; more basic systems list locations of materials. Benefits of a computer catalog of resource materials include improved access to materials, increased awareness of available materials, and ease of updating the catalog.

The University of Missouri Hospital and Clinics employs an on-line computer system that offers indexing, order entry, and documentation of patient education materials.[27] This centralized on-line system features:

- An index of all approved patient education materials (print and audiovisual)
- A listing of patient data
- Documentation of the distribution of educational materials to patients
- The on-line and hard-copy documentation of the staff member's educational transactions
- An annotated brief of each indexed material
- An on-line inventory of all materials developed
- A mechanism to generate a patient charge for materials
- A summation report of transactions by staff members, materials, or units/areas[28]

According to Kruckenberg Schofer and Ward, benefits of this system include on-unit access to an education materials catalog, ease of updating the index, reduction of paperwork, provision of a permanent record of educational interactions, and generation of a patient charge.

The documentation features of this system promote integration of materials into the educational plan by requiring users to enter educational objectives and outcome/evaluation of the educational encounter. Thus, this feature also facilitates compliance with JCAHO and legal requirements for documentation. The University of Missouri system exemplifies the potential of computers to promote effective use of patient education materials.

☐ Expanding the Patient Education Manager's Role in Quality Improvement

Patient education managers have several roles in ensuring the quality of patient education efforts. First, they can sometimes function more effectively by shifting their primary emphasis to that of internal consultant rather than materials producer. They can also evaluate materials for effectiveness and suggest ways to improve them.

Materials Consultant versus Materials Producer

How do staff within the organization perceive the role of the patient education department and the PEM? Many patient education departments and PEMs find that they are viewed as materials producers. If that is the perception, the next step is to either decide that is appropriate or work to alter that definition of roles.

Altering the perception of roles may be a matter of expanding awareness of the focus and range of current services. On the other hand, that perception may accurately reflect the patient education staff's emphasis on function and services up to that point. The patient education staff may determine that they exert a greater impact within the hospital by redefining their primary role to that of internal consultants versus materials producers. If the intent is to move away from a materials production role, the patient education staff must: (1) clearly delineate their new role, (2) set service priorities that are consistent with that new role, (3) establish a procedure for handling materials development requests, (4) market the department's new service image within the hospital, and (5) employ a range of strategies to support effective use of patient education materials.

One strategy for helping to accomplish the PEM's shift in role to that of internal consultant is to develop a resource packet on materials development for health care professionals. The Department of Patient and Community Health Education at the University of Virginia Health Sciences Center offers the following resources in its packet:

- An overview of the program development process
- A checklist for evaluating materials
- Information on conducting a needs assessment
- Writing guidelines
- Readability formula
- Tips for layout and design
- Guidelines for pretesting
- A list of sources of health information

When a health care professional requests assistance with materials development, a patient education staff person arranges a one- to two-hour consultation session to review the packet and walk through the planning phase of materials development with the health professional. The latter may recontact the department for brief consultation at any point during the materials development process.

Other strategies that enable the department to focus on process consultation rather than materials production are:

- Delivering training programs on the effective use of patient education materials
- Helping staff easily access materials by identifying sources and providing copies
- Providing a resource room for health care professionals that contains materials directories and catalogs, samples of print materials, camera-ready artwork, and development guidelines
- Encouraging recognition for materials development in the Division of Nursing's career ladder system and performance evaluation process

The Patient Education Manager's Role as an Advocate for Quality

PEMs can assert strong leadership in improving the quality of print materials. Professional exchange is one mechanism that helps advance the quality of patient education tools. Conferences, journals, and professional organizations provide excellent forums for sharing strategies for evaluating materials, criteria for assessing appropriateness of print materials, and expertise in developing materials for special populations.

Another avenue for promoting quality is providing feedback to producers on ways to improve the quality of their materials. Despite the abundance of materials on the market, there is a shortage of patient education tools that appropriately address human diversity. PEMs should contact materials producers and communicate their expectation that materials will be responsive to the needs of special populations. Although field-testing is essential to development of effective materials, few materials producers indicate that they field-test their patient education materials. PEMs can encourage producers to make field-testing standard practice by asking whether their materials have been field-tested, and whenever possible, by informing producers that they will purchase only field-tested materials.

By the same token, colleagues and producers who do develop and field-test materials that are sensitive to patients' diversity should be applauded. Providing feedback to producers on the strengths and deficiencies of their materials is another step that promotes effective use of patient education materials.

□ Conclusion

Print materials can be valuable tools for patient education managers. When used effectively, print materials can help staff maximize limited teaching time and enable patients to better manage their health. However, apparently many PEMs have difficulty tapping into the full potential of print materials.

One key to effective use of print tools bears repeating: Effective use of print tools starts with defining the need. Definition of need includes developing a profile of the target population and its needs, specifying the need to be addressed, and determining whether print materials represent an appropriate tool for helping to meet that need. The next steps are to identify, obtain, and assess existing materials. In summary, it cannot be assumed that print materials are the answer to every problem; time needs to be taken to explore all the "trees in the forest."

It is important to learn from what is already available. That is key not only to effective use of print materials but, more broadly, to effectiveness as a patient education manager. In addition to its abundance of good and not-so-good materials, the field of patient education is blessed with a wealth of excellent PEMs, programs, and research. Drawing on the richness of those resources is one of the most important steps that PEMs can take to promote effective use of print materials.

References

1. Gibson, P. A., Ruby, C., and Craig, M. D. A health/patient education database for family practice. *Bulletin of the Medical Library Association* 79(4):357–69, 1991.

2. Doak, C. C., Doak, L. G., and Root, J. H. *Teaching Patients With Low Literacy Skills.* Philadelphia: J. B. Lippincott Co., 1985.

3. National Cancer Institute, Department of Health and Human Services, Office of Cancer Communications. *Making Health Communications Work: A Planner's Guide.* Washington, DC: NIH Publications No. 89-1493, Apr. 1989.

4. Zimmermann, M., Newton, N., Frumin, L., and Wittet, S. *Developing Health and Family Planning Print Materials for Low Literate Audiences: A Guide.* Washington, DC: PATH (Program for Appropriate Technology in Health), 1989.

5. Adapted from A. L. Mason, *Developing Patient Communications,* unpublished resource sheet. Charlottesville, VA: University of Virginia Health Sciences Center, 1990.

6. Doak and others, p. 103.

7. National Cancer Institute, p. 39.

8. Doak and others.

9. National Cancer Institute.

10. Zimmermann and others.

11. National Cancer Institute.

12. National Cancer Institute.

13. Doak and others.

14. Ontario Public Health Association and Frontier College: The Literacy and Health Project, Making the World Healthier and Safer for People Who Can't Read, Phase One (report). Toronto: Ontario Public Health Association and Frontier College, 1989, pp. 22–32.

15. Ontario Public Health Association and Frontier College, p. 24.

16. Centers for Disease Control, Center for Chronic Disease Prevention and Health Promotion. *Literacy And Health In The United States: Selected Annotations.* Atlanta, GA: CDC, 1991.

17. Doak and others.

18. Zimmermann and others.

19. Meade, C. D., and Smith, C. F. Readability formulas: cautions and criteria. *Patient Education and Counseling* 17(2):153–58, 1991.

20. Pichert, J. W., and Elam, P. Readability formulas may mislead you. *Patient Education and Counseling* 7(1):181–91, 1985.

21. Hall, T. A. Designing culturally relevant educational materials for Mexican American clients. *The Diabetes Educator* 13(3):281–85, 1987.

22. Hall, p. 284.

23. Hall, p. 285.

24. Hall, pp. 281–85.

25. Hall, pp. 281–85.

26. González, V. M., González, J. T., Freeman, V., and Howard-Pitney, B. *Health Promotion in Diverse Cultural Communities.* Palo Alto, CA: Stanford Health Promotion Resource Center, 1991.

27. Kruckenberg Schofer, K. K, and Ward, C. J. The computerization of the patient education process. *Computers in Nursing* 8(3):116–22, 1990.

28. Kruckenberg Schofer and Ward, p. 117.

☐ Appendix. Guides to Locating Print Patient Education Materials

Combined Health Information Database (CHID)

The Combined Health Information Database (CHID) is a computerized bibliographic data base developed and managed in a collaborative effort by several federal agencies. It contains references to health information and health education resources, and serves health educators, health care professionals, and consumers. This data base includes bibliographic citations and abstracts for journal articles, reports, books, pamphlets, audiovisuals, and health education and health promotion programs.

At present, there are 21 subfiles on CHID:

- AIDS education
- AIDS school health education
- Alzheimer's disease
- Arthritis and musculoskeletal and skin diseases
- Asthma education
- Blood resources
- Cancer patient education
- Cancer prevention and control
- Cholesterol, high blood pressure, and smoking education
- Deafness and other communication disorders
- Diabetes
- Digestive diseases
- Disease prevention/health promotion
- Eye health education
- Health promotion and education
- Heart attack
- Kidney and urologic diseases
- Maternal and child health
- Oral health
- Posttraumatic stress disorder
- VA patient health education

The CHID is available through BRS/Maxwell Online, Inc. Many public, university, and hospital libraries subscribe to BRS, so those wishing to search CHID should check with their local libraries first. Information on subscribing directly to CHID can be obtained by contacting:

BRS Information Technologies
Maxwell Online, Inc.
8000 Westpark Drive
McLean, VA 22101
Phone: 800/468-0908

For additional specific information on CHID, contact:

Combined Health Information Database
Attention: Mr. Richard Pike
National Institutes of Health
Box CHID
9000 Rockville Pike
Rockville, MD 20892
Phone: 301/468-6555
FAX: 301/770-5164

Consumer Health Information Sourcebook, 3rd ed., 1990, by Alan M. Rees and Catherine Hoffman

This publication contains descriptions of books, magazines and newsletters, pamphlets, health information clearinghouses, organizations, toll-free hotlines, and other sources of health information. Descriptions cover more than 30 diseases and topics. This sourcebook also includes a directory of publishers and authors, subjects, and titles.

The _Consumer Health Information Sourcebook_ can be purchased from:

Oryx Press
4041 North Central, Suite 700
Phoenix, AZ 85012
Phone: 602/265-2651

Consumer Health and Nutrition Index

This publication provides ready access to articles in health magazines, general magazines, and newsletters. Subjects include nutrition, specific diseases, drugs, exercise, and other health areas. The end of the index includes a separate section of citations to articles containing book and audiovisual reviews.

The _Consumer Health and Nutrition Index_ is available from:

Oryx Press
4041 North Central, Suite 700
Phoenix, AZ 85012
Phone: 602/265-2651

Health Reference Center

The Health Reference Center is a comprehensive compact disc-based system that provides current information on hundreds of health topics, including diseases, drugs, medical treatments and advances, fitness, nutrition, and others. The Center includes information from a wide variety of periodicals and numerous reference books as well as custom-written background information on more than 300 diseases and medical conditions.

The Health Reference Center is available on compact disc through subscription. Contact:

Information Access Company
362 Lakeside Drive
Foster City, CA 94404
Phone: 800/227-8431

Health Resource Builder: Free and Inexpensive Materials for Libraries and Teachers

This reference is a guide to free and low-cost print materials available from government departments and associations, foundations, and institutions involved in health. Among the numerous areas covered are cancer, sexuality, health education, mental illness, heart disease, and diabetes. This guide also provides information on national health observances, health hotlines, and regional and state offices of public agencies.

Health Resource Builder: Free and Inexpensive Materials for Libraries and Teachers can be purchased from:

McFarland and Company, Inc.
Box 611
Jefferson, NC 28640
Phone: 919/246-4460

Office of Disease Prevention and Health Promotion, National Health Information Center

The National Health Information Center assists the public in locating health information by identifying resources and through an inquiry and referral system. Questions are referred to appropriate sources who then respond to inquiries. This office prepares and distributes invaluable publications and directories on disease prevention and health promotion topics. Among those excellent publications are the *Directory of Health Information Resources in the Federal Government*, the *Healthfinders* series of resource lists, and *Staying Healthy: A Bibliography of Health Promotion Materials*.

Access this resource by writing or calling:

ODPHP National Health Information Center
P.O. Box 1133
Washington, DC 20013-1133
Phone: 800/336-4797
Maryland residents only should phone 301/565-4167.

Office of Minority Health Resource Center

This office responds to inquiries from consumers and professionals regarding minority health-related topics. It distributes materials, provides referrals, identifies sources of technical assistance, and coordinates a network of professionals involved in the field of minority health and related areas. Among the excellent resources offered by this resource center are *Guide to Health Materials for Black Americans* and *Sources of Spanish Language Health Materials*.

Access this resource by calling or writing:

Office of Minority Health Resource Center
P.O. Box 37337
Washington, DC 20013-7337
Phone: 800/444-6472

Chapter 18

Enhancing the Role of Families in Patient Education

Bobby Heagerty, M.A.

□ Objectives

The reader will be able to:

- Describe various roles of the family in patient care and education
- Discuss the benefits and challenges of involving families in patient care and education
- Define the goals for involving families in patient care and education
- Identify specific strategies for involving families in patient care and education
- Describe a process for developing family support programs
- Describe an example of a comprehensive model program of family involvement and education

□ The Relationship of Families to Patient Wellness

Families play a critical role in the recovery and rehabilitation of hospital patients. In all aspects of patient care, the family's involvement can make the difference between readjustment and recovery *and* a worsened condition that requires readmission to the hospital. The values and beliefs of the family are the true context in which the patient will or will not thrive, both in the hospital and outside. The family's informational, educational, and support needs must be addressed by health care providers in all care settings, or optimal health outcomes for the patient will not be achieved.

This chapter defines the characteristics of family dynamics and involvement related to patient care and education. It offers useful tips and resources to assist in the development and enhancement of family education and support services. In addition, it examines general approaches to involving families and specific examples of successful programs in a variety of settings.

☐ Definition of the Family and Its Roles in Patient Care

A family may be formally defined as those persons related by blood or marriage, but a broader and more accurate definition also includes individuals tied by emotional bonds, such as significant others or friends. A family can also be described as an interactive, interdependent system: What affects one family member affects the other(s).

In the context of patient care, the focus is on that family member who is the patient's primary care giver. Although children, parents, spouses, siblings, extended family, and friends all have a bearing on the patient's health and well-being, it is the primary care giver who has the most effect and in turn is most affected. Thus, although the whole family is affected by a diagnosis or an incident, it is the primary care giver who is the one the health care team is most responsible to for the good of the patient.

In addition to defining the people included in the term *family,* a family can be further described by its various roles in patient care. Although providing care is a major role, the less tangible roles of providing social and emotional support are also vital.

In the care-giver role, families may assist patients both in the hospital and after discharge. Family members may need to help with care as a patient recovers from a short-term condition, or they may need to provide ongoing assistance for a chronic condition. Families may also provide assistance with activities of daily living, such as bathing, dressing, walking, and other functions. Additionally, the role of care giver has become increasingly important as the numbers of elderly have grown and as these individuals need more assistance.

Another of the family's roles is to provide a social milieu and support system for the patient: heritage, values, educational level, and economic status. The family often dictates the life-style, access to health care services, expectations of the health care system, and ability to pay for services.

Finally, the family's role as an emotional support system further defines and complicates the picture. As the family provides emotional support for the patient, it develops its own emotional needs, which need to be addressed by health care staff.

The family's active participation in the provision of care, social milieu, and emotional support underscore the hospital's need to consider the task of family education and support separate from that of traditional patient education. Health care can no longer focus solely on patient care; it must also address the needs and contributions of the family.

To further complicate the issue, the roles of patient, primary (family) care giver, other family members, and assorted medical professionals fluctuate and interweave. As society changes, the traditional roles of the family are redefined. Self-care has taken over many areas of care previously designated solely to nurses or physicians. Family care givers also provide more and more home health care. Also, in many cases the process of making decisions about care becomes a joint one between the medical professionals and the patient and family. Of necessity, health care in which patients and families participate has transcended traditional health care.

☐ The Changing Health Care Environment and Family Involvement

Certain changes in the health care environment are important to understanding why families are playing a greater role in patient care and recovery. Demographic, social, and economic factors, as well as a philosophical shift in the focus of care, have led hospitals to depend more on family members in ensuring the well-being of patients.

In addition, the aging of the U.S. population has had a tremendous impact on the health care system. Because the crest of the baby-boomer wave has just hit middle age and because these individuals can look forward to a long life span, the need for greater resources and ways to care for the aging population will continue.

Despite the common perception about the routine nature of institutionalized care for the elderly,[1] American families place relatives in nursing facilities less often than families in other Western countries.[2] Families in this country provide more than 80 percent of the day-to-day care for the chronically impaired or frail elderly. For this reason, health care organizations must continue to find better ways to sustain the family's commitment to care.

Social policies and economic pressures will continue to squeeze the health care system to do more for less. This generally means shorter inpatient lengths of stay and greater use of outpatient services. As this happens, health care providers will need to involve families and care givers even more to fill the gaps in care.

Traditional, biological families are less available; they are scattered, already busy with full-time employment, and preoccupied with a wider variety of responsibilities. Family groups are smaller, more women are in the work force, and divorce and remarriage are blurring the lines of family responsibility. Thus, involving families in patient care has become more complex.

A philosophical shift in the focus of care is another significant factor in family involvement. Like the term *family*, which has been radically redefined, the terms *quality of life* and *wellness* are being reexamined and refocused. To be sure, achieving a good quality of life for patients has always been the goal of the health care system, and wellness has been the underpinning of this definition. However, with the explosion of medical advances, an aging society, and the concurrent increase in chronic disease, the terms *quality of life* and *wellness* have taken on entirely different connotations. Being well is no longer synonymous with being healthy; *being well* implies a wholeness and integrity of self in the face of a variety of predicaments, including disease. This shift to a more philosophical holistic approach to quality of life and wellness has come with the shift to chronic disease management in medicine—an increased emphasis on care versus cure. The emerging strategies for working with families strongly reflect this transition. For example, families must now be involved at an earlier stage of patient care and must be prepared to provide ongoing care and monitoring after the patient is discharged.

Finding, involving, helping, and ultimately empowering families is the most effective way to adjust to the changing health care scene. It will also help address the problems brought about by reduced length of stay, higher acuity, more technology in home care, and other challenges of modern medicine. The next section describes some of the clear benefits to the hospital when patients and families are involved in patient care and can be a constituency to lend hospital support.

☐ The Benefits of Family Involvement in Cultivating a Constituency

There are many benefits to involving families in patient care and education. Patients and their families are not only consumers of health care, they are also constituents of the individuals and institutions that provide those services. Just as voters are politicians, families are a powerful force in numbers that can make a big difference to the health care institution within the context of its relationship to the community it serves. Therefore, involving families in an ongoing way is critical for good constituency relations.

Whether for cross-selling in the marketplace, advocacy for more favorable policies, or support in times of crisis, a constituency can provide hospitals with a powerful and effective advocate in the community. If patients and their families feel that the hospital and providers are there when they need them, they too will be there when needed. Strategic positioning in the community comes with good constituency relations, a force that can be instrumental in helping shape community opinion and future developments. Institutions thus benefit from better market penetration, a heightened image as a socially responsible institution, and improved leverage and influence.

The public relations benefits of strong family education and support programs are also very important. Family opinion can help shape public opinion. Families who leave the hospital feeling as if they still have control of their lives—that they have not just handed the reins over to those who know better—are more likely to advocate for the hospital, refer friends and family to affiliated providers, and express less frustration over the cost of their health care. The image of a hospital as being there for the whole family and caring as well as curing is a very positive one.

Involving and supporting families also creates a fabric of care in society—a safety net for changing times—that enables a community to take care of its own, in partnership with its medical providers. Such societal problems as elder abuse, premature nursing home placement, and care-giver burnout are alleviated by educating and supporting families.

Unlike a continuum of care (figure 18-1), a fabric of care is more a network, with more access points, services used, and movement between and among services (figure 18-2). It is less linear than the continuum concept. A fabric of care prevents the need for crisis planning after the family falls apart and the patient falls through the gaps in the system.

Physician constituency relations are also enhanced when the hospital helps with the time-consuming job of educating and supporting families. Families turn almost unilaterally to their physicians for information on community resources. However, most physicians are focused on the medical management of the patient's problem and do not have the time or capacity to stay current on the various community resources and education available. As a result, physicians do not refer and patients and families may complain that physicians did not provide the information they needed. If physicians and their office staff can direct families to one place for this information—especially a hospital-based resource, which has medical credibility and does not appear to be a social service—their burden is significantly reduced.

☐ Challenges to Involving Families and Providing Care-Giver Services

Many of the challenges to involving and working with families arise because consumers have higher expectations for health care services than other kinds of services. Health care is an intensely interpersonal and intimate phenomenon. As a result, health care providers are expected to utilize communication and compassion in order to enhance the consumer perspective of quality of service delivered. People can become dissatisfied if the communication is ineffective or if they perceive a lack of caring on the part of staff. The following factors need to be understood, acknowledged, and managed.

Increasing Medical Specialization

Increasing medical specialization among physicians, which has accompanied the great advances in providing care, has added to the sense of dissatisfaction among patients and their families. It is harder for patients to work with different providers, many of whom do not know personal preferences or family dynamics. Education and support strategies must compensate for this lack of familiarity.

Heightened Consumer Awareness and the Shift to Patient-Centered Care

Patients and families, as consumers, are demanding more involvement in health care decision making. However, the traditional model of care delivery is seen by many as a paternalistic system. Historically, medical care has been defined by the health care professional, with the physician totally in control. This system has not traditionally involved other family members in decisions. It also tends to treat patients strictly as patients and not as participants in their own care. Although some patients and professionals still prefer this traditional approach, more and more patients are demanding their right to participate in the decision-making process and be treated as people.

The shift to patient-centered care involves the family even more. Family members are expected to provide input for patient care, and they have their own expectations of care for their loved one. What family members expect, from the process as well as the outcome, is an important factor in the dynamic of health care delivery. Recent efforts to refocus health care delivery to address patient expectations, or at least to find out what they are, have altered many of the clinical, informational, and educational approaches of hospital services. Studies show that discrepancies in expectations create much of the

Figure 18-1. Traditional Model of a Continuum of Care

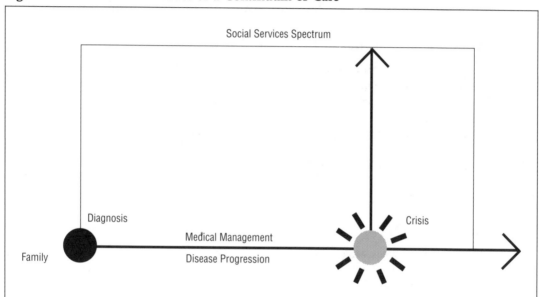

Figure 18-2. Family Support Model for a Fabric of Care

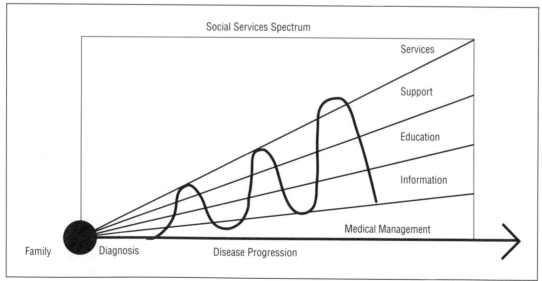

dissatisfaction.[3,4] This seems to indicate that this communication must be in the form of a dialogue and not just didactics.

The Evolution of Roles

Patient–provider and family–provider relationships, like patient–family relationships, are continually evolving. This natural evolution has been broken into three stages:[5] (1) naive trusting (dependence on the goodwill of the professionals); (2) disenchantment (angry aggression, dissatisfaction with care, frustration, and fear); and (3) guarded alliance (purposeful activity promoting cooperation, humanizing, and evaluating according to informed criteria). Though not distinct in their borders nor applicable to all relationships, these phases do apply to many families, especially those dealing with chronic illness. This conceptualization helps develop the rationale for careful assessment and sequential tailoring of educational and support efforts. The challenge for health care providers and educators lies in moving the family rapidly through the first two phases and into the alliance phase as soon and as efficiently as possible. This helps ensure the success of patient education efforts.

The Need for Families to Return to Normalcy

The professional health care system is organized around the medical model of disease, in which medical management focuses on intervening with regard to the disease process. Often left out of that equation is the family's or patient's desire to maintain or return to "normalcy." The subjective experience of living with a disease is as important as the objective process of medical management. Recognition of this desire for normalcy is important if care providers and patient educators are to work with families as they journey, along with the patients, through difficult times. Very often, in order to achieve successful outcomes for patients, patient educators and others must work to reshape relationships, at least temporarily, among family members.

The Need to Prevent Adversarial Relationships

It is critical to prevent adversarial relationships from developing between families and health care providers. Families may fluctuate between assertive and passive behavior, depending on the situation and the dynamics of the family. The family's desire to maintain the goodwill of the provider so that the care of the patient will be optimal often sets up a frustration within the family. If families are too assertive, they fear irritating the clinician and jeopardizing the patient's care. If they are too compliant, they worry about becoming victims of the process of the care or the disease itself. Lack of information increases internal emotional conflict, and surprising outbursts, later regretted, can happen. Family members must continually assess their perception of what is happening in order to prevent such dilemmas.

The Increasing Desire for Empathy

Other intangibles, such as the desire for hope or empathy from the provider, are expectations that, if not met, can cause great frustration. Encouragement and hope need not be equated with promise. To many families, *hope* does not necessarily mean "free of disease," but rather the potential that life can still be meaningful, comfortable, and manageable—the newer definition of quality of life. When these expectations are clarified among care providers and families, communication is enhanced and outcomes are improved.

☐ Why Meeting These Challenges Is Important

Understanding and recognizing these challenges is a precursor to developing the best relationship—that of guarded alliance. This relationship acknowledges the strengths and limitations of both provider and receiver of care and the evolution the relationship must go through to provide a flexible basis for the assessment of informational, educational, or support needs. This relationship can also provide a goal for both family and provider to work toward; a partnership, however guarded, is always superior to a relationship based on blind trust or disenchantment.

Once these challenges are understood, the next step is to examine the underlying goals of involving families in patient care and education. After that, an approach for involving families can be developed.

☐ The Goals of Involving Families in Patient Care and Education

The task of involving families in health care has classically been handled within the familiar scenario of the nurse or physician turning to the spouse (or other family care giver) and asking, "And how are *you*?" Such an approach can be inadequate and usually fails to meet the real needs of families. Family needs are often not the same as patient needs. When treated as only another patient care mechanism, families become part of the background. However, when family needs are appropriately acknowledged and their fears and frustrations validated, family members come forward—to be helped and to offer their help with the patient. The following goals can be part of a strategy to foster family involvement.

Differentiate Family Educational Needs from Patient Needs

Historically, in most inpatient settings, family support has been provided by social workers and pastoral services, whereas patient education has been the domain of nursing practice. Family education was addressed in terms of posthospitalization patient care, especially in cases where the patient was limited in his or her capacity for understanding or physically following through with the physician's recommendations.

Today, with the increase in outpatient treatment and family involvement, it has become apparent that there are three kinds of educational needs that affect both patient and family, specifically with regard to the patient's medical condition:

- Acute educational needs, when a lack of understanding is causing anguish and/or physical danger
- Maintenance educational needs, where a medical condition has altered a life and ongoing skill building is needed to cope and manage a situation
- Preventive educational needs, when a condition or life change is likely to occur to a person and both the person and the family are not prepared to deal with it

Careful assessment of both the patient and the family is necessary to determine where their respective needs arise from. Of course, acute needs must be addressed first, and these should be closely aligned with the medical and nursing assessment. Maintenance and preventive education are more and more often provided in a follow-up systematic way, with special clinics, classes, materials, and counseling sessions.

Encourage Independence

The most important goal of education is empowerment, which is the precursor of independence for both the family and the patient. The efforts of the health care provider should go toward promoting independence—not dependence—of families as well as patients. Medical problems and institutions are often intimidating, and it is often up to health care professionals to initiate the partnership with the families to enable them to make good decisions and reach a level of comfort with their interaction. Unfortunately, it is much easier to overwhelm the family with information (and with the professional knowledge behind the information) than it is to simplify, clarify, and illustrate the pertinence of the information to the family's goals. However, the latter approach is necessary to foster family and patient independence.

Create Productive Collaborations with Families

The family is a valuable and necessary resource for the patient education manager (PEM). From chance comments overheard to input from more formal focus or support groups, families provide feedback on educational needs, timing, perceptions of services provided, communication styles and techniques of providers, and a wide variety of other useful information. By treating families as partners who bring their own expertise to the situation, the PEM can build a foundation for a working collaboration between the family and the health care provider. The following elements of collaboration are useful to keep in mind while developing this approach:

- Mutual respect for skills and knowledge
- Honest and clear communication
- Mutually agreed-upon goals
- Shared planning and decision making
- Open and two-way sharing of information
- Accessibility and responsiveness
- Joint evaluation of progress
- Absence of labeling and blaming

As time pressures (for example, shorter hospital stays) compress opportunities for inpatient teaching, innovative approaches to patient and family education and support are being tried. The truest test of success is responding to feedback from patients and families to determine which of the methods for collaboration work best and how these methods can be constantly improved. This reflects the shift of the health care industry closer to a service industry mode, where feedback is important in shaping services.

☐ Strategies for Involving Families

At discharge, hospital patients are often frail and less able to physically and mentally absorb information and education. Shorter lengths of stay and earlier discharge exacerbate the problem. Thus, family members become an extension of the health care team, often finding themselves overwhelmed by a job for which they feel ill-prepared. Because patients are so often not ready for self-care information at discharge, patient education typically becomes *family education,* and this affects the strategies used for involving families.

Caring for a frail relative is both emotionally and physically draining. The goal of family education should be not only to assist the patient, but also to help relieve some of the stress care givers experience, ultimately helping them to provide higher-quality care at home. The next section offers some practical strategies and key steps that can be used to provide families and patients with education and support.

Recognize Barriers

It is important to understand some of the barriers that prevent families from seeking or using educational or support services. Some of these were described in the previous section on challenges, but recognition of these barriers is an important step toward involving families in patient care and education.

All too often, services are promoted according to the perspective of health care providers (that is, they focus on patient care outcomes) rather than to how family care givers see their needs. Family care givers are more interested in balancing patient care against an array of issues, other responsibilities, role changes, and a variety of care-giving burdens—emotional, financial, and so on. Successful outreach to, and integration of, families into patient education requires an understanding of how care givers view their roles.

Being a care giver may require redefinition of the individual's role in the family and assuming responsibilities not usually thought of as part of ordinary family relationships. In some families, seeking formal help or services for family problems is not perceived as "normal" or may be regarded as an admission of weakness or failure. In terms of home health or respite services, many families hesitate to use paid care givers and/or are reluctant to have strangers providing personal care to a loved one.

An additional barrier is lack of knowledge about care-giver services, from care-giver classes—behavior management, legal and financial planning—to support groups, home care, and other services. Confusion about services and how to acquire them is often a problem for families. The variety and scope of services can seem complex and overwhelming, especially to the elderly care giver. In addition, family members may not perceive a need for education or services and thus may tend to focus more on the needs of their ill relatives than their own needs. For example, when asked whether she used respite care service, one care giver replied, "My husband doesn't need it yet," which illustrates a common form of denial. Family members may not make a distinction between services intended to meet their needs and those intended to help the ill family member.

Learn Ways to Find and Involve Families

The family education model presented later in this chapter incorporates the family as integral to patient education, so much so in fact that in caring for the patient, the family becomes the "patient." As the care-giving family acquires the skills, knowledge, and strength to provide optimum care to the patient, it is also promoting its own self-care. In this context, then, several suggestions are presented herein on how to involve families in education and support services.

Family education and care-giver support programs should be described or portrayed as a positive option, not as coming to the rescue. Care givers are often fully aware of the problems and are looking, instead, for positive solutions or at least guidelines on how to cope. A few key points must be kept in mind when developing a campaign or promotion to reach care givers; the PEM must:

- Provide specific examples of how education will benefit both the care giver and the care recipient
- Start with the care giver's expressed concern and then move to other needs; validate their feelings if not their actions
- Recognize and acknowledge the barriers and then get around them
- Offer choices and options, not direction; help them maintain a sense of control
- Be specific and precise in a holistic concept; explain how information applies or fits into the context of the day-to-day life of the family and what else might be affected; help families apply information and learning to actual day-to-day situations
- Make information and education seem easy, concrete, achievable, practical, and pertinent; help families get "unstuck" (if one strategy doesn't work, try another); provide handy tools, tips, fact sheets, handbooks, and hotlines
- Use common language to describe programs and services; avoid jargon
- Present programs in a nonthreatening way (for example, use the term *education program* instead of *support group*)
- Use words that build self-esteem (for example, describe a home care provider as a companion rather than as someone to watch over the patient)

- Help family care givers define themselves as care givers, with needs, rights, and responsibilities; give them a vocabulary to work with beyond the medical diagnosis
- Give tribute and recognition to what they are already doing as care givers; treat them as partners
- Build in rewards and reinforcers (refreshments, peer support, and praise are all effective); use verbal assurances such as "You're doing a good job," "I can see that you're trying," and "We're glad you care—it will help a lot"
- Establish benchmarks, such as the number of hours of respite, appropriate classes attended, sharing of experiences and ideas, getting out of the house more
- Work with, through, and for natural support networks—support groups, churches, neighborhood associations, and informal groups of neighbors
- Use a variety of access mechanisms—physician referral, direct referral, support group referral, agency referral; reinforce word-of-mouth referral; enhance a speakers bureau and a strong community education program
- Provide a good referral system, because many care givers lack the time and energy to enter the service delivery system

Enlist Physician Support

Families learn about educational services and resources through physicians and other health care providers, as well as via word of mouth. To assist with physician outreach, packets should be developed for care givers that deal with specific illnesses. These materials can be supplied to medical offices for distribution, and targeting certain specialties will help reach specific groups of care givers. The offices of gynecologists and family practitioners, for example, will reach women at mid-life, those most likely to be care givers of elderly persons. Work with medical societies or associations to educate physicians and health care staff through newsletters, conferences, and any other appropriate mechanisms.

Network within the Community and Develop Collaborations

There are a variety of community organizations that can help locate families and care givers in need of education and support. Free presentations and information should be offered to churches, community colleges, schools, service clubs, and other community organizations as well as the aging services network. The PEM should meet with corporate assistance staff (such as employee assistance program counselors) or human resource managers, as well as others such as family and work issues consultants and elder care counselors.

Developing collaborations with groups outside the hospital furthers the goals of patient/family education by building a broader base of support. Working with these groups also creates bonds with the community. Working with outside groups shows the public that the hospital is interested in meeting community needs without strictly pursuing the policy of an individual institution. Public and private funding organizations as well as individuals appreciate collaborative efforts and are usually more supportive of grant proposals that involve collaboration. Nurturing a collaboration for a specific purpose can lead to other productive partnerships that will, in turn, lend momentum to successful outreach efforts.

There are literally dozens of potential partners for coalition and collaboration. The following are just a few:

- Agencies dealing with aging and long-term care issues and services
- Adult and community education programs
- College or university geriatric, gerontology, social work, and nursing departments
- Interfaith councils
- Nonprofit organizations, such as social services organizations, those that are health or disease specific, and even some cultural groups

In addition, informal networks within the hospital, such as nursing staff and others, could be used. They should be given something tangible (for example, a newsletter or a "prescription" for education and family support services) that, in turn, they can give to friends or other people they know who are involved in care giving. Low-cost media campaigns can be effective, particularly when a program is able to get the support of a local television station to produce and air public service announcements. Radio stations will usually read prepared scripts for public service announcements.

Advocate for Social Change

Educational services are much more effective and will reach many more people if the hospital is perceived as an innovator that cares about family support issues. An important way to illustrate this leadership to the public is to demonstrate expertise and concern for public policy issues involving care givers. Emphasis in this area will result in enhanced credibility for the hospital and ultimately attract the support of families.

Advocacy on behalf of family care givers is also productive in terms of involving families in education. At least one designated staff member in a given hospital should be aware of some of the legislative or public policy issues related to care giving. This staff person can become a valuable resource to public officials and a key resource for information on the issues facing the frail and chronically ill.

Finance a Family Support Program

Another way to involve families is to provide a family support program. The broader the base of funding for a family support program, the more secure and effective it can be. Charging modest fees for classes, booklets, newsletters, memberships, and such services as respite, day care, care planning, and billing assistance is appropriate. Grants and contracts with other institutions, agencies, and clinics for the provision of education and training can also produce revenue for a program. As with any highly interactive and personal program or service, donations can and should be sought. Foundations and corporations look upon such services as meeting a societal need and should be approached. The hospital should see this type of service as helping with a variety of strategic and business needs—recruiting and supporting physicians, preventing inappropriate readmissions, community relations, to name a few—and provide some support for it.

☐ A Practical Process for Developing Family Support Programs

The pragmatic aspects of family education follow many of the same principles as good patient education programs and practice. These include assessment followed by analysis and planning, then implementation, documentation and evaluation, and follow-up.

Assessment

Assessment begins with identification of who needs the teaching. Because of a patient's acuity, frailty, cognitive competence, or role changes, family members are often the primary targets of educational programming. Assessing what information is needed comes next; immediate, need-to-know, pertinent educational needs are weighed against the long-range needs that will evolve later in the care process, taking into account what the learner perceives is important, useful, and/or desirable to know. Determining how to educate follows; learning readiness comes into play at this stage, as does learning style. Assessing the stress/anxiety level and working to alleviate it is critical at this point; learning is achieved better by both the patient and the family if fear and anxiety are well managed. Patient and family coping mechanisms should be evaluated at this point to adapt teaching strategies appropriately. These mechanisms can include minimization (reducing or attempting to ignore the significance of a problem), intellectualization (adopting an overly rational attitude and deemphasizing emotions), repetition, acting strong, and remaining near the patient.[6]

Analysis and Planning

After assessment comes the analysis and planning phase. At this point, the educational goals are determined jointly with the health care professional and patient and/or family. The education is tailored to meet the needs and capabilities of the patient and the family separately. During this phase, it is important to consider the humanistic approach to education—that of preserving as much patient and family autonomy and control as possible. Offering choices through education is a good technique to help maintain a sense of shared control.

Implementation

Implementation of family education takes place in a variety of ways. Workshops, practice settings, family conferences, one-on-one instruction, audiotapes and videotapes, and educational television channels are good mechanisms for instruction. Forms, checklists, resource lists, behavioral contracts, visual aids such as charts and pictures, and published handbooks are all good tools to use in the process. The newest technique of computerized learning is developing some interesting approaches, such as interactive video use in shared decision-making situations.

The more educational tools patients and families have, the better, as long as they are pertinent, clear, and perceived as valuable and usable. Special touches, such as lists of questions to ask the physician or nurse while in the hospital, "hot tips" handouts, and journal-writing assignments, can increase the family's interest and participation, which in turn increases learning, compliance, and satisfaction. It is important to remember that just because something was said does not mean it was heard. The more humanistic the educational approach (reflected in materials, settings, and interactions), the greater the possibility of improving educational outcomes.

A hallmark of most of the model education programs in hospitals is a notebook that can go home with the family. These notebooks have been developed to help compensate for shorter hospital stays. In the past, verbal teaching could be reinforced several times; now the printed medium must help. The notebook usually includes standard information with opportunities for individualizing case by case. The notebooks deal mostly with self-care, but they vary widely in format and depth. Most *do* have space for practitioners' comments, specifications, and admonitions. Some books are put together around individual needs—selecting only certain articles, chapters, lists, guidelines, and so on.

Documentation and Evaluation

With increasing attention being paid to documentation, evaluation has become a critical component of patient and family education. (See chapter 9 for a thorough discussion of documentation issues.) Evaluation can encompass how clearly or how thoroughly information was given or how pertinent the information was. It can also look only at the teaching or can examine how well or whether learning took place.

Quality and outcome assessments are being emphasized, not just from the provider perspective but also from the consumer perspective. This reinforces the imperative to involve families and patients in planning and goal setting and in the process of education. Informal methods of evaluation (such as conversations that bedside nurses have with patients) can be as useful as formal documentation done by PEMs in continually fine-tuning even the best educational program. Feedback can be solicited in a variety of ways: surveys, interviews, and focus groups are only a few.

Evaluation opportunities also can enhance patient and family satisfaction with the information and education provided—a side benefit. When patients and families are given a chance to comment, praise, or vent, they do not leave the hospital with frustrations or gratitudes left unexpressed. Both feelings provide important information to health care providers.

Follow-up

Follow-up is the final phase of the process of involving families in patient care and education. It can be seen as the key to keeping the family as a constituent of the hospital. Referral to other resources for care, services, and education is an important part of follow-up, especially when evaluation shows that more learning is necessary to help ensure a successful outcome. Other methods include discharge counseling, telephone follow-up to patients one to two weeks later, letters, and linkages with outpatient support systems, such as support groups, resource centers, counselors, and educational programs.

□ A Comprehensive Model of Family Support Services

As hospitals struggle to provide services that will keep the family and the patient functioning and coping adequately, family support services provide an invaluable service to the lay as well as the medical community. Research has shown that the services that best help the family in the face of chronic disease are information, education, respite care, and support.[7]

These services have been incorporated into an effective program at Good Samaritan Hospital and Medical Center, one of five hospitals in the Legacy Health System, Portland, Oregon. During the past decade, the Family Support Center at Good Samaritan Hospital and Medical Center has been a national leader in developing care giver and family support services for chronic disease. The motto "You're Not Alone" embodies the philosophy of the center, which provides families with the tools they need to be active and respected partners in the care of their affected family member, empowered to maximize the quality of all their lives in the process.

Family Support Services

Information is the most important commodity provided by Good Samaritan's resource center. Receiving over 800 calls a week for information and referral to other resources, the center stocks more than 1,000 volumes, numerous audiotapes and videotapes, extensive reference reprint files, and original booklets on a broad range of care-giving issues. The center's speakers bureau offers more than 50 presentations to the community annually, and quarterly publications go to families and health care professionals, with an active mailing list of nearly 18,000. The Family Support Center has produced a variety of how-to books on family support programs (figure 18-3).

Educational programs include a wide variety of topics and formats:

- A monthly series of lectures for care givers that draws an average audience of approximately 150 each time
- Specific disease-related community education programs
- Quarterly "Helping You Care" classes teaching hands-on skills to family care givers, including managing stress, understanding the aging process, managing medications, giving personal care, understanding body mechanics, and using adaptive devices for patient care

Figure 18-3. Resources Provided by the Family Support Center at Good Samaritan Hospital and Medical Center, Portland, Oregon

---

Resources for Program Planners

Developing Communication Tools
Developing In-Home Respite Services
Developing a Caregiver Education Program
Developing a Caregiver Training Program
Developing Caregiver Information Services
Developing a Support Group Organization
Developing a Caregiver Listing Service
Developing Health Education Programs
Developing Legal/Financial Planning
Reaching the Employed Caregiver
Administrative Manual
Caring That Makes a Difference (respite provider training manual)

Resources for Families

Carebook
Helping You Care (care-giver training manual)
Caregiving Handbook
Legal/Financial Planning Guide for Families
Guide to Hiring In-Home Help
You're Not Alone: A Planning Guide for Families
POPS: Polishing Our People Skills (peer counseling training guide)
Family Support Center CARE Club membership

Note: These titles can be ordered from the Family Support Center, Good Samaritan Hospital and Medical Center, 1015 NW 22nd Avenue, Portland, OR 97210.

- Monthly legal/financial planning classes
- Small group sessions that cover management issues for family members dealing with specific chronic diseases
- A number of other classes, including peer-counseling training, health promotion, billing assistance training, insurance selection and evaluation, care options evaluation and selection, and advance directives decision making

Center staff members provide training for most Portland-area workers in respite care (supervised companionship to relieve care givers temporarily) and foster care (residence in private homes where three to five impaired adults are cared for by a resident care giver). In addition, the Family Support Center plans conferences and workshops for medical and scientific professionals to rapidly inform them of new findings in the field, such as care-giver dynamics, needs, and interventions.

One of the most important services provided by the center is the Caregiver Respite Program. It was developed in 1984 as a result of an early care-giver needs assessment that indicated that "a break now and then" was the service most needed. Several grants and contracts later, the Caregiver Respite Program is now one of the best known and most successful in the country. It provides more than 8,000 hours of respite care annually and trains more than 100 private providers for the Caregivers Listing Service (for those families who wish to contract for services on their own). Most recently, the Caregiver Respite Program has developed a day-care program for Alzheimer's patients.

Support is provided by the 23 support group organizations founded, assisted, or supported by the Family Support Center. These organizations have more than 100 support groups around the state, with total participation estimated at more than 10,000, addressing a range of conditions from Alzheimer's disease to Parkinson's disease to sleep disorders. Center staff provide leadership training, information sharing among groups, and opportunities for collaboration in many activities, from fund-raising to workshop planning and political relations.

The Family Support Center supports not only community-based providers, but also hospital inpatient services. Discharge planners and floor nurses refer families to the Center to assist in the transition from hospital to home. Home medical care staff, provided by Legacy's Visiting Nurse Association, often work with the Family Support Center to help both patient and family facing the burden and challenge of home care. Physicians' offices refer to the Family Support Center as an extension of their care, often "prescribing" a visit to the center. The Family Support Center is available to families of inpatients as well as the community. The outcome is that Good Samaritan's family support services successfully bridge the gap between medical and social services in the community.

Family support services through the Center have played another important role for the hospital. Along with Good Samaritan's emphasis and support for chronic disease management clinics—especially in the areas of neurological, heart, and kidney disease, cancer, and diabetes—the Family Support Center has helped position the hospital as a strong, involved, and responsive partner in the health of the community. Constituency relations has become a priority, and this form of community service has proved to be a very effective marketing tool.

Chronic Care Management

Another of Good Samaritan's approaches to involving families is its chronic care management programs, or clinics, including both clinical and educational interventions. Each disease area that is a major focus of the hospital involves extensive patient and family education in the process. Each program has an ongoing relationship with its constituency and has a strong presence in the community as a result. The chronic care clinics do not replace primary medical care but, rather, enhance or supplement the physician's care. Interestingly, these programs did not develop out of a visionary centralized plan, but grew up independently in order to meet the growing needs of patients and families to be more involved in their own health care. These clinics work hand in hand with the Family Support Center to provide the fabric of support for the family coping with chronic disease.

Heart Patient Program
It has been shown that heart surgery patients and families have benefited from structured teaching programs. Because of the cardiac patient's decreased length of stay, the family is being turned to more and more for patient care education, and it is frequently the family who has a major role in the patient's readjustment during convalescence. Thus, their behavior can determine the rate and extent of the patient's recovery. The health of the family unit has been shown to be a key factor in patient outcome, and spouse/partner counseling and education appears to have a strong effect on rehabilitation outcome.

Because of shorter stays and because some families travel many miles for heart surgery, special strategies for disseminating information and providing support are being developed at Good Samaritan. Good Samaritan provides an extensive library of information and comprehensive bedside education for both patient and family, and continually develops and provides educational tools, such as videotapes and written materials, that address issues important to elderly heart patients and their families.

Mechanisms that draw from the best-produced information and personalize it for patient and family are the most effective. As already mentioned, a notebook that can be individualized and added to by both the health care provider and the family is a valuable guide to ongoing education after the hospital stay. Good Samaritan provides such a notebook and also utilizes some of the philosophical approach and materials of Heart-Mates Cardiac Family Recovery Program.[8] Cardiac rehabilitation program staff stress the fact that the crisis is over, that the family will be able to manage, and that there are resources to help. Family meetings, materials, and counseling all provide both validation and reassurance to the patient as well as the family. The importance of life-style changes to prevent recurrence is stressed, and it is clearly stated that the entire family owns the risk factors and needs to address them. Helping the family to develop the momentum to move forward, even if only one step at a time, is the goal of the program.

Cancer Program

Families affected by cancer have their own unique needs. Diagnostic improvements, increased variety and complexity of treatments, and longer life spans have all added to the information base available to patients and families. There are longer time periods involved in key management issues, both functional and environmental, and more rehabilitation research and service information has been developed in response to longer survival rates. Research on educational and support strategies for cancer families has shed light on many aspects of living with cancer, from coping strategies and cancer archetypes to immune system response. Autonomy, dignity, and "humanness" are key qualities that have become part of cancer care and education. Along with the patient, the family must redefine itself, both as a unit and in relation to the patient. Therefore, information and education is as essential for the family as it is for the patient.

Good Samaritan's outpatient cancer rehabilitation program staff provide education related to the cancer, the patient's functional needs, and the social and emotional needs of patients and families. This education is based on careful assessment of the patient's and the family's needs. The goal of patient education is to maximize independence and control as well as to emphasize wellness. Patient-centered care is a feature of the cancer program, because patient and family goals, not just provider goals, are considered carefully. Prioritization, timing, and appropriate sequence are important factors in providing education to patients and families.

Family education and support needs vary widely with different diagnoses, but flexibility is a key trait of the program and educational strategies. Education is provided both individually and in group settings, and the latter setting offers the additional benefit of peer support.

Good Samaritan's cancer program recognizes the importance of having a cancer rehabilitation team that is able to adapt and shift to changing needs and use all the available literature and community supports. The team uses resources from the American Cancer Society and the National Cancer Institute.

Kidney Program

Kidney disease can also affect the family in a variety of ways. Although independence and self-management are stressed, the family is often in a hands-on care-giving role. Living with dialysis and diet restrictions is a day-to-day stressor, for both patient and family.

Good Samaritan's dialysis program involves several educational and support approaches for both patient and family. An individualized self-care notebook, a published handbook on kidney disease, training sessions, and support groups are provided in addition to newsletters, materials, and educational forums provided by the local Kidney Association. Spouses are encouraged to contact each other for support, and living one day at a time is strongly emphasized. In the kidney program, as well as the diabetes program, the use of the best available literature, patient and family tracks for education and support, and ongoing involvement with the patients are key components of the program.

Diabetes Program

Diabetes poses another chronic disease management challenge for health care providers and hospitals. Patients and families must learn to live with a long-term alteration of their health condition, which is usually diagnosed after their life-style patterns have been firmly established. Changing eating patterns, daily exercise regimens, regular glucose monitoring, insulin administration, and frequent health care visits affect the family almost as much as the individual. In turn, the family's knowledge and support may be the key motivating factor in the patient's compliance with his or her everyday regimens.

At Good Samaritan's Diabetes Institute, education for both patients and families has been a hallmark tradition for decades. A manual and a handbook developed locally accompany the team approach to teaching, with opportunities for both individual counseling and peer support. Healthy choices in diet and exercise are considered a family affair, and an innovative five-day education program has been developed with special components that specifically address family issues. The Diabetes Institute has successfully empowered a large and loyal constituency.

Neurological Disease Program

Neurological disease presents its own challenges, because cognition and behavior are central definitions of being; alterations in either domain pose major challenges for coping and managing. Patient learning may be severely limited, emphasizing the importance of the family's role.

The Neurology Continuing Care Clinics have developed around specific disease focuses (Alzheimer's, multiple sclerosis, amyotrophic lateral sclerosis, stroke, and so on), providing ongoing care to patients and families living with a neurological disease. The clinics focus on the impact of the disease—usually chronic and degenerative and sometimes dementing—on the patient and the family. They provide support to primary and specialty physicians in care coordination, behavior and symptom management consultation, counseling, education on the disease process, medication management and information, and referral to community resources.

The neurological disease program is much different from the other chronic care clinics. Because most of the problems affect the patient's cognition and behavior, the family is the primary client. Responses to disease and individual changes vary widely, and a flexible program model is appropriate.

The clinic staff make a special effort to address concerns patients and families see as most important. This validation establishes trust, and once this trust is established the provider can move on to teaching and counseling issues. A care plan is developed jointly, and the number of sessions varies from family to family.

Roles within the family are acknowledged in order to utilize family dynamics, which are very powerful and can facilitate or undermine a care plan. Creativity is stressed in identifying solutions to such situations as problem behaviors. *The Carebook,*[9] developed by the founder of the Continuing Care Clinics, helps families accumulate and document important information, both objective and subjective, that is helpful in the care-giving role.

An important strategy used by the experts in continuing care is *reverse guilt*. If the care giver is not doing well, the patient certainly is not: "They depend on you, so you have to take care of yourself!"

Decision making is addressed by clinic staff, but the staff consider themselves teachers of options and consequences, not directors of lives. By having staff provide them with choices and information, the family maintains control. Clinic staff encourage the seeking of additional information and peer support; they introduce topics that primary care providers, other family members, and friends cannot or will not, such as advance directives or placement, and then work to develop a comfort level with them. "There's always something you can do" is an operational philosophy of the clinics; a solution orientation is much more helpful than a problem orientation.

☐ Conclusion

Because patients leave the hospital earlier than ever before, and in a more frail condition, care givers are more vulnerable to excessive stress and burnout. Understanding some of the reasons families do not immediately respond to educational efforts helps patient education managers develop better strategies for reaching those people with information that will empower them. When PEMs take an active leadership role in issues facing care givers, both the image and the quality of the hospital are strengthened.

Although the health care industry is being compressed and distressed by less time to do more, increasing expectations, decreasing funding, and the resulting frustrations, it can look to the family as a potential ally and supporter. When empowered by education and support, families can be effective and powerful partners of practitioners and hospitals.

References

1. Rabin, D. L., and Stockton, P. *Long-term Care for the Elderly: A Factbook.* New York City: Oxford University Press, 1987, p. 239.

2. Brody, E. The family at risk. In: E. Light and B. D. Liebowitz, editors. *Alzheimer's Disease Treatment and Family Stress: Directions for Research.* Washington, DC: U.S. Government Printing Office, 1989, DHHS Publ. No. (ADM) 89-1569.

3. Goulart, D. T. Educating the cardiac surgery patient and family. *Journal of Cardiovascular Nursing* 3(3):1-9, May 1989.

4. Kernich, C., and Robb, G. Development of a stroke family support and education program. *Journal of Neuroscience Nursing* 20(3):193-97, June 1988.

5. Thorne, S. E., and Robinson, C. A. Health care relationships: the chronic illness perspective. *Research in Nursing and Health* 11:293-300, 1988.

6. Wyness, M. A. Patient and family education: a key component of neuroscience nursing. *AXON* 8(4):95-98, June 1987.

7. Heagerty, B., Dunn, L., and Watson, M. A. They are not alone: lending support to family caregivers. *Health Progress* 69(11):55-75, Dec. 1988.

8. Levin, R. F. *The Cardiac Family Recovery Program Training Manual.* Minneapolis: HeartMates, Inc., 1990.

9. Beedle, J. *The Carebook: A Workbook for Caregiver Peace of Mind.* Portland, OR: Lady Bug Press, 1991.

Bibliography

Print Materials

Alexander, R., and Tompkins-McGill, P. Parent checklist. *Social Work* 32(4):361-62, 1987.

Barusch, A. S. *Eldercare: Family Support Training.* Newberry Park, CA: Sage Publications, 1991.

Brock, M. J. Uncertainty, information needs, and coping effectiveness of renal families. *American Nephrology Nursing Association Journal* 17(3):242-47, June 1990.

Evans, B. S. The family as a unit in the management of diabetes. *Home Healthcare Nurse* 6(5):10-13, Sept.-Oct. 1988.

Fleming, S. Supporting the family's role in patient recovery, rehabilitation. *Promoting Health* (special suppl.), Jan.-Feb. 1987, pp.1-12.

Frymark, S. Cancer rehabilitation in the outpatient setting. *Oncology Issues* 5(1):12-17, Winter 1990.

Goldfarb, L. A., Brotherson, M. J., Summers, J. A., and Turnbull, A. P. *Meeting the Challenge of Disability or Chronic Illness: A Family Guide.* Baltimore: Paul H. Brooks Publishing, 1986.

Goulart, D. T. Educating the cardiac surgery patient and family. *Journal of Cardiovascular Nursing* 3(3):1-9, May 1989.

Grieco, A. J., Garnett, S. A., Glassman, K. S., Valoon, P. L., and McClure, M. L. Current perspectives: strategies to promote patient self-management. *Patient Education and Counseling* 15:3-15, 1990.

Hill, M. Teaching after CABG surgery: a family affair. *Critical Care Nurse* 9(8):58-72, Sept. 1989.

Jennings, B., Callahan, D., and Caplan, A. L. Ethical challenges of chronic illness. *Hastings Center Report* (special suppl.), Feb.–Mar. 1988.

Johny, A., and Bille, D. A. On the scene wellness promotion. *Nursing Administration Quarterly* 11(3):13–60, Spring 1987.

Kernich, C., and Robb, G. Development of a stroke family support and education program. *Journal of Neuroscience Nursing* 20(3):193–97, June 1988.

Levin, R. F. *Heartmates: A Survival Guide for the Cardiac Spouse.* New York City: Prentice-Hall Press, 1987.

McKelvey, J., and Borgersen, M. Family development and the use of diabetes groups: experience with a model approach. *Patient Education and Counseling* 16:61–67, 1990.

McKinney, E., and Beedle, J. Continuing care clinics meet needs of patients with chronic disease. *Outreach* 11(1):5–7, Jan.–Feb. 1990.

Meissner, H. T., Anderson, M., and Odenkirchen, J. D. Meeting information needs of significant others: use of the cancer information service. *Patient Education and Counseling* 15:171–79, 1990.

Ruzicki, D. A. Realistically meeting the educational needs of hospitalized acute and short-stay patients. *Nursing Clinics of North America* 24(3):629–37, Sept. 1989.

Simpson, T. Needs and concerns of families of critically ill adults. *Focus on Critical Care* 16(5):388–97, Oct. 1989.

Staib, C. Why parents should become allies with professionals. *Focal Point* 2(3):10, Spring 1988.

Thompson, R., and Weisberg, S. Families as educational consumers: what do they want? what do they receive? *Health and Social Work* 15(3):221–27, Aug. 1990.

Wright, L. M., and Leahey, M. *Families and Chronic Illness.* Springhouse, PA: Springhouse Corporation, 1987.

Videos

Empowering the Elderly Caregiver of a Heart Patient. Portland, OR: Legacy Heart Services, 1992.

Portrait of the HeartMate: The Challenge of Recovery. Minneapolis: HeartMates, Inc., 1989.

Portrait of the HeartMate: Family Concerns. Minneapolis: HeartMates, Inc., 1989.

Chapter 19

Supporting Patient Learning through Consumer Health Information Resource Centers

---

Salvinija G. Kernaghan

□ Objectives

The reader will be able to:

- Describe the benefits of consumer health information resource centers to hospitals, individual hospital departments and their staffs, and consumers
- List the types of services that a typical consumer health information resource center can provide
- Relate these services to the range of support that a resource center can provide to the patient education and information function of various hospital departments
- Identify the possible organizational relationships that consumer health information resource centers can maintain with other institutional units
- Summarize the basic elements that must be considered in planning a new consumer health information resource center

□ How Consumer Health Information Resource Centers Provide New Support for Patient Learning

Consumer health information resource centers are not a new phenomenon on the health care scene. However, although a handful of the earliest models date back to the 1970s, it has taken two decades for the majority of hospitals to recognize the full potential of the consumer health information center movement. From both the patient's and the hospital's perspective, this recognition has come not a moment too soon.

In fact, consumer health information resource centers have given hospitals one effective alternative to the patient education gap that resulted from several concurrent developments:

- Restricted inpatient stays, which in turn diminished inpatient teaching time
- The shift of many services that were traditionally provided in the acute care setting to a variety of outpatient settings, long-term care facilities, and home care,

compromising the potential for continuity and complicating patients' ability to fully understand both the course of their care and the system that attempts to provide it

- An increased understanding of the critical influence of prevention and active self-management on patients' ability to avoid life-threatening conditions and the often-severe complications of long-term chronic illness

As a result of these developments, the mechanisms for health care delivery have become more complicated and diverse, demanding that patients become better-informed consumers and more active participants in their own care. Ironically, many of these changes either have minimized the patients' opportunity to learn new health care consumer skills or have not yet made good use of a new set of "teachable moments."

Consumer health information resource centers are helping hospitals to respond to both of these challenges. Although they can take many forms and provide a range of information services, resource centers are typically separate rooms or larger facilities that house a collection of print, audio, and audiovisual media devoted to providing health information to patients, their families, other community members, and members of the hospital staff. In this way, centers have filled many of the information/education gaps that resulted from shifts in service settings, and have also put enormous health information resources directly into the hands of consumers themselves, to be used when they need information and can profit from it most.

A 1987 survey by the American Hospital Association identified 693 such resource centers, representing 21.4 percent of responding hospitals.[1] It is no exaggeration to say that since that survey, interest in and actual development of such centers among other hospitals has been explosive. This level of interest stems not only from the hospitals' potential to maintain and strengthen their capabilities in patient education and consumer information. The fact that consumer health information resource centers can become the entry point for referrals to physicians and many other hospital services also generates great interest among hospitals as they seek a wider network of connections with community residents. Finally, few other ongoing hospital programs can rival consumer health information resource centers in terms of either sheer numbers of community residents served or the daily visibility and valuable help that they offer to both the sick and the well. This point may be of critical importance to hospitals as they evaluate their community benefit and tax-exempt status.

Awareness of these community and organizational benefits can be valuable input as patient education professionals review their changing roles and strive to make adjustments that serve both their patients and their institution. Whether they assume direct responsibility for developing a consumer health information resource center or cooperate with another hospital division that manages such a center, patient education managers (PEMs) can expect a range of valuable support for organizing and providing patient learning opportunities.

Understanding the Goals and Services of the Typical Resource Center

Every consumer health information resource center intends to help consumers by providing information relevant to their health or their health care. However, depending on the types of information that are offered, this overarching goal can have three subordinate objectives:

1. *To inform* consumers by providing current materials on health, disease, and wellness in language and media that consumers can understand and use
2. *To teach* the skills of self-care, self-management, and coping by offering one-on-one learning opportunities, video-assisted learning, and group classes and support groups

3. *To promote the hospital* in general and hospital services in particular by helping consumers make more positive and appropriate linkages with other hospital services, the medical staff, and other community-based agencies and providers

A hospital's emphasis on any one of these three objectives naturally colors the range and depth of service that its resource center can provide. Some hospitals have made a commitment to all three objectives with equal vigor, using the consumer health information resource center as the hub of their information and education effort.

Whatever the choice, every resource center includes the following elements:

- *A mechanism by which consumers can access information.* Depending on space available, the size of the collection, staff size, the community's ease of access to the site, and the type of population served, a resource center can choose to provide its services:
  - To anyone who visits the center and does a self-serve information search or asks for staff help. The resource center user can include: outpatients and inpatients (although the latter are not typical users of such centers) who either use it on their own initiative or are referred by a health care provider; family members of patients and other community residents who are not currently under anyone's care; hospital or medical staff in search of information for either professional or personal reasons; and hospital employees.
  - To anyone who telephones the center and asks a specific question of a professional staff member. The staff member offers a brief answer during the telephone conversation or mails follow-up materials to the person making the inquiry, or does both.
  - To both walk-in and telephone queries.
  - Off-site through other cooperating agencies, such as a local public library that houses and manages the collection in return for hospital staff's developing a set of resources that are appropriate for the community's information needs.
- *A collection of books, pamphlets, current periodicals, and audiovisual materials related to health.* A consumer health information resource center that intends to serve the general health information needs of a community will cover a broad range of topics. Because every hospital population includes individuals with a range of information-seeking styles, such a collection usually includes materials from the most basic to the most complex—from pamphlets that essentially summarize information on a given subject to journal articles that discuss it at greater length to medical textbooks that analyze its every aspect. Resource centers serving special populations, such as cancer patients, children, women, or older adults, usually focus their collection on topics that relate to the health of these groups, while also including some materials on health in general.
- *A mechanism by which consumers can be referred to other appropriate sources.* The degree to which a collection emphasizes certain types of materials often reflects the center's major purpose. In general, centers that favor large collections of pamphlets and AV materials rather than more in-depth sources typically tie this basic level of information to referrals to other learning opportunities, such as group classes, counseling, and the like. These centers are often staffed by either nurses or health educators, and they are frequently managed by, or in cooperation with, the hospital's marketing division.

    This is not to say that resource centers with a more traditional library approach and a wider range of print materials do not also have the ability to make linkages to other services. However, these centers tend to be managed by professional librarians whose initial charge is to develop a collection that will quickly respond to a wide variety of information requests, from patients as well as from staff who need support in teaching patients. If these librarians understand early on the

401

connection between the resource center's success and the linkages it can make with other services, they quickly learn the value of developing networks of referral and support. As a result, it is a rare resource center that does not refer its users to other appropriate services.

Realizing That Resource Centers Are in Flux

Apart from describing these resource center basics, it is difficult to be specific about the way such centers interact with the patient education function in most hospitals. In large part, because these centers are assuming information and education responsibilities that are becoming restricted or revised as other hospital services change, consumer health information resource centers are—like much of the rest of the health care delivery system—still in flux.

In addition to filling information and education vacuums created by organizational changes, resource center development is also responding to a watershed in the way the majority of hospitals and health care professionals regard the sharing of information with the community. As individual institutions become more responsive to consumers' need for more information and education, they are increasing the resources they commit to such services, often shifting some resources from other areas and generally experimenting with the best organizational configuration for resource delivery. Because these developments are so new in so many hospitals, there may currently be almost as many different divisions of labor in the cooperative efforts of patient education and consumer information resource centers as there are centers themselves.

Even at this relatively early phase of resource center metamorphosis, however, it is possible to point to several different kinds of support that consumer health information resource centers can offer in particular institutions. As the following examples demonstrate, the best strategy for implementing a given type of support invariably depends on the formal organizational tie between the resource center and patient education and on the resources each can bring to bear on a particular information/education task.

Managing Materials

Perhaps the most common type of support a resource center can provide to any patient education task or program is to assume responsibility for acquiring, storing, and managing the distribution of information/education materials. This is also the most typical service focus of a resource center organized by a hospital's medical library, which tends to emphasize the information function almost exclusively, consciously avoiding the role of interpreter or teacher. Therefore, although its relationship with patient education functions throughout the hospital may be very close, in this scenario the resource center quite clearly takes a supportive role—someone else assesses learning needs and does the teaching while the resource center provides the learning materials and tools.

For example, the medical library staff at the Catherine McAuley Health System in Ann Arbor, Michigan, who developed the McAuley Health Information Library took advantage of its location in the physicians' office building to solicit input on patient learning needs from everyone in the facility who would be responsible for patient education and information. This included the physicians themselves, members of their office staff, and those health care professionals who provide service in the facility's several specialty testing laboratories and other clinics.

The initial survey of learning needs helped to shape the Health Information Library's collection and also to suggest to the library's staff the kinds of new materials that particular providers would appreciate seeing. A periodic listing of new materials organized by subject is just one tool that library staff can use to update their practitioner colleagues about current developments in information and teaching resources. This kind of exchange of information about user needs and available library resources to meet those needs serves both the providers and the resource library well. Those who teach can depend on the library to acquire and manage materials and keep track of current resources; in return, the library develops a solid network of professional referrals and consumer patrons.

At the National Jewish Center for Immunology and Respiratory Diseases in Denver, patient education is one of the four primary areas of service that all patients receive (the other three being diagnosis, treatment, and psychological counseling). Because this institution deals exclusively with severe chronic disease, and therefore has a strong emphasis on patient education, most of its primary patient care providers are expected to teach patients as part of treatment, to a degree that may not always be true in other general medical facilities. This is one reason why Rosalind Dudden, director of library services, does not include direct patient education services in the relatively new consumer health library under her direction. Her major thrust is to support the staff who teach the patients, stocking and providing the written and audiovisual resources that may be needed, but also providing direct patient information services for those patients and families who choose to use the library. To support the staff, the library purchases scientific and medical publications, many of which incorporate patient teaching methods. In addition, the library stocks all the pamphlets the Center produces—approximately 85 different topics—and distributes them to patients free of charge. Additional resources, including pamphlets, books, newsletters, and audiovisual materials, that are produced by others also are available.

Beyond this circumscribed role of information distribution, however, Dudden believes that the process of planning and developing the consumer library has helped to better integrate the variety of hospitalwide teaching efforts and certainly to make more efficient and wider use of already available teaching and information resources. By bringing together representatives of many of the services that could benefit from a centralized support for patient teaching, Dudden recalls, the planning effort also became an information exchange.

For example, the Center operates a nationwide telephone service—the Lungline—to provide information on respiratory diseases. Nurse educators who staff this service mail follow-up information pamphlets developed by the hospital to help answer callers' questions. However, various clinics and subspecialty areas were not always aware that such pamphlets existed and often felt the lack of such appropriate handouts; for example, the skin-testing lab did not know about the brochure on skin testing that was being mailed to Lungline callers. Discussing the efficient distribution of information to patients through a consumer health library helps to inform all the disciplines about the wealth of resources available through different Center services and thus to better coordinate many of the patient information and education efforts already in place.

Centralizing Answers to Patients' Questions

A major function that consumer health information research centers serve—and which in turn supports patient education—is to centralize access to a wide range of information for patients and families with health-related questions.

For example, in the Veterans Administration Medical Center, in Sepulveda, California, the patient education resource center (PERC) is an organizational unit of the library service, but is not physically located in the medical library. Instead, it is considered one of the "clinic stops" available to outpatients who use the Medical Center's ambulatory care clinic. As Marianne Davis, chief of the patient services division of library service and PERC coordinator, reports, the Resource Center "sits smack-dab in the middle of the clinic," and is the centralized support for the teaching efforts of the clinic's three multidisciplinary care teams.

Clinic outpatients visit the Center, either on their own or sent by a care provider for further information, education, or counseling. Although clinic providers can choose to give patients basic information and/or materials during the outpatient encounter, for more intensive teaching or extensive information, providers can use a PC-based patient information system to review a menu of all the patient education activities offered in the hospital, including a listing for the PERC. An ambulatory care team member may opt to send a patient to group-learning activities conducted in the PERC's two classrooms. These classrooms are also used for individual counseling, especially on cholesterol nutrition, behavior modification, and impotence. Finally, the primary care provider can also use the PC menu to send patients to the PERC for further information. Sometimes the referral is quite specific, for example, to view a particular videotape, but it may also be more general, for example, to request current literature on effective alternatives to prostate surgery, information that is not easily found in pamphlet form.

To fill this kind of request, Davis often depends on a CD-ROM–based health information program called the Health Reference Center,™ which provides comprehensive abstracts or full text of pamphlets, journal articles, and excerpts from books, and other health information sources. This program is so user-friendly, says Davis, that several outpatients "have become hard-wired to it," consulting it themselves when they have a question.

Given that most hospitals need to carefully manage their resources and avoid duplication, it is most efficient to provide access to such new and relatively expensive technology through a centralized source, such as the PERC. The same principle also holds for other equipment and hardware, such as audio and video recorders/players and computers. These provide access to information/education through the audiovisual media and through internal and external data bases, and can greatly simplify the task of information resource acquisition, management, and distribution.

Another example of how a resource center can help streamline a multitude of patient education activities is the ongoing development of patient and family support and information services at Good Samaritan Hospital, in Portland, Oregon. Although the initial charge of this service was to provide information and education services to patients with neurological diseases, reports Yvonne Ross, director of education and information for the support center, the hospital's desire for more efficient assignment of staff resources has been the catalyst in widening the center's scope of service to include other chronic conditions, such as cardiopulmonary disease and cancer. As a result, what used to be a network of decentralized information resource centers will slowly become centralized, with some of the teaching and many of the support resources being located in one space. For example, the library collections of the cancer service, the "heart" library, and a portion of the diabetes collection will be combined with the resources on neurological diseases to make one centralized print and audiovisual collection; and this will be further expanded with materials on a broader range of health issues, so that the resource center can serve a wider audience.

Individual teaching will continue to be provided by nurses in the various services, Ross says, but they will depend on the centralized resource center to take on some of their teaching tasks and much of their library function. In turn, Ross continues, the resource center will depend on the institution's medical library staff to provide the collection management functions that her own staff are not trained to do, such as cataloguing and computerized information searching.

A somewhat different version of centralized information support can be reached by telephone. Unlike the telephone service by which nurses offer callers both information and advice according to an approved protocol, a telephone service managed by an information resource center usually offers only that—information. However, this information covers as broad a range of subjects as do most consumer health information collections. Callers can usually receive answers to questions on normal physiological functions; pharmacology and medication; medical-testing functions and procedures; treatment options; local mutual aid (support) groups; and health care agencies, organizations, and other resources related to specific health care problems. Packets of written information in answer to specific questions are mailed to the caller following the conversation with the resource staff person, always including a statement that the contents are not to be construed as medical advice and recommending that callers consult their physician for further information or interpretation.

Such a telephone information service can be one part of a resource center that also serves walk-in visitors, or it may provide information exclusively by telephone. Either option is a significant benefit to those patients who need information, but find it either inconvenient or difficult to visit a resource center in person. A service of this kind can be especially useful in an inpatient setting for patients who are bedridden or for those who are preparing for discharge and may benefit from a comprehensive set of discharge information that the primary nurse cannot provide.

Finally, another aspect of centralized support that a resource center can provide to a hospital's patient education activities is to act as the information and entry point—frequently by telephone—for the variety of community health education and health promotion classes that a hospital may offer. For example, a diabetic looking for nutritional guidance may call the resource center asking for written information and be told that a series of classes is available through the hospital's dietary department, a refresher class is offered by the health promotion staff, and/or one-on-one nutritional counseling can be arranged. A computerized link between the resource center and the course listing of each of these departments can then offer the caller one-stop registration.

☐ Adding Opportunities to Learn

In addition to pointing consumers to learning opportunities elsewhere in the hospital, the resource center can also offer them on-site. As this chapter explained earlier, teaching activities do not commonly occur in a resource center managed by its hospital's medical library, because its professional service focus is on information rather than teaching. In contrast, consumer health information resource centers managed by nursing, patient education, or marketing in cooperation with either one of these typically add patient teaching to their range of services.

For example, the resource center that is managed by a hospital's marketing division—a frequent organizational arrangement that reflects a hospital's institutional promotion goals—frequently combines information and education with appropriate referral of resource center users to other hospital services. It both acts as the entry point for patients attempting to identify the source of the service they need, including referrals to physicians; and provides self-learning opportunities through written and audiovisual resources and patient education through part- or full-time staffing by nurses and/or health educators.

One such facility is Wadley LifeSource, in Texarkana, Texas, which is Wadley Regional Medical Center's (off-site) resource center, located in a nearby shopping mall. In addition to a general health library, LifeSource offers ongoing health screenings, related counseling by nurses and health educators on the management of chronic diseases such as high blood pressure and diabetes, guest lectures by medical staff members and other health care professionals, and referrals to longer-term education programs provided in the hospital.

One example of this resource center's strategy for linking potential clients with appropriate hospital-based education services is when Wadley LifeSource acts as the pickup point for packets for the March of Dimes campaign, which is intended to encourage pregnant teens to consult a physician for prenatal care. Such a highly visible event in a shopping mall ensures that both teens and campaign volunteers become aware of the resource center's information material on teen pregnancy and of the medical center's educational programming for parents-to-be.

One of the most comprehensive and oldest examples of a resource center that incorporates patient education into its services can be found in the Kaiser Permanente Medical Center, in Oakland, California. Its Health Education Center is one of the activities of the health education department. The facility not only houses a large collection of learning tools (including books, pamphlets, and many audiovisuals that may be viewed on-site or borrowed for home viewing), it also is the site of various teaching activities. Among these are instruction in breast self-examination, counseling to prepare patients for HIV testing, counseling and teaching related to cholesterol and high blood pressure, and instruction in home blood pressure monitoring.

According to Barbara Christianson, health education coordinator, these Center activities support the health education department's efforts to achieve one of its major goals—to provide appropriate direct clinical education services. "Our medical center physicians have told us that about 30 percent of the time patients come to the Medical Center for physician services, but what they really need is health education," Christianson reports. "Direct clinical education services" are meant to more appropriately take the place of this 30 percent of physician visits. In this way, the Health Education Center is not just an adjunct to care—not an opportunity to learn something beyond the basic—but, rather, the clinical education service is actually part of the treatment plan.

Statistics indicate that the department is very much on the right track in its efforts to achieve this goal, says Christianson. Several years ago, approximately 75 percent of the department's patients were self-referred. Currently, more than 50 percent come to use the department's education services—including the health education center—with a professional referral in hand. In addition to providing learning opportunities at Kaiser Permanente's Health Education Center, its staff also help to plan and support a range of teaching activities that are provided throughout the Kaiser Permanente Medical Center.

For example, staff routinely provide preoperative education to patients of the ophthalmology service, which is located one floor above and which does not have space for audiovisual equipment. Patients scheduled for cataract surgery need relevant information to prepare them for the procedure and to help them through a successful and timely recovery; for the majority of patients this information can be standardized. The ophthalmology service staff, with the help of the Resource Center, identified what this preoperative information should contain and found an appropriate audiovisual program that would present the information to every patient, therefore relieving staff of a repetitive, albeit important, task. Every patient who is scheduled for the cataract procedure is now required to view the videotape in the Resource Center, which has both the space and the equipment for this activity and is only a few steps away from the ophthalmology service.

Identifying the Need for Programming

A resource center that does not assume any direct teaching tasks can also be a great help in identifying possible new opportunities for patient education. *Consumer Health Information: Managing Hospital-Based Centers* describes one such example from the Bronson Methodist Hospital's (Kalamazoo, Michigan) telephone information service.

> When Bronson's medical library began to offer this service to consumers, it realized how useful the content of callers' questions would be to other departments in the hospital who were providing health care to patients. Library staff soon began to pass this information on to the marketing department as well as to service line administrators and patient education staff. Such information can often provide the last piece of evidence to support a management decision about reorganizing a current program or launching a new service.[2]

For example, when the library passed on repeated requests for information on the risks of high cholesterol, the hospital was encouraged to launch monthly cholesterol screening and information sessions at one of its sites.

As this and all the other examples in this chapter demonstrate, the education/information task itself is an essential determinant of the manner in which a consumer health information resource center can help define programming and support the patient education function. Christianson of the Kaiser Permanente Health Education Center offers a number of examples. If the patient simply needs to view a videotape related to a specific clinical problem, she says, and this videotape is frequently prescribed by one service, helping that clinical service to develop a small patient education resource area may be the most effective way to ensure that the patient actually watches the tape. The further away a clinical service is from the resource center, the less often its patients tend to make the trip to the center to access necessary materials, Christianson suggests. In this arrangement, the central resource center can act as a backup, a source of further information, and a gatekeeper to other sources of material as they are developed in the field.

In contrast, if the same information and education about an issue must be available to all hospital clients, a central resource center is probably the most appropriate provider. For example, the Kaiser Permanente Medical Center's response to recent legislation on advance directives is to have the Resource Center be the site of information on this issue. Patients can come to the Resource Center to view or borrow a videotape on the subject, pick up a durable power of attorney form, have Resource Center staff explain the form and its use, and return it for filing. It would have been very inefficient for the Medical Center to train all staff to routinely provide this information, Christianson explains, and it has been a valuable service to point patients to one source of information and material on this critical issue.

The ultimate question for the resource center to ask itself in making a determination about its participation in patient education, Christiansen concludes, is: "If we shouldn't be providing it, how can we help someone else do it?"

☐ Taking Steps toward Support

PEMs who wish to take advantage of the many possible links with resource centers can ask themselves the reverse: "If the patient education staff cannot provide this service or take on this activity, given current circumstances, can the resource center help?"

The answer to this question clearly depends on whether the hospital already has a consumer health information resource center in place. If it does, the PEM can follow Christianson's advice: Let the nature of the task guide the collaboration between patient education and the resource center.

On the other hand, if no resource center exists, the PEM must carefully assess whether such a center promises to significantly improve the department's ability to provide high-quality patient education services. The following questions should be considered:

- Is the current level of print and audiovisual resources in the hospital sufficient to meet the information/education needs of hospital users?
- Do the patient education department and those who teach find much of their time being devoted to the task of acquiring and managing materials rather than teaching patients?
- Do outpatients and the hospital community in general have a clearly identifiable and accessible source of information on health-related issues in general and on available opportunities for learning self-care/self-management skills?
- Does the department have a dependable source of information to help identify patients' information and education needs and interests?
- Would centralizing some of the department's information and education functions in a resource center facilitate the department's operations and make more efficient and effective use of its resources?

If the answers to these questions suggest that a consumer information resource center could indeed be beneficial, this chapter has achieved its purpose but also reached its limits. It is far beyond the scope of this chapter to describe the process of consumer health information resource center development; for such information, the reader is referred to the list of resources at the close of this chapter.

Considering the significant benefits that consumer health information resource centers can offer, PEMs should not be discouraged from further investigating what may seem to be a massive organizational undertaking. An informal poll of hospital colleagues and providers—not least of them, the physician community—will likely uncover a strong interest in such an undertaking and a willingness to at least discuss its feasibility. Many a successful resource center has been developed through collaboration among several hospital interest groups who have both shared in the labor and reaped the benefits of centralized consumer information and education services.

□ Conclusion

Regardless of whether consumer health information resource centers provide actual patient teaching or serve as a centralized place where patients and families can obtain prepared patient education materials, they play an important role. Many hospitals have come to depend on them to manage the distribution of materials, provide referrals, and support the hospitalwide patient education function. Their example is good evidence that such services are a significant new phase in the way hospitals keep their communities informed and well.

References

1. Kernaghan, S. G., and Giloth, B. E. *Consumer Health Information: Managing Hospital-Based Centers.* Chicago: American Hospital Association, 1991.

2. Kernaghan and Giloth, pp. 37–38.

Resources

Kernaghan, S. G., and Giloth, B. E. *Consumer Health Information: Managing Hospital-Based Centers.* Chicago: American Hospital Association, 1991.

(American Hospital Association, 840 North Lake Shore Drive, Chicago, IL 60611; Tel. 312/280-6000; AHA Catalog No. 070200)

This work contains a comprehensive discussion of the organizational and community benefits of hospital-based centers; a description of the major operational elements of consumer health information services, with examples taken from contemporary hospital-based centers across the United States; and a special section on telephone information services, with recommendations on risk management strategies. It includes illustrations and samples of referral, promotional, and evaluation materials and a resource list.

Medical Library Association, 6 North Michigan Avenue, Suite 300, Chicago, IL 60602; Tel. 312/419-9094.

In addition to the fee for membership in the MLA, a small fee affords members access to its Section on Consumer and Patient Health Information, which produces a quarterly newsletter, provides a directory of members who are information service managers, and offers networking and continuing education opportunities related to managing consumer and patient health information services.

Rees, A. M., editor. *Managing Consumer Health Information Services.* Phoenix: Oryx Press, 1991.

(Oryx Press, 4041 North Central, Suite 700, Phoenix, AZ 85012; Tel. 1-800-279-ORYX)

An update of an earlier version, *Developing Consumer Health Information Services* (Bowker, 1982), this volume includes case studies of information services in both community and hospital settings, discusses trends in medical consumerism, and provides an overview of international developments in consumer health information. It includes comprehensive lists of resources appropriate for small and large collections.

Steele, B., and Willard, C. *Guidelines for Establishing a Family Resource Library.* 2nd ed. Washington DC: Association for the Care of Children in Hospitals, 1989.

Intended for agencies serving the needs of parents and children, this publication discusses planning, staffing, financing, policy and procedure development, appropriate services, promotion and outreach, and evaluation. It includes a variety of sample forms useful in many library activities and a list of resources relevant to family library development.

Part Three

Additional Resources

Appendix

National Patient Education and Health Promotion Organizations

This listing was prepared by staff in the AHA's Division of Ambulatory Care and the Hospital Research and Educational Trust.

American Association of Diabetes Educators (AADE)
444 North Michigan Avenue, Suite 1240
Chicago, IL 60611-3901
312/644-2233

AADE has three major purposes: (1) to provide educational opportunities for the professional growth and development of its members; (2) to promote development of high-quality diabetes education for the diabetic consumer; and (3) to foster communication and cooperation among individuals and organizations involved in diabetes education. Its members include nurses, dietitians, social workers, physicians, pharmacists, podiatrists, and others. Members receive the monthly *AADE Newsletter* and a bimonthly journal, *The Diabetes Educator.* AADE has established a separately incorporated body, the National Certification Board for Diabetes Educators, to develop and implement the certification process for diabetes educators. To be certified, a health care professional must meet eligibility requirements and pass a national examination every five years.

American Association of Retired Persons (AARP)
601 E Street, NW
Washington, DC 20049
202/434-2277

AARP is a national organization responsible for advocating the needs of older people. Services provided to its members include group health insurance programs and sponsorship of community service programs such as crime prevention and defensive driving. Through its Andrus Foundation, AARP awards grants to colleges and universities for research projects in applied gerontology. It provides on-line bibliographical retrieval services through AGE-LINE and publishes the monthly AARP *News Bulletin* and the bimonthly journal *Modern Maturity.* AARP has recently formed the Healthy Older Adults Action Alliance to encourage health promotion among older adults as part of Healthy

People 2000. The organization also runs The National Resource Center on Health Promotion and Aging, which publishes the newsletter *Perspectives in Health Promotion and Aging.*

American Public Health Association (APHA)
1015 15th Street, NW, Suite 300
Washington, DC 20005
202/789-5600

APHA is a nongovernmental professional membership organization representing all disciplines and specialties of public health. Its mission is to protect and promote personal and environmental health by exercising leadership in the development and dissemination of health policy. The organization conducts an annual meeting and publishes monthly *The Nation's Health* and *The American Journal of Public Health.* Members can select a primary specialty section with which to affiliate; the Public Health Education and Health Promotion and School Health Education and Services sections are of particular interest to practitioners in patient education and health promotion.

Association for the Advancement of Health Education (AAHE)
1900 Association Drive
Reston, VA 22091
703/476-3437

AAHE is a professional organization for health educators that spans all practice settings but with an emphasis on school and university settings. In addition to special-interest areas and a large annual convention, members receive the *Journal of Health Education.* AAHE is a member of the American Alliance for Health, Physical Education, Recreation and Dance, whose other constituent organizations include the National Association for Sport and Physical Education; the National Association for Girls and Women in Sport; the Association for Research, Administration, Professional Councils and Societies; and the National Dance Association.

Association for Fitness in Business (AFB)
342 Massachusetts Avenue
200 Marott Center
Indianapolis, IN 46204
317/636-6621

AFB is a not-for-profit professional and educational association organized for the purpose of advancing the field of worksite wellness. AFB supports and assists in the development of health and fitness programs in the workplace by:

- Publishing current information and essential data
- Developing programs of continuing education
- Stimulating research
- Facilitating career development

Members receive the membership newsletter *Action* and the bimonthly *American Journal of Health Promotion,* which provides professional information on health and fitness programs in business, hospitals, and community-based facilities.

Centers for Disease Control (CDC)
Center for Chronic Disease Prevention and Health Promotion
Division of Chronic Disease Control and Community Intervention
1600 Clifton Road, NE
Atlanta, GA 30333
404/639-3311

The CDC's Center for Chronic Disease Prevention and Health Promotion has developed a technical assistance process, with supporting print materials for implementing community-based health promotion programs. PATCH (Planned Approach to Community Health), a program of the CDC, assists state and local health departments and other community organizations in planning communitywide health promotion activities focusing on local health problems.

International Patient Education Council (IPEC)
P.O. Box 1438
Rockville, MD 20849
301/948-1863

The mission of IPEC is "To advance the science and practice of patient education, in order to promote educationally-centered health care at the local, regional and international levels." The organization publishes *Patient Education RX* for its members, and the *Journal of Patient Education and Counseling* is published in collaboration with IPEC. Each year, IPEC sponsors National Patient Education Week in the first week of November, and produces a how-to planning packet for the week.

National Center for Health Education (NCHE)
72 Spring Street, Suite 208
New York, NY 10012
212/334-9470

NCHE is a private not-for-profit organization whose purpose is to expand the practice of health education. A major focus is on integrating health education into community programs targeted to children and adolescents. In 1990, NCHE was awarded a cooperative agreement with the Centers for Disease Control to work with 16 cities in creating coalitions to provide school-based health education. The Center also manages and disseminates *Growing Healthy*, a comprehensive health education curriculum for elementary-school children.

National Commission for Health Education Credentialling (NCHEC)
475 Riverside Drive, Suite 740
New York, NY 10115
212/870-2047

NCHEC is an independent organization that certifies and recertifies health education professionals. It is composed of a Board of Commissioners and three boards. The Division Board for Certification is responsible for the certification test preparation. Health educators who wish to become certified must now complete professional training programs in health education as well as sit for the certification examination. The Division Board for Professional Development is responsible for the annual renewal and recertification processes, which include requirements for continuing education. This board is also responsible for the designation of providers of Category I continuing education contact hours in health education. The Division Board for Professional Preparation is responsible for reviewing the professional preparation activities of college and university programs with a health education emphasis.

The National Wellness Association (NWA)
1319 Fremont, South Hall
Stevens Point, WI 54481
715/346-2172

NWA is a not-for-profit organization of professionals working in all areas of health and wellness promotion. Its mission is to meet the growing needs of health promotion professionals for information, services, and networking. NWA members represent many of the settings where health promotion and wellness programs are incorporated, including hospitals, corporations, colleges and universities, community service agencies and school districts, fitness clubs, private consulting firms, insurance companies, public health departments, small businesses, and allied health organizations. The organization publishes a quarterly membership newsletter and conducts national wellness conferences and institutes.

Office of Disease Prevention and Health Promotion (ODPHP)
Public Health Service
U.S. Department of Health and Human Services
Switzer Building, Room 2132
330 C Street, SW
Washington, DC 20201

ODPHP is located within the U.S. Department of Health and Human Health Services. Its mission is to promote health and prevent disease among Americans through programs such as Healthy People 2000, a national initiative to set health promotion and disease prevention objectives for the year 2000. ODPHP is responsible for a number of other national initiatives including nutrition, preventive services, school health, worksite health promotion, and community/media health promotion. The Office also sponsors a National Health Information Center.

ODPHP National Health Information Center
P.O. Box 1133
Washington, DC 20013-1133
800/336-4797
301/565-4167

A service of ODPHP, the National Health Information Center responds directly to requests for health information through its on-site library and data base or by forwarding information requests to other organizations. The Center publishes *Healthfinders*, a series of publications listing information resources on a variety of health topics including national health observances, women's health, and family care.

Society for Public Health Education (SOPHE)
2001 Addison Street, Suite 220
Berkeley, CA 94704
415/644-9242

SOPHE is the national professional organization for public health educators in community, medical, international, worksite, university, and school settings. The organization has 18 chapters and publishes a newsletter, *News and Views*, and a journal, *The Health Education Quarterly*. It sponsors an annual meeting in the fall in conjunction with the American Public Health Association and a midyear scientific meeting in late spring.

Wellness Councils of America (WELCOA)
Historic Library Plaza
1823 Harney Street, Suite 201
Omaha, NE 68102
402/444-1711

WELCOA is a national umbrella organization dedicated to providing direction and support services to community-based wellness councils and to furthering their mission to promote healthier life-styles for all Americans. A Wellness Council is a group of employers who have joined together voluntarily to provide programs at the worksite to help their employees pursue more healthful life-styles.

In promoting wellness programs at the worksite, the Council acts as a catalyst in gaining the support of chief executive officers in the business community to provide health promotion programs. The organization provides consultation to individual businesses seeking to establish wellness programs, serves as a clearinghouse in making available health information and related resources to the business community, and coordinates and sponsors communitywide wellness activities.

Bibliography

This bibliography covers journal articles from 1990 to 1992 and the major books of the past 10 years that deal with patient education. The journal section is divided into four parts: general education topics; patient education and advance directives; print/technology options for patient education; and target population patient education programs.

☐ Journal Articles

General Patient Education Topics

Arndt, M. J., and Underwood, B. Learning style theory and patient education. *Journal of Continuing Education in Nursing* 21(1):28–31, Jan.–Feb. 1990.

Barrett, C., and others. Nurses' perceptions of their health educator role. *Journal of Nursing Staff Development* 6(6):283–86, Nov.–Dec. 1990.

Beisecker, A. E., and Beisecker, T. D. Patient information-seeking behaviors when communicating with doctors. *Medical Care* 28(1):19–28, Jan. 1990.

Belcher, D. W. Implementing preventive services. Success and failure in an outpatient trial. *Archives of Internal Medicine* 150(12):2533–41, Dec. 1990.

Bertakis, K. D. Impact of a patient education intervention on appropriate utilization of clinic services. *Journal of the American Board of Family Practice* 4(6):411–18, Nov.–Dec. 1991.

Bourgeois, P. Statistics, CPT, ICD-9, CDM, and level III codes: what are they and how did I get this job? *Diabetes Educator* 17(5):351–52, Sept.–Oct. 1991.

Bransome, E. D., Jr. Improving the financing of diabetes care in the 1990s. Recommendations of the 1989 conference. *Diabetes Care* 15 Supplement 1:66–72, Mar. 1992.

Degeling, D., and others. Patient education policy and practice in Australian hospitals. *Patient Education and Counseling* 15(2):127–38, Apr. 1990.

Fahrenfort, M. Patient education in Dutch hospitals: the fruits of a decade of endeavors. *Patient Education and Counseling* 15(2):139–50, Apr. 1990.

Fleming, V. E. Client education: a futuristic outlook. *Journal of Advanced Nursing* 17(2):158–63, Feb. 1992.

Gibson, P. A., and others. A health/patient education database for family practice. *Bulletin of the Medical Library Association* 79(4):357–69, Oct. 1991.

Giloth, B. E. Management of patient education in US hospitals: evolution of a concept. *Patient Education and Counseling* 15(2):101–11, Feb. 1990.

Giloth, B. E. Promoting patient involvement: educational, organizational, and environmental strategies. *Patient Education and Counseling* 15(1):29–38, Apr. 1990.

Green, L. W. Hospitals and health care providers as agents of patient education. *Patient Education and Counseling* 15(2):169–70, Apr. 1990.

Greenberg, J. S. Competencies necessary to conduct patient and self-care education in the medical setting. *Healthcare Education and Training* 6(1):6–12, 1991.

Grieco, A. J., and others. New York University Medical Center's Cooperative Care Unit: patient education and family participation during hospitalization—the first ten years. *Patient Education and Counseling* 15(1):3–15, Feb. 1990.

Grueninger, U. J., and others. A conceptual framework for interactive patient education in practice and clinic settings. *Journal of Human Hypertension* 4 Supplement 1:21–31, Feb. 1990.

Hafstad, L. Outcome factors in patient education. *Physician Assistant* 16(2):37–38, 40–41, Feb. 1992.

Hanks, A. The patient's patient. *Nephrology News and Issues* 5(12):22–36, Dec. 1991.

Harrison, L. L. Strategies to facilitate inpatient education. *MCN: American Journal of Maternal Child Nursing* 15(4):255, July–Aug. 1990.

Informed consent. Opening the doors to physician–patient communication (1). *Minnesota Medicine* 73(10):35–39, Oct. 1990.

Jenny, J. Nursing patient education: a Canadian perspective. *Patient Education and Counseling* 16(1):47–52, Aug. 1990.

Kruger, S. A review of patient education in nursing. *Journal of Nursing Staff Development* 6(2):71–74, Mar.–Apr. 1990.

Kruger, S. The patient educator role in nursing. *Applied Nursing Research* 4(1):19–24, Feb. 1991.

Lindner, K. A piece of my mind. Encourage information therapy. *JAMA: Journal of the American Medical Association* 267(19):2592, May 20, 1992.

Lipetz, M. J., and others. What is wrong with patient education programs? *Nursing Outlook* 38(4):184–89, Jul.–Aug. 1990.

McCann, D. P., and Blossom, H. J. Residents' and faculty members' views of and skills in patient education. *Academic Medicine* 67(2):134, Feb. 1992.

Morra, M. E. Future trends in patient education. *Seminars in Oncology Nursing* 7(2):143–45, May 1991.

Muller, R. J., and Agre, P. Patient education: a multidisciplinary approach to influence patient compliance. *Topics in Hospital Pharmacy Management* 10(4):50–58, Jan. 1991.

Noble, C. Are nurses good patient educators? *Journal of Advanced Nursing* 16(10):1185–89, Oct. 1991.

O'Connor, C. T. Patient education with a purpose. *Journal of Nursing Staff Development* 6(3):145–47, May–June, 1990.

Padilla, G. V., and Bulcavage, L. M. Theories used in patient/health education. *Seminars in Oncology Nursing* 7(2):87–96, May 1991.

Porter, Y. Evaluation of nursing documentation of patient teaching. *Journal of Continuing Education in Nursing* 21(3):134–37, May–June, 1990.

Rakel, B. A. Interventions related to patient teaching. *Nursing Clinics of North America* 27(2):397–423, June 1992.

Redman, B. K., and Braun, R. Courses in patient education in master's programs in nursing. *Journal of Nursing Education* 30(1):42–43, Jan. 1991.

Reducing patient stays and improving satisfaction take one giant step. *Hospital Patient Relations Report* 6(5):5, May 1991.

Rivers, R. Staff nurses' perception of responsibility to provide patient education in hospital setting. *Journal of Healthcare Education and Training* 6(2):8–12, 1991.

Robinson, J. Patient education: opportunity and necessity. *Journal of Nursing Staff Development* 7(2):97–98, Mar.–Apr. 1991.

Simonds, S. K., and Kanters, H. W. Comparative analysis of patient education by four professions in The Netherlands and the United States. *Patient Education and Counseling* 15(2):151–67, Apr. 1990.

Smoothing the transition from hospital to home. Patient Learning Center increases quality of care. University of Minnesota Hospital and Clinic. *Profiles in Healthcare Marketing* (47):14–18, May–June 1992.

Speros, C. I., and Sol, N. Health promotion in hospitals. *WHO Regional Publications European Series* 37:267–81, 1991.

Spotting reading problems among patients can help ensure they receive proper care. *Hospital Patient Relations Report* 5(12):4, Dec. 1990.

Stevenson, E., and Crosson, K. Patient education: history, development, and current directions of the American Cancer Society and the National Cancer Institute. *Seminars in Oncology Nursing* 7(2):135–42, May 1991.

Third-party reimbursement for outpatient diabetes education and counseling. *Diabetes Care* 13 Supplement 1:36, Jan. 1990.

This medical library is not for doctors only. *Profiles in Healthcare Marketing* (46):48–50, Mar.–Apr. 1992.

Tobin, C. T. Third-party reimbursement coverage for diabetes outpatient education programs. *Diabetes Care* 15 Supplement 1:41–43, Mar. 1992.

Van Doren, D. C., and Blank, K. M. Patient education: a potential marketing tool for the private physician. *Journal of Health Care Marketing* 12(1):71–77, Mar. 1992.

Walker, L. M. Patient education: do it right, and everyone wins. *Medical Economics* 69(13):155–58, 160–63, July 6, 1992.

Webber, G. C. Patient education. A review of the issues. *Medical Care* 28(11):1089–103, Nov. 1990.

Wheeler, M. L., and Warren-Boulton, E. Diabetes patient education programs. Quality and reimbursement. *Diabetes Care* 15 Supplement 1:36–40, Mar. 1992.

Patient Education and Advance Directives

Blossom, H. J., and McCann, D. P. A revolution in understanding: how ethics has transformed health care decision making: the role of patient education. *QRB: Quality Review Bulletin* 18(4):118, Apr. 1992.

Colvin, E. R., and Hammes, B. J. "If I only knew": a patient education program on advance directives. *ANNA Journal* 18(6):557–60, Dec. 1991.

Educating patients about advanced directives. *QRC Advisor* 7(9):1, 7, June 1991.

Havens, D. M., and Greenberg, P. Talk about death and dying: it's the law. *Journal of Pediatric Health Care* 6(3):158–60, May–June 1992.

Hospitals explore ways of educating patients about advanced directives. *Hospital Patient Relations Report* 6(2):3, 7, Feb. 1991.

Iserson, K. V. Getting advance directives to the public: a role for emergency medicine. *Annals of Emergency Medicine* 20(6):692–96, June 1991.

Koska, M. T. Can outcomes data help patients make end-of-life decisions? *Hospitals* 65(11):42, 44, June 5, 1991.

Miles, J. Protecting patient self-determination. New legislation requires healthcare providers to inform patients of rights regarding advance directives. *Health Progress* 72(3):26–30, Apr. 1991.

Program reduces hospital stays and maintains patient satisfaction; creator earns cash prize and fellowships. *Hospital Patient Relations Report* 5(10):7, Oct. 1990.

Sachs, G. A., and others. Empowerment of the older patient? A randomized, controlled trial to increase discussion and use of advance directives. *Journal of the American Geriatrics Society* 40(3):269–73, Mar. 1992.

Teschke, D. A. Living will center, videotapes help hospitals meet regulation. *Healthcare Financial Management* 45(11):103, Nov. 1991.

Print/Technology Options for Patient Education

Andrews, J. How we do it. Sexual assault aftercare instructions. *Journal of Emergency Nursing* 18(2):152–57, Apr. 1992.

Aukerman, G. F. Developing a patient education newsletter. *Journal of Family Practice* 33(3):304–5, Sept. 1991.

Barnes, L. P. The illiterate client: strategies in patient teaching. *MCN: American Journal of Maternal Child Nursing* 17(3):127, May–June, 1992.

Biermann, E., and Mehnert, H. DIABLOG: a simulation program of insulin–glucose dynamics for education of diabetics. *Computer Methods and Programs in Biomedicine* 32(3–4):311–18, July–Aug. 1990.

Brown, S. A., and others. Diabetes education in a Mexican-American population: pilot testing of a research-based videotape. *Diabetes Educator* 18(1):47–51, Jan.–Feb. 1992.

Card, poster ready to assist with patient talk. *American Nurse* 23(10):18, Nov.–Dec., 1991.

Clarke, S. E., and others. Information for patients and staff concerning nuclear medicine. *Nuclear Medicine Communications* 13(4):271–81, Apr. 1992.

Davis, S. W., and others. Clinical trials booklet evaluation. *Progress in Clinical and Biological Research* 339:409–17, 1990.

Davis, T. C., and others. The gap between patient reading comprehension and the readability of patient education materials. *Journal of Family Practice* 31(5):533–38, Nov. 1990.

Early, P. Asthma workbook airs first for adults. *Profiles in Healthcare Marketing* (43):80–83, July 1991.

Early, P. One-minute spots teach and earn. *Profiles in Healthcare Marketing* (43):29–33, July 1991.

Firby, P. A., and others. Nurses' opinions of the introduction of computer-assisted learning for use in patient education. *Journal of Advanced Nursing* 16(8):987–95, Aug. 1991.

Former drug addicts, family members talk about disease in hospital video. *Hospital Patient Relations Report* 5(9):7, Sept. 1990.

Frank-Stromborg, M., and Cohen, R. Evaluating written patient education materials. *Seminars in Oncology Nursing* 7(2):125–34, May 1991.

Gibbs, S. Prescription information leaflets for patients. *European Respiratory Journal* 5(1):140–43, Jan. 1992.

Goldsmith, M. F. Vaccine information pamphlets here, but some physicians react strongly. *JAMA: Journal of the American Medical Association* 267(15):2005–7, Apr. 15, 1992.

Holmes, P. Telephone translators. *Nursing Times* 86(28):21–23, July 11–17, 1990.

Holt, G. A., and others. Patient interpretation of label instructions. *American Pharmacy* NS32(3):58–62, Mar. 1992.

Holzman, D. Interactive video promotes patient–doctor partnership. *Business and Health* 10(4):42,46–49, Mar. 15, 1992.

Isaacman, D. J., and others. Standardized instructions: do they improve communication of discharge information from the emergency department? *Pediatrics* 89(6 Pt 2):1204–8, June 1992.

Jackson, R. H., and others. Patient reading ability: an overlooked problem in health care. *Southern Medical Journal* 84(10):1172–75, Oct. 1991.

Larson, I., and Schumacher, H. R. Comparison of literacy level of patients in a VA arthritis center with the reading level required by educational materials. *Arthritis Care and Research* 5(1):13–16, Mar. 1992.

Lerman, C., and others. The impact of mailing psychoeducational materials to women with abnormal mammograms. *American Journal of Public Health* 82(5):729–30, May 1992.

Lilliott, N. Discharge instructions. Advice for knee, shoulder arthroscopy outpatients. *AORN Journal* 54(5):1015–28, Nov. 1991.

Masten, Y., and Conover, K. P. Automated continuing education and patient education. *Computers in Nursing* 8(4):144–50, Jul.–Aug. 1990.

Meade, V. Patient drug information hotlines multiply. *American Pharmacy* NS31(8):29–31, Aug. 1991.

Meissner, H. I., and others. Meeting information needs of significant others: use of the Cancer Information Service. *Patient Education and Counseling* 15(2):171–79, Apr. 1990.

Petryshen, P., and others. Multimedia applications in nursing for computer-based staff training and patient education. *Journal of Continuing Education in Nursing* 23(3):140–42, May–June 1992.

Poirier, T. I., and Giudici, R. A. Evaluation of patient counseling microcomputer software programs. *Hospital Pharmacy* 27(5):408, 411–15, May 1992.

Rohret, L., and Ferguson, K. J. Effective use of patient education illustrations. *Patient Education and Counseling* 15(1):73–75, Feb. 1990.

Snider, J. Creating and implementing an online patient education catalog. *Bulletin of the Medical Library Association* 79(3):321–23, July 1991.

Street, D., and Popkess, A. Patient education: instruction cards for i.v. antibiotics. *Hospital Pharmacy* 25(4):360, 366, Apr. 1990.

Taira, F. Individualized medication sheets. *Nursing Economics* 9(1):56–58, Jan.–Feb. 1991.

Tongue, B., and Stanley, I. A video-based information system for patients. *Health Trends* 23(1):11–12, 1991.

Touch cards trace breast lumps. *Profiles in Healthcare Marketing* (43):24–28, July 1991.

Vargo, G. Computer assisted patient education in the ambulatory care setting. *Computers in Nursing* 9(5):168–69, Sept.–Oct. 1991.

What are your patients reading? *Hospital Food and Nutrition Focus* 7(10):6–7, June 1991.

Whiteley, M. "So you're going to have an operation?" The making of a video. *British Journal of Theatre Nursing* 2(1):4–7, Apr. 1992.

Target Population Patient Education Programs

A patient review of the ESRD program: part I. *Nephrology News and Issues* 5(4):22–27, Apr. 1991.

Agre, P., and others. How much time do nurses spend teaching cancer patients? *Patient Education and Counseling* 16(1):29–38, Aug. 1990.

Alkhawajah, A. M., and Eferakeya, A. E. The role of pharmacists in patients' education on medication. *Public Health* 106(3):231–37, May 1992.

Allen, M., and others. Effectiveness of a preoperative teaching programme for cataract patients. *Journal of Advanced Nursing* 17(3):303–9, Mar. 1992.

Andrew, C. Treatment information and the radiotherapy patient. *Radiography Today* 57(652):25–29, Sept. 1991.

Avigne, G., and Phillips, T. L. Pediatric preoperative tours. Successful hospital program expands to community. *AORN Journal* 53(6):1458–65, June 1991.

Baker, J., and Muma, R. D. Counseling patients with HIV infection. *Physician Assistant* 15(7):40–42, 47–48, July 1991.

Barnes, L. P. Teaching self-care to children. *MCN: American Journal of Maternal/Child Nursing* 16(2):101, Mar.–Apr. 1991.

Bartholomew, L. K., and others. Development of a health education program to promote the self-management of cystic fibrosis. *Health Education Quarterly* 18(4):429–43, Winter 1991.

Beresford, S. A., and others. Evaluation of a self-help dietary intervention in a primary care setting. *American Journal of Public Health* 82(1):79–84, Jan. 1992.

Berwick, M., and others. The role of the nurse in skin cancer prevention, screening, and early detection. *Seminars in Oncology Nursing* 7(1):64–71, Feb. 1991.

Boswell, E. J., and others. Negotiating independent practice in diabetes education. *Diabetes Educator* 18(4):288, 290, July–Aug. 1992.

Boyd, M. A., and others. For those left behind. An educational inpatient rehabilitation program. *Journal of Psychosocial Nursing and Mental Health Services* 29(1):24–29, Jan. 1991.

Caffery, L., and Claussen, D. S. Inpatient education for fiberoptic/videoptic diagnostic and therapeutic procedures for gastroenterology. *Gastroenterology Nursing* 14(2):106–9, Oct. 1991.

Caldwell, L. M. The influence of preference for information on preoperative stress and coping in surgical outpatients. *Applied Nursing Research* 4(4):177–83, Nov. 1991.

Calsyn, D. A., and others. Ineffectiveness of AIDS education and HIV antibody testing in reducing high-risk behaviors among injection drug users. *American Journal of Public Health* 82(4):573–75, Apr. 1992.

Carpenter, L. C., and others. Facilitating community breast cancer detection and screening. *Oncology Nursing Forum* 19(1):93, Jan.–Feb. 1992.

Carpentier, W. S., and others. Efficacy of diabetes education: classroom versus individualized instruction. *HMO Practice* 4(1):30–33, Jan.–Feb. 1990.

Carson, D. K., and others. The effectiveness of a family asthma program for children and parents. *Children's Health Care* 20(2):114–19, Spring 1991.

Clary, C., and others. Psychiatric inpatients' knowledge of medication at hospital discharge. *Hospital and Community Psychiatry* 43(2):140–44, Feb. 1992.

Cobb, N., and others. "Burn repeaters" and injury control. *Journal of Burn Care and Rehabilitation* 13(3):382–87, May–June 1992.

Coker, M., and Lampert, A. Teaching checklist for home infusion therapy. *Oncology Nursing Forum* 17(6):923–26, Nov.–Dec. 1990.

Collins-Colon, T. Do it yourself. Medication management for community based clients. *Journal of Psychosocial Nursing and Mental Health Services* 28(6):25–29, June 1990.

Comi, R. J. A unique collaborative network for diabetes education. *Diabetes Educator* 17(6):442–43, 445, Nov.–Dec. 1991.

Cypress, M., and others. The scope of practice of diabetes educators in a metropolitan area. *Diabetes Educator* 18(2):111–14, Mar.–Apr. 1992.

Daltroy, L. H., and Liang, M. H. Advances in patient education in rheumatic disease. *Annals of the Rheumatic Diseases* 50 Suppl. 3:415–17, June 1991.

Davis, E. D., and others. Implementing a nursing care quality program to improve diabetes patient education. *Journal of Nursing Care Quality* 6(3):67–77, Apr. 1992.

Davis, J. Diabetes Management Center: a dream come true. *Health Progress* 71(1):106–9, Jan.–Feb. 1990.

Depies, M., and others. MRI anxiety reduction. *Administrative Radiology* 10(7):43–44, 48, July 1991.

Dulaney, P. E., and others. A comprehensive education and support program for women experiencing hysterectomies. *Journal of Obstetric, Gynecologic, and Neonatal Nursing* 19(4):319–25, July–Aug. 1990.

Duryee, R. The efficacy of inpatient education after myocardial infarction. *Heart and Lung* 21(3):217–25, May 1992.

Eddy, M. E., and Coslow, B. I. Preparation for ambulatory surgery: a patient education program. *Journal of Post Anesthesia Nursing* 6(1):5–12, Feb. 1991.

Elder-Tabrizy, K. A., and others. AIDS and competing health concerns of blacks, Hispanics, and whites. *Journal of Community Health* 16(1):11–21, Feb. 1991.

Eng, K., and Emlet, C. A. SRx: a regional approach to geriatric medication education. *Gerontologist* 30(3):408–10, June 1990.

Everheart, C. Taking care of yourself for life: health promotion and education for child-cancer survivors. *Journal of Pediatric Oncology Nursing* 8(2):58–59, Apr. 1991.

Factors related to cholesterol screening and cholesterol level awareness—United States, 1989. *Patient Education and Counseling* 17(1):79–83, Feb. 1991.

Farkas, M. Utilizing the nursing process in the development of a medication group on an inpatient psychiatric unit. *Perspectives in Psychiatric Care* 26(3):12–17, 1990.

Field, P. A., and Renfrew, M. Teaching and support: nursing input in the postpartum period. *International Journal of Nursing Studies* 28(2):131–44, 1991.

Fitzpatrick, S. B., and others. A novel asthma camp intervention for childhood asthma among urban blacks. The Pediatric Lung Committee of the American Lung Association of the District of Columbia (ALADC) Washington, DC. *Journal of the National Medical Association* 84(3):233–37, Mar. 1992.

Fletcher, S. W., and others. How best to teach women breast self-examination. A randomized controlled trial. *Annals of Internal Medicine* 112(10):772–79, May 15, 1990.

Fox, S. A., and others. Improving the adherence of urban women to mammography guidelines: strategies for radiologists. *Radiology* 174(1):203–6, Jan. 1990.

Freda, M. C., and others. Lifestyle modification as an intervention for inner city women at high risk for preterm birth. *Journal of Advanced Nursing* 15(3):364–72, Mar. 1990.

Freda, M. C., and others. A "PROPP" for the Bronx: preterm birth prevention education in the inner city. *Obstetrics and Gynecology* 1 Supplement 76:93S-96S, July 1990.

Freda, M. C., and others. What do pregnant women know about preventing preterm birth? *Journal of Obstetric, Gynecologic, and Neonatal Nursing* 20(2):140–45, Mar.–Apr. 1991.

Fredette, S. L. A model for improving cancer patient education. *Cancer Nursing* 13(4):207–15, Aug. 1990.

Frey, M. A., and Fox, M. A. Assessing and teaching self-care to youths with diabetes mellitus. *Pediatric Nursing* 16(6):588, 597–99, Nov.–Dec. 1990.

Funnell, M. M., and others. Empowerment: an idea whose time has come in diabetes education. *Diabetes Educator* 17(1):37–41, Jan.–Feb. 1991.

Galuk, D. The nurse (as) diabetes educator. *Advancing Clinical Care* 5(5):27–29, Sept.–Oct. 1990.

Galuk, D. L. Classes for the diabetic patient. A five day format. *Advancing Clinical Care* 5(6):29–31, Nov.–Dec. 1990.

Gardner, C. Role of nurses in the education, treatment, and prevention of occupational HIV transmission. *Journal of Intravenous Nursing* 3 Supplement P 14:S8-S12, May–June 1991.

Gelbaum, I. Circumcision. To educate, not indoctrinate—a mandate for certified nurse-midwives. *Journal of Nurse-Midwifery* 2 Supplement 37:97S–113S, Mar.–Apr. 1992.

Gillette, Y., and others. Hospital-based case management for medically fragile infants: results of a randomized trial. *Patient Education and Counseling* 17(1):59–70, Feb. 1991.

Glavassevich, M., and others. An educational program to improve quality of life for individuals with acoustic neuroma. *Journal of Neuroscience Nursing* 23(4):231–34, Aug. 1991.

Gleavy, D. The nursing role in epidemiology, risk management, and patient–public education. *Journal of Ophthalmic Nursing and Technology* 9(5):215–19, Sept.–Oct. 1990.

Gleichmann, S., and others. Physician–patient workshops. *Journal of Human Hypertension* 4 Supplement 1:73–76, Feb. 1990.

Good-Reis, D. V., and Pieper, B. A. Structured vs. unstructured teaching. A research study. *AORN Journal* 51(5):1334–39, May 1990.

Greenberg, L. W. Pediatric patient education: the unanswered challenge to medical education. *Patient Education and Counseling* 17(1):3–7, Feb. 1991.

Grueninger, U. J. Objectives for teaching patient education. *Journal of Human Hypertension* 4 Supplement 1:93–97, Feb. 1990.

Grueninger, U. J. Practice organization and management for patient education. *Journal of Human Hypertension* 4 Supplement 1:55–62, Feb. 1990.

Grupp, K., and Albert, M. Teaching wound care in the home. *Home Health Care Services Quarterly* 11(3–4):157–95, 1990.

Haines, N. Same day surgery. Coordinating the education process. *AORN Journal* 55(2):573–80, Feb. 1992.

Harvey, C. V., and Hanchek, K. Interdisciplinary patient teaching plans: design and implementation. *Orthopedic Nursing* 10(2):55–62, Mar.–Apr. 1991.

Hayes, N., and Lovetang, R. Home infusion therapy options for patients with AIDS. *Caring* 10(7):20–24, 26, July 1991.

Hetherington, S. E. A controlled study of the effect of prepared childbirth classes on obstetric outcomes. *Birth* 17(2):86–90, June 1990.

Heyduk, L. J. Medication education: increasing patient compliance. *Journal of Psychosocial Nursing and Mental Health Services* 29(12):32–35, Dec. 1991.

Heyman, E. and others. Is the hospital setting the place for teaching breast self-examination? *Cancer Nursing* 14(1):35–40, Feb. 1991.

Hirsch, S. H., and others. Medication education for an elderly black and Hispanic population in the United States. *Hygie* 10(4):36–39, 1991.

Hodge, R. L., and others. Patient education and public education: separate, overlapping or complementary? *Journal of Human Hypertension* 4 Supplement 1:79–83, Feb. 1990.

Holt, L., and Maxwell, B. Pediatric orientation programs. Hospital tours allay children's fears. *AORN Journal* 54(3):530–32, 534–36, 538–40, Feb. 1990.

Hough, D., and others. Patient education for total hip replacement. *Nursing Management* 22(3):80I–80J, 80N, 80P, Mar. 1991.

Irvine, A. A., and Mitchell, C. M. Impact of community-based diabetes education on program attenders and nonattenders. *Diabetes Educator* 18(1):29–33, Jan.–Feb. 1992.

Johannsen, J. M. Self-care assessment: key to teaching and discharge planning. *Dimensions of Critical Care Nursing* 11(1):48–56, Jan.–Feb. 1992.

Karl, S. B., and Eck, E. K. Living healthy with HIV. A patient education program whose time has come. *Group Practice Journal* 39(1):31–35, Jan.–Feb. 1990.

Kass, N. E., and others. Pregnant women's knowledge of the human immunodeficiency virus: implications for education and counseling. *Women's Health Issues* 2(1):17–25, Spring 1992.

Kelly, G. R., and others. Medication compliance and health education among outpatients with chronic mental disorders. *Medical Care* 28(12):1181–97, Dec. 1990.

Kessler, D. A. Communicating with patients about their medications. *New England Journal of Medicine* 325(23):1650–52, Dec. 5, 1991.

Kirk, J. K., and Grabenstein, J. D. Interviewing and counseling patients about immunizations. *Hospital Pharmacy* 26(11):1006–10, Nov. 1991.

Kirwan, J. R. Patient education in rheumatoid arthritis. *Current Opinion in Rheumatology* 2(2):336–39, Apr. 1990.

Kistin, N., and others. Breast-feeding rates among black urban low-income women: effect of prenatal education. *Pediatrics* 86(5):741–46, 1990.

Kramer, R. F., and others. Patient–family education: enhancing nursing involvement. *Journal of Pediatric Oncology Nursing* 7(2):62, Apr. 1990.

Koska, M. T. Health care innovators and entrepreneurs, 1991. A staff nurse brings Peanuts cancer special to life. *Hospitals* 65(10):50–51, May 20, 1991.

Legion, V. Health education for self-management by people with epilepsy. *Journal of Neuroscience Nursing* 23(5):300–5, Oct. 1991.

Libbus, M. K., and Sable, M. R. Prenatal education in a high-risk population: the effect on birth outcomes. *Birth* 18(2):78–82, June 1991.

Lilley, P. The educational needs of radiotherapy patients. *Radiography Today* 57(655):13–14, Dec. 1991.

Locke, J. A. Establishing an education program for non-English-speaking families. *Journal of Pediatric Nursing* 7(3):227–28, June 1992.

Lovejoy, N. C., and others. Potential predictors of information-seeking behavior by homosexual/bisexual (gay) men with a human immunodeficiency virus seropositive health status. *Cancer Nursing* 15(2):116–24, Apr. 1992.

Magyari, T. The role of the genetic counselor in a unique preconception substance-use education program for low-literate minority women. *Birth Defects* 26(3):179–184, 1990.

Mahon, S. M. Screening and early detection in high-risk families. *Oncology Nursing Forum* 19(1):91, Jan.–Feb. 1992.

Marcus, A. C., and others. Improving adherence to screening follow-up among women with abnormal pap smears: results from a large clinic-based trial of three intervention strategies. *Medical Care* 30(3):216–30, Mar. 1992.

Maycock, J. A. Role of health professionals in patient education. *Annals of the Rheumatic Diseases* 50 Supplement 3:429–34, June 1991.

McFarland, P. H., and Stanton, A. L. Preparation of children for emergency medical care: a primary prevention approach. *Journal of Pediatric Psychology* 16(4):489–504, Aug. 1991.

McKelvey, J., and Borgersen, M. Family development and the use of diabetes groups: experience with a model approach. *Patient Education and Counseling* 16(1):61–67, Aug. 1990.

Mickle, T. R., and others. Evaluation of pharmacists' practice in patient education when dispensing a metered-dose inhaler. *DICP* 24(10):927–30, Oct. 1990.

Miner, D. Preoperative outpatient education in the 1990s. *Nursing Management* 21(12):40, 44, Dec. 1990.

Molzon, J. A. What kinds of patient counseling are required? *American Pharmacy* NS32(3):50–57, Mar. 1992.

Monroe, D. Patient teaching for X-ray and other diagnostics. Cardiac catheterization. *RN* 54(2):44–46, Feb. 1991.

Morisky, D. E., and others. A patient education program to improve adherence rates with antituberculosis drug regimens. *Health Education Quarterly* 17(3):253–67, Fall 1990.

Niewenhous, S. S. Cardiovascular education programs in the home health arena. *Caring* 10(1):34–40, Jan. 1991.

Oldaker, S. M. Live and learn: patient education for the elderly orthopaedic client. *Orthopedic Nursing* 11(3):51–56, May–June 1992.

O'Neil, C. K. Pharmacist-managed medication training in personal-care homes. *American Journal of Hospital Pharmacy* 48(7):1530–31, July 1991.

Orr, P. M. An educational program for total hip and knee replacement patients as part of a total arthritis center program. *Orthopedic Nursing* 9(5):61–69, 86, Sept.–Oct. 1990.

Pasquarello, M. A. Developing, implementing, and evaluating a stroke recovery group. *Rehabilitation Nursing* 15(1):26–29, Jan.–Feb. 1990.

Patient education in selected countries. *Journal of Human Hypertension* 4 Supplement 1:107–16, Feb. 1990.

Pearsey, T. We teach all our patients about AIDS. *RN* 54(11):17–18, Nov. 1991.

Piloian, B. B. Alternative staffing strategies for community hospital-based diabetes education programs. *Diabetes Educator* 18(4):293, 295–96, July–Aug. 1992.

Price, S. Preparing children for admission to hospital. *Nursing Times* 87(9):46–49, Feb. 27–Mar. 5, 1991.

Richards, D. Perinatal education to improve birth outcomes. *Home Healthcare Nurse* 9(5):35–39, Sept.–Oct. 1991.

Roccella, E. J. Measures for developing education of the hypertensive patient. *Journal of Human Hypertension* 4 Supplement 1:9–12, Feb. 1990.

Rogers, L. Q., and others. Primary prevention of coronary artery disease through a family-oriented cardiac risk factor clinic. *Southern Medical Journal* 83(11):1270–72, Nov. 1990.

Rose, B. K. Informed consent and hysterectomy: enhancing the right to know. *American Journal of Public Health* 82(4):609–10, Apr. 1992.

Roter, D. L., and others. Routine communication in sexually transmitted disease clinics: an observational study. *American Journal of Public Health* 80(5):605–6, May 1990.

Satterfield, D., and Kling, J. Diabetes educators encourage safe needle practice. *Diabetes Educator* 17(4):321–55, July–Aug. 1991.

Scherer, Y. K., and others. A time-series perspective on effectiveness of a health teaching program on chronic obstructive pulmonary disease. *Journal of Healthcare Education and Training* 6(3):7–13, 1992.

Schulmeister, L. Establishing a cancer patient education system for ambulatory patients. *Seminars in Oncology Nursing* 7(2):118–24, May 1991.

Shibutani, S., and Iwagaki, K. Self-management programs for childhood asthma developed and instituted at the Nishinara-Byoin National Sanatorium in Japan. *Journal of Asthma* 27(6):359–74, 1990.

Shields, M. C., and others. The effect of a patient education program on emergency room use for inner-city children with asthma. *American Journal of Public Health* 80(1):36–38, Mar. 1990.

Sidel, V. W., and others. Controlled study of the impact of educational home visits by pharmacists to high-risk older patients. *Journal of Community Health* 15(3):163–74, June 1990.

Simon, W. H., and others. Back to school relieves patients' pain. *Pennsylvania Medicine* 93(1):40–44, Jan. 1990.

Skipper, A., and Rotman, N. A survey of the role of the dietitian in preparing patients for home enteral feeding. *Journal of the American Dietetic Association* 90(7):939–44, July 1990.

Sluijs, E. M. A checklist to assess patient education in physical therapy practice: development and reliability. *Physical Therapy* 71(8):561–69, Aug. 1991.

Small, R. E., and Moherman, L. J. Geriatric education: a fundamental requirement for pharmacy practice. *American Pharmacy* NS30(11):42–44, Nov. 1990.

State-specific changes in cholesterol screening and awareness—United States, 1987–1988. *MMWR: Morbidity and Mortality Weekly Report* 39(18):304–5, 311–14, May 11, 1990.

Stewart, J. V., and Sheehan, A. M. Permanent pacemakers: the nurse's role in patient education and follow-up care. *Journal of Cardiovascular Nursing* 5(3):32–43, Apr. 1991.

Sullivan, M., and others. AADE guidelines. Infection control guidelines for patient education as a means of preventing blood-borne disease transmission during diabetes self-care procedures. *Diabetes Educator* 17(4):259, July–Aug. 1991.

Swenson, I., and others. Nurses counseling patients about smoking cessation—why, when, and how. *Hospital Topics* 69(4):27–29, Fall 1991.

Taggart, V. S., and others. You can control asthma: evaluation of an asthma education program for hospitalized inner-city children. *Patient Education and Counseling* 17(1):35–47, Feb. 1991.

Taren, D. L., and Graven, S. N. The association of prenatal nutrition and educational services with low birth weight rates in a Florida program. *Public Health Report* 106(4):426–36, July–Aug. 1991.

Terry, P., and others. The result of an educational intervention for physicians providing HIV-antibody testing and counseling. *Minnesota Medicine* 75(4):37–39, Apr. 1992.

Waitkoff, B., and Imburgia, D. Patient education and continuous improvement in a phase 1 cardiac rehabilitation program. *Journal of Nursing Quality Assurance* 5(1):38–48, Nov. 1990.

Walsh, K. C. Communication: the heart of patient education. *Plastic Surgical Nursing* 10(4):171–72, Winter 1990.

Wenler, E., and others. Establishing a self-medication program within an institution. *Perspectives* 14(4):17–19, Winter 1990.

White, K. S., and others. Patient awareness of health precautions after splenectomy. *American Journal of Infection Control* 19(1):36–41, Feb. 1991.

Wiederholt, J. B., and others. Verbal consultation regarding prescription drugs: findings from a statewide study. *Medical Care* 30(2):159–73, Feb. 1992.

Wild, J. Dialysis without tears. *Nursing Times* 88(18):50–51, Apr. 29–May 5, 1992.

Wix, A. R., and others. Drug–food interaction counseling programs in teaching hospitals. *American Journal of Hospital Pharmacy* 49(4):855–60, Apr. 1992.

Wong, J., and others. Effects of an experimental program on post-hospital adjustment of early discharged patients. *International Journal of Nursing Studies* 27(1):7–20, 1990.

Woolery-Antill, M. Granulocyte-macrophage colony-stimulating factor: a teaching program for staff and patients. *Journal of Pediatric Oncology Nursing* 7(2):61, Apr. 1990.

Worcester, M. I. Tailoring teaching to the elderly in home care. *Home Health Care Services Quarterly* 11(1–2):69–120, 1990.

Wuest, J. Trying it on for size: mutual support in role transition for pregnant teens and student nurses. *Health Care for Women International* 11(4):383–92, 1990.

Zappa, S. C. Education program for hematology–oncology patients and siblings. *Journal of Pediatric Oncology Nursing* 8(2):88, Apr. 1991.

□ Books

Adult Patient Education in Cancer. Bethesda, MD: U.S. Department of Health and Human Services, Public Health Service, National Institutes of Health, 1982.

Anderson, C. *Patient Teaching and Communicating in an Information Age.* Albany, NY: Delmar Publishers, 1990.

Bille, D. A. *Practical Approaches to Patient Teaching.* Boston: Little, Brown, 1981.

Bisbee, C. C. *Educating Patients and Families About Mental Illness: A Practical Guide.* Gaithersburg, MD: Aspen Publishers, 1991.

Blitzer, A. *Communicating With Cancer Patients and Their Families.* Philadelphia: Charles Press, 1990.

Breckon, D. J. *Hospital Health Education: A Guide to Program Development.* Rockville, MD: Aspen Systems Corp., 1982.

Chatcham, M., and Knapp, B. *Patient Education Handbook.* Barvel, MD: Robert J. Brody Co., 1982.

DeBoskey, D. S., Hecht, J. S., and Calub, C. J. *Educating Families of the Head Injured: A Guide to Medical, Cognitive, and Social Issues.* Gaithersburg, MD: Aspen Publishers, 1991.

Diabetes Nutrition Teaching Tools: A Resource Guide for Dietitians: Diabetes Nutrition Education Materials, a Selected Description for Use with American Indians and Alaska Natives. Albuquerque, NM: Indian Health Service Diabetes Program, 1989.

Doak, C. C., Doak, L. G., and Root, J. H. *Teaching Patients with Low Literacy Skills.* Philadelphia: Lippincott, 1985.

Falvo, D. R. *Effective Patient Education: A Guide to Increased Compliance.* Rockville, MD: Aspen Systems, 1985.

Ford, R. D. *Patient Teaching Manual.* Springhouse, PA: Springhouse Corp., 1990, looseleaf.

Fried, R. A., Iverson, D. C., and Nagle, J. P. *The Clinician's Health Promotion Handbook.* Denver: Mercy Medical Center, 1985.

Gerteis, M., Edgman-Levitan, S., Daley, J., and DelBanco, T., eds. *Through the Patient's Eyes.* San Francisco: Jossey-Bass, 1993.

Glanz, K., and others. *Health Behavior and Health Education: Theory, Research, and Practice.* San Francisco: Jossey-Bass Publishers, 1990.

Griffith, H. W. *Instructions for Patients.* Philadelphia: Saunders, 1989.

Green, L. W., and Kreuter, M. W. *Health Promotion Planning: An Educational and Environmental Approach.* Mountain View, CA: Mayfield Publishing Co., 1991.

Haggard A. *Handbook of Patient Education*. Rockville, MD: Aspen Publishers, 1989.

Hanak, M. *Patient and Family Education: Teaching Programs for Managing Chronic Disease and Disability*. New York City: Springer Publishing Co., 1986.

How to Teach Patients. Springhouse, PA: Springhouse Corp., 1989.

Jackson, J. E., and Johnson, E. A. *Patient Education in Home Care: A Practical Guide to Effective Teaching and Documentation*. Rockville, MD: Aspen Publishers, 1988.

Karig, A. W., and Hartshorn, E. A. *Counseling Patients on Their Medications: One of the Principal Responsiblities of the Health Care Practitioner*. Hamilton, IL: Drug Intelligence Publications, 1991.

Lawrence, K. E., and Di Lima, S. N. *Geriatric Patient Education Resource Manual*. Gaithersburg, MD: Aspen Publishers, 1991, looseleaf.

Lawrence, K. E., and Painter, S. J. *Chiropractic Patient Resource Manual*. Gaithersburg, MD: Aspen Publishers, Inc., 1992.

Lorig, K. *Patient Education: A Practical Approach*. St. Louis: Mosby-Year Book, 1992.

Medication Teaching Manual: A Guide for Patient Counseling. Bethesda, MD: American Society of Hospital Pharmacists, 1991.

Metz, R. J. S., and Benson, J. W. *Management and Education of the Diabetic Patient*. Philadelphia: Saunders, 1988.

Minton, P. N., and McKrell, J. L. *Patient/Family Education: Making It Work in a Rehabilitation Setting*. Pittsburgh, PA: Harmarville Rehabilitation Center, 1988.

Murphy-Black, T., and Faulkner, A. *Antenatal Group Skills Training: A Manual of Guidelines*. Chichester, NY: Wiley, 1988.

Patient Teaching. Springhouse, PA: Springhouse Corp., 1987.

Patient Teaching Loose-Leaf Library. Springhouse, PA: Springhouse Corp., 1990, looseleaf.

Priest, J., and Schott, J. *Leading Antenatal Classes: A Practical Guide*. Boston: Butterworth Heinemann, 1991.

Rankin, S. H., and Duffy, K. L. *Patient Education: Issues, Principles, and Guidelines*. Philadelphia: Lippincott, 1983.

Rankin, S. H., and Stallings, K. D. *Patient Education: Issues, Principles, Practices*. Philadelphia: Lippincott, 1990.

Redman, B. K. *Patterns for Distribution of Patient Education*. New York City: Appleton-Century-Crofts, 1981.

Redman, B. K. *The Process of Patient Education*. St. Louis, MO: Mosby-Year Book, 1992.

Smith, C. E. *Patient Education: Nurses in Partnership with Other Health Professionals*. Orlando, FL: Grune & Stratton, 1987.

Spicer, M. R. *How to Design and Use a Patient Teaching Module.* Atlanta: Pritchett & Hull, 1986.

Squyres, W. D., and Associates. *Patient Education: An Inquiry into the State of the Art.* New York City: Springer Publishing Co., 1980.

Squyres, W. D. *Patient Education and Health Promotion in Medical Care.* Palo Alto, CA: Mayfield Publishing Co., 1985.

Teaching Patients With Acute Conditions. Springhouse, PA: Springhouse Corp., 1992.

Teaching Patients With Chronic Conditions. Springhouse, PA: Springhouse Corp., 1992.

Tillman, P. S. *Patient Education for Self-Care: The Role of Nurses.* Bethesda, MD: U.S. Department of Health and Human Services, National Library of Medicine, 1990.

Wenger, N. K. *The Education of the Patient with Cardiac Disease in the Twenty-first Century.* New York City: Le Jacq Publishing, 1986.

Wilson, R. A. *Consumer-Centered Health Education.* Gaithersburg, MD: Aspen Systems Corp., 1985.

Woldum, K. M. *Patient Education: Tools for Practice.* Rockville, MD: Aspen Systems Corp., 1985.

ADDITIONAL BOOKS OF INTEREST

Progressive Health Care Management Strategies

by Donald N. Lombardi, Ph.D.

This ground-breaking book provides new insight and, more importantly, practical strategies for incorporating twenty organizational values into leadership techniques, personnel recruitment and development, service planning, and business interactions.

1992. 383 pages, 13 figures, 1 table.
Catalog No. E99-088300 $49.95 (AHA members, $39.95)

Measuring and Managing Patient Satisfaction

by Steven R. Steiber and William J. Krowinski

Directed to marketing, planning, and quality assurance professionals, the text describes how patient satisfaction fits into the overall management and research strategies of the health care provider, and presents step-by-step strategies for the design and implementation of telephone and mail questionnaires that will provide practical and useful information.

1990. 191 pages, 63 figures, 11 tables, 1 appendix, bibliography, index.
Catalog No. E99-136106 $45.00 (AHA members, $35.00)

Bridging the Communication Gap with the Elderly: Practical Strategies for Caregivers

by Barbara J. Cox and Lois Lord Waller

Designed for inservice or independent study, this book provides insight into the nature of inter-personal communication problems between caregivers and the frail elderly and presents strategies to overcome the roadblocks to effective interaction. The authors provide straightforward advice to every professional in the hospital, home, or long-term care setting, including how to respond to depression, grief, and spiritual questions and the need to deal sensitively with questions about advance directives.

1991. 126 pages.
Catalog No. E99-130104 $25.95 (AHA members, $19.95)

To Order, call TOLL FREE
1-800-AHA-2626